Cardiac CT, PET and MR

Cardiac CT, PET and MR

EDITED BY

Vasken Dilsizian MD

Professor
Department of Medicine and Radiology
University of Maryland School of Medicine
Director, Cardiovascular Nuclear Medicine and
Cardiac Positron Emission Tomography
University of Maryland Medical Center
Baltimore, Maryland

and

Gerald M. Pohost MD

Professor
Chief, Division of Cardiovascular Medicine
Department of Medicine
Keck School of Medicine
University of Southern California
Los Angeles, California

FOREWORD BY

Robert O. Bonow, MD

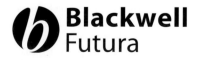

Futura, an imprint of Blackwell Publishing

© 2006 by Blackwell Publishing
Blackwell Futura is an imprint of Blackwell Publishing

Blackwell Publishing, Inc., 350 Main Street, Malden, Massachusetts 02148-5020, USA
Blackwell Publishing Ltd, 9600 Garsington Road, Oxford OX4 2DQ, UK
Blackwell Publishing Asia Pty Ltd, 550 Swanston Street, Carlton, Victoria 3053, Australia

First published 2006

3   2007

Library of Congress Cataloging-in-Publication Data
Cardiac CT, PET, and MRI / edited by Vasken Dilsizian and Gerald M. Pohost.
        p. ; cm.
    Includes bibliographical references and index.
    ISBN: 978-1-4051-2447-8 (alk. paper)
    1. Cardiovascular system–Imaging.   2. Cardiovascular system–Tomography.
3. Cardiovascular system–Magnetic resonance imaging.   4. Tomography, Emission.
I. Dilsizian, Vasken.   II. Pohost, Gerald M.
    [DNLM: 1. Diagnostic Techniques, Cardiovascular.   2. Coronary Vessels–
radionuclide imaging.   3. Diagnostic Imaging–methods.   4. Heart–radionuclide
imaging.   WG 141 C264764 2006]

RC683.5.I42C33 2006
616.1′0757–dc22

                                                                    2005031968

A catalogue record for this title is available from the British Library

ISBN: 978-1-4051-2447-8

Set in Minion 9.5/12pt
by Graphicraft Limited, Hong Kong

Printed and bound by COS Printers Pte Ltd, Singapore

Commissioning Editor: Gina Almond
Development Editor: Mirjana Misina
Production Controller: Kate Charman

For further information on Blackwell Publishing, visit our website:
www.blackwellcardiology.com

The publisher's policy is to use permanent paper from mills that operate a sustainable forestry
policy, and which has been manufactured from pulp processed using acid-free and elementary
chlorine-free practices. Furthermore, the publisher ensures that the text paper and cover board
used have met acceptable environmental accreditation standards.

Notice: The indications and dosages of all drugs in this book have been recommended in the
medical literature and confirm to the practices of the general community. The medication
described does not necessarily have specific approval by the Food and Drug Administration for
use in the diseases and dosages for which they are recommended. The package insert for each
drug should be consulted for use and dosage as approved by the FDA. Because standards for
usage change, it is advisable to keep abreast of revised recommendations, particularly those
concerning new drugs.

Contents

v

Contributors

Stephen L. Bacharach, PhD
Visiting Professor of Radiology
University of California, San Francisco
Center for Molecular and Functional Imaging
and Senior Tenured Research Scientist
National Institutes of Health
Bethesda, MD

Frank M. Bengel, MD
Director of Cardiovascular Nuclear Medicine
John Hopkins University Medical Institutions
Baltimore, MD

Henning Braess, MD
Senior Scientist
Philips Research
Department of Molecular Imaging Systems
Aachen, Germany

Patrick M. Colletti, MD
Professor of Radiology
Professor of Biokinesiology
University of Southern California
Keck School of Medicine
Director Nuclear Medicine Fellowship
Chief of MRI
LAC+USC Imaging Science Center
Los Angeles, CA

Robert Detrano, MD, PhD
Professor of Medicine
Department of Medicine
Los Angeles Biomedical Research Institute
University of California at Los Angeles
Los Angeles, CA

Marcelo F. Di Carli, MD
Chief of Nuclear Medicine/PET
Co-Director Cardiovascular Imaging
Brigham and Women's Hospital
Associate Professor of Radiology
Harvard Medical School
Boston, MA

Vasken Dilsizian, MD
Professor
Department of Medicine and Radiology
University of Maryland School of Medicine
Director, Cardiovascular Nuclear Medicine and
Cardiac Positron Emission Tomography
University of Maryland Medical Center
Baltimore, MD

Jane M. Francis, DCRR DNM
Superintendent Radiography
University of Oxford Centre for Clinical Magnetic
Resonance Research
John Radcliffe Hospital
Oxford, United Kingdom

Krishna S. Nayak, PhD
Assistant Professor
Department of Electrical Engineering
Viterbi School of Engineering
Division of Cardiovascular Medicine
Keck School of Medicine
University of Southern California
Los Angeles, CA

Stephan G. Nekolla, PhD
Senior Physicist
Nuklearmedizinische Klinik und Poliklinik
Technische Universität München
München, Germany

Stefan Neubauer, MD
Professor of Cardiovascular Medicine
Clinical Director
University of Oxford Centre for Clinical Magnetic
Resonance Research
John Radcliffe Hospital
Oxford, United Kingdom

Patricia Nguyen, MD
Chief Fellow
Department of Medicine, Cardiovascular
Stanford University School of Medicine
Stanford, CA

Koen Nieman, MD, PhD
Clinical Fellow
Department of Cardiology
Research Fellow
Cardiovascular Imaging Unit
Departments of Cardiology and Radiology
Erasmus Medical Center
Rotterdam, The Netherlands

Gerald M. Pohost, MD
Professor
Chief, Division of Cardiovascular Medicine
Department of Medicine
Keck School of Medicine
University of Southern California
Los Angeles, CA

Subha V. Raman, MD, MSEE
Assistant Professor
Department of Medicine, Cardiovascular
Department of Biomedical Informatics
Medical Director, CMR/CT
The Ohio State University
Columbus, OH

Matthew D. Robson, PhD
Chief Cardiac MR Physicist
University of Oxford Centre for Clinical Magnetic
Resonance Research
John Radcliffe Hospital
Oxford, United Kingdom

Markus Schwaiger, MD
Professor and Director
Nuklearmedizinische Klinik der TU Munchen
Klinikum rechts der Isar Munchen
Munich, Germany

Jospeh B. Selvanayagam,
MBBS (Hons) DPhil
Cardiologist
British Heart Foundation
Intermediate Research Fellow
University of Oxford Centre for Clinical Magnetic
Resonance Research
John Radcliffe Hospital
Oxford, United Kingdom

Karam Souibri, MD
Assistant Professor
Division of Cardiovascular Medicine
Caen University Hospital
Normandy, France

Padmini Varadarajan, MD
Assistant Professor of Medicine
Division of Cardiovascular Medicine
Keck School of Medicine
University of Southern California
Los Angeles, California

Nathan D. Wong, PhD
Professor of Medicine
Department of Medicine
University of California at Irvine
Irvine, CA

Philip C. Yang, MD
Assistant Professor of Medicine
Division of Cardiovascular Medicine
Department of Medicine
Stanford University School of Medicine
Stanford, CA

Foreword

Cardiovascular imaging has become a cornerstone in the diagnosis and management of virtually all patients with established heart disease and is also an essential component of the diagnostic evaluation of those in whom heart disease is suspected. Noninvasive imaging of cardiac structure and function, myocardial perfusion and viability, and non-coronary vascular pathology has thus become intimately entwined in routine clinical practice. Building upon the previous decades of technologic advances and imaging experience, the advanced imaging techniques – positron emission tomography (PET), cardiovascular magnetic resonance (CMR), and cardiac computed tomography (CT) – are now poised to deliver noninvasive coronary angiograms, to delineate the coronary artery wall in exquisite detail, and to complement these detailed anatomic images with corresponding functional data regarding perfusion, metabolism, and viability. While these highly promising methods have created great excitement among physicians, their patients and the public, they have also created uncertainties regarding their indications and their role relative to diagnostic angiography and standard stress testing, as well as uncertainties regarding physician training and credentialing. In this context, Dilsizian and Pohost's authoritative text *Cardiac CT, PET and MR* is a timely, valuable resource for all physicians involved in the diagnosis and treatment of patients with heart disease, including imaging subspecialists, both beginner and expert, as well as the clinicians referring patients for diagnostic and physiologic imaging procedures. Drs. Dilsizian and Pohost have recruited a "Who's Who" of expert authors, who are well known, internationally recognized authorities in their respective disciplines.

The book provides in depth, comprehensive discussion of the technical characteristics and clinical applications of each of the advanced imaging modalities. Beginning with the essential reviews of imaging physics and instrumentation underlying PET, CMR, and CT technology and the protocols used to create anatomic and functional images, *Cardiac CT, PET and MR* courses through the broad applications of each of the imaging technologies. The rapidly evolving evidence base supporting the current state of the art is presented in detail, and future directions are explored. The final chapters focus on the concurrent assessment of anatomy and physiology, using CMR or fusion imaging with combined PET/CMR and PET/CT systems. These latter combined techniques have the potential to deliver both the exquisite anatomic detail of CMR or CT and the corresponding unique physiologic information provided by PET tracers that track perfusion, metabolism, innervation, and receptor activity.

PET and CMR are contributing to the steady progress in detecting and tracking fundamental biologic processes at the cellular and subcellular level. In the current era of genomic research, molecular biology, and stem cell therapies, these methods have great potential to accelerate understanding of basic pathophysiologic processes in animals and humans and to develop new tools for early diagnosis, drug development, and precise assessment of the efficacy of new therapies. These advances in molecular imaging will undoubtedly converge in the near future with the parallel advances in anatomic macroscopic imaging. An understanding of the current and future capabilities of noninvasive imaging is essential to fully achieve this potential. *Cardiac CT, PET and MR* has arrived at precisely the right time to contribute importantly to this progress.

Robert O. Bonow, MD

PART I

Instrumentation, imaging techniques, and protocols

CHAPTER 1

Positron emission tomography

Stephen L. Bacharach

The goal of all cardiac nuclear imaging is to trace the fate of radioactively labeled biochemical compounds (tracers) within the body, usually in the myocardium or blood pool. One usually either makes a static image of the distribution of the radio tracer (e.g. ^{18}FDG (fluorodeoxyglucose) or ^{201}Tl (thallium)), or follows the uptake and clearance of the tracer with time. In the former case, static imaging is all that is required, while in the latter a series of images, acquired dynamically over time, is necessary. Positron emission tomography (PET) has these same goals. Although PET works in a manner very similar to conventional tomographic nuclear imaging techniques (e.g. single-photon emission computed tomography—SPECT), there are some very significant differences. It is these differences that make PET of great potential value in nuclear cardiology, and it is these differences we will emphasize in this chapter.

Positron decay

PET tracers, as their name implies, decay by emission of a positron. Except for their opposite charge, positrons are nearly identical to ordinary negatively charged electrons (which in fact are often called "negatrons"). They have the same mass, and behave similarly when passing through the body. Positrons, however, are the "antimatter" of electrons. When a positron and an electron are in close proximity for more than the briefest interval, both will disappear (called "annihilation"), and their masses will be converted into energy in the form of two gamma rays traveling in almost exactly opposite directions. The energy of each photon is 0.511 meV (exactly the equivalent energy corresponding to the mass of the electron or positron). These pho-

tons are sometimes called "annihilation" photons. The two photons travel in nearly exactly opposite directions in order to conserve momentum. The entire process is illustrated in Fig. 1.1. In this figure it is assumed that a positron emitter (in this case carbon-11 (^{11}C)) is emitted by a tracer somewhere in the body (e.g. the myocardium). When the positron is emitted from the nucleus it is traveling at very high speed—nearly the speed of light. It moves through the tissue just as an electron would, bouncing off many of the atoms and losing energy as it does so. Eventually (typically within a mm or so, depending on the radionuclide) it slows down enough to spend a significant time near an electron. As soon as this happens the two annihilate and the two gamma

POSITRON EMISSION AND ANNIHILATION

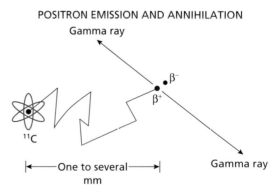

Fig. 1.1 A positron is shown being emitted from the nucleus of ^{11}C. It is assumed that the ^{11}C atom is located in tissue. The positron is initially emitted at a speed which is a significant fraction of the speed of light. As it passes through the tissue, it gradually slows down, as it bounces off the atoms in the tissue. Eventually it slows down sufficiently so that it spends significant time near an atomic electron—its anti-matter equivalent. When this happens the electron and the positron both annihilate—their mass being converted to energy in the form of two photons traveling in opposite directions, as shown.

Table 1.1 Positron Energies and Ranges (in tissue).

Isotope	Max. Energy (meV)	Avg. Energy (meV)	Avg. Distance Positrons Travel (mm)	Max. Distance Positrons Travel (mm)
^{18}F	0.635	0.250	0.35	2.3
^{11}C	0.96	0.386	0.56	4.1
^{13}N	1.19	0.492	0.72	5.2
^{15}O	1.72	0.735	1.1	8.1
^{88}Ga	1.90	0.836	1.1	9.4
^{82}Rb[a]	3.35 (83%)	1.52	2.4	16.7

[a] Rb emits two different positrons. Eighty-three percent of the time it emits a 3.35 MeV maximum energy positron, and 12% of the time a 2.57 MeV positron.

rays (each with 0.511 meV) are emitted, as shown in Fig. 1.1, each going in nearly the exact opposite direction. Although in Fig. 1.1 the annihilation photons are shown traveling in exactly opposite directions, occasionally photons are emitted a few tenths of a degree more or less than *180°* apart.

PET scanners detect pairs of gamma rays resulting from annihilation. By determining where these two gamma rays (and all other pairs of gamma rays) originated, the PET scanner can produce an image showing the location in the body where the positrons have annihilated. However, if the positron has traveled far from its parent atom, the image will be inaccurate—the locus of the annihilating positron will not correspond to the locus of the radioactive atom. For this reason the initial speed (i.e. energy) of an emitted positron will affect the capacity of the PET scanner to accurately define the position of radioactive atoms within the myocardium. This in turn affects the ultimate spatial resolution of the images that can be obtained with a PET scanner.

There are many radioisotopes that emit positrons, and so would be suitable for use with a PET scanner. Several of the most important ones are listed in Table 1.1, along with their half-lives and some characteristics of the positron that is emitted [1]. One of the reasons PET has played such an important role in basic research is that several of the radioisotopes that are positron emitters (carbon, nitrogen and oxygen) are the basic building blocks of all physiologically important biochemical compounds. This has permitted researchers to label amino acids, glucose, and a host of other biochemical compounds. Unlike the case with technetium-99m (^{99m}Tc), the labeling can often be done without making any alterations to the biochemical structure of the compound of interest. That is, a non-radioactive ^{12}C atom can be replaced with a ^{11}C atom, so that the resultant radiolabeled biochemical compound behaves just like the unlabeled one. The difficulty with ^{11}C, nitrogen-13 (^{13}N) and oxygen-15 (^{15}O) is that their half-lives are very short. This means they must be produced locally with an on-site cyclotron. It also means that the chemist in charge of labeling the biochemical compound of interest has very little time to do so. For these reasons (and others discussed below), the two most clinically important positron emitting isotopes for cardiology are the last two on the list, fluorine-18 (^{18}F) and Rubidium-82 (^{82}Rb). ^{18}F has a two hour half-life. This is long enough to allow production at a site up to a few 100 Km away. The recent dramatic increase in the use of ^{18}F labeled deoxyglucose (FDG) for tumor imaging has resulted in a large number of such commercial production sites in the US (and to a lesser extent abroad). One can easily arrange for delivery of daily unit doses of ^{18}FDG. ^{18}FDG has proven very valuable in assessing myocardial viability [2]. Its use for this purpose has in the past been limited to large research institutions because of the lack of availability of ^{18}FDG and a PET scanner. This situation has changed dramatically in the past year or two. As mentioned, FDG is now widely available commercially, and there are a huge number of new PET scanners which have been installed, the majority in non-research hospitals. Although most of these scanners were installed for oncology imaging, the machines are often suitable for cardiac imaging as well.

The other clinically important radiopharmaceutical in Table 1.1 is ^{82}Rb. This is a potassium analog and can be used to measure myocardial perfusion [3], see chapter 4. No labeling is required. Although it has a very short half-life (76 s), it can be produced from a longer lived ^{82}Sr generator, with a half-life of 25 days. At the moment such generators are fairly expensive, but the cost is expected to drop substantially if demand increases.

Aside from half-life, two other factors must be considered when determining the utility of a positron emitting isotope. First, it is important that nearly all the decays are by positron emission, rather than by other forms of decay whose emissions cannot be imaged with a PET scanner. ^{11}C, ^{13}N, and ^{15}O all decay nearly 100% of the time by positron emission. ^{18}F and ^{82}Rb decay about 97% and 95% of the time by positron emission, respectively [4]. The remaining fraction of the decays are by electron capture—a process that can produce radiation and be imaged with a PET scanner, without causing significant radiation exposure to the patient. In addition, for ^{82}Rb a small fraction (~11%) of the positrons are accompanied by an additional high energy gamma ray (1.16 meV) which can produce some interference with imaging the 0.511 meV annihilation photons. There are other positron emitters (e.g. ^{94}Tc, several isotopes of Cu and many others) that have an even larger number of other emissions and significant other modes of decay. This often results in poorer dosimetry for the patient because these emissions may increase the patient's radiation exposure, but do not produce useful imaging information. None the less many of these isotopes have been used successfully in PET imaging.

The second factor one must consider when evaluating a radioisotope is the energy of the positron that is emitted. As mentioned above, this is important because what one images with a PET scanner is not the distribution of the radiotracer, but rather the distribution of the annihilation photons. Positrons are not emitted with a single characteristic energy as are gamma rays. Instead they have a range of possible energies from 0 up to a characteristic maximum energy. Each positron-emitting radio-

nuclide has its own characteristic maximum and average energy of positron emission, as shown in Table 1.1. Because of this, and because the path of the positron as it slows down is quite tortuous (e.g. Fig. 1.1), not all the positrons emitted by a given type of atom travel the same distance—some travel quite far and others do not. Table 1.1 also shows the average distance from the parent atom each positron travels in tissue. The positrons emitted by fluorine-18 (^{18}F) have a very low energy. Thus, on average they travel only a very small distance away from the parent atom (about 0.35 mm). In contrast, oxygen-15 (^{15}O) emits positrons that are considerably more energetic and travel an average of 1.1 mm. Positrons from ^{82}Rb travel an average of 2.4 mm. Because the spatial resolution in a typical cardiac PET image is about 7 mm, the extra blurring caused by the range of travel in tissue can be significant for isotopes such as ^{82}Rb, and to a lesser extent, ^{15}O.

Before we can further discuss the characteristics of PET scanners, it is necessary to understand how tomographic images are made and how they are "reconstructed" from the radioactivity seen by the ring of detectors surrounding the patient. Many treatises have been written dealing with the mathematical steps necessary to produce cross-sectional images with emission tomographs [5]. Here we will describe the reconstruction process in a physical, rather than a mathematical, way.

To define the three-dimensional shape of an object, one must first be able to look at the object from all sides. This may be an evolutionary advantage of binocular vision (two eyes, not one). Each eye's slightly different view of the same object, when processed by the brain, allows formation of a three-dimensional image of the object's surface. Because our eyes are not placed very far apart we cannot see all sides of an object at once, and so we must extrapolate (often incorrectly) using the information from the two angles we can see in order to visualize the object's full appearance. In a similar manner, a physician may wish to examine several planar ^{201}Tl scans, each taken at a different angle, in an effort to mentally reconstruct the three-dimensional distribution of ^{201}Tl in the myocardium. The situation in this case is more complex because nuclear medicine images portray not just the surface of an object, but its interior as

Need to Know <u>WHERE</u> Photons Came From

<u>EXTRINSIC COLLIMATION</u>

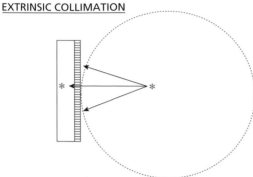

Collimator tells us where gamma ray came from

<u>Problem:</u> Collimators block about 999/1000 photons. VERY low sensitivity device.

Fig. 1.2 In single photon tomography (SPECT) a collimator is needed to tell the direction from which the gamma ray came. The camera must then rotate around the patient (the dashed line shows the rotation) in order to measure the projection images at every angle.

well. That is, the object is transparent (except for attenuation) to its radiation.

Just as all sides of an object must be seen by the eye and brain to appreciate its three-dimensional surface, many 2D planar views, each taken at a differ-

ent angle, are necessary to allow determination of the 3D interior activity concentration of an object. Each of these 2D views at a particular angle is referred to as a "projection". The reconstruction process (i.e. the method for producing tomographic slices) is based on acquiring these projections. PET, SPECT and even CT must all acquire projection images, and in fact all use the same method for reconstructing the 2D projection images into tomographic slices. The only difference is in how each modality obtains its projection images. In SPECT these "projection" images are obtained by rotating a gamma camera around the object being imaged, as in Fig. 1.2. In CT the views are obtained by rotating an x-ray tube around the patient and measuring how many photons are able to get through the body (so each projection is just a planar x-ray image—see Fig. 1.3). We will see shortly how PET accomplishes the same thing—creating a planar image of the positron annihilation radiation at each angle.

In theory, an infinite number of projections are necessary to define the three-dimensional distribution of activity in an object. In practice, cardiac SPECT images are usually reconstructed from fewer than 100 angles, while several hundred different views, each at a different angle are usually acquired for PET.

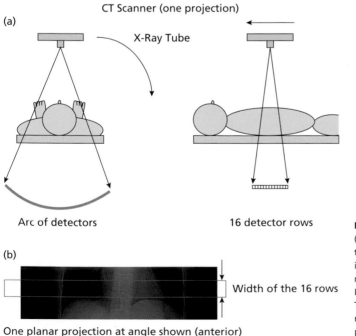

Fig. 1.3 In x-ray computed tomography (CT) the x-ray tube must move around the body (a) to acquire projection images just as the gamma camera must move around the body in SPECT. Image (b) shows one planar projection. The tomographic image can be reconstructed from a set of these projections at all angles.

Once the PET (or SPECT or CT) scanner has collected data from all these projections, or views, several steps are necessary to create a tomographic slice. The details of these steps [5] are unimportant for understanding the rest of this chapter. They may be considered simply as mathematical operations that convert the many projection images into a single tomographic section or slice.

PET scanners can simultaneously obtain all the views necessary to reconstruct a tomographic image with the use of a ring (or multiple rings) containing hundreds or thousands of detectors that encircle the patient. The mechanical assembly holding all these detectors is called the "gantry". The means by which the ring of detectors acquires data for the many views required can be explained by first remembering the basic information that is needed to perform the reconstruction, i.e. the projection images. A projection image is made up of all the photons that came from a certain direction (projection angle). In the SPECT example of Fig. 1.2 the camera is able to tell from which direction the photons have come by using a collimator [6]. All photons that do not strike the camera perpendicular to its face are blocked by the collimator. So in Fig. 1.2 the number of gamma rays detected at each point on the gamma camera face must have come only from 270 degrees. Unfortunately, blocking all the photons arriving from other angles is a very inefficient way to make a projection image. Many collimators block more than 999 out of every 1000 photons emitted by the radioactive atoms in the patient. Such a SPECT device would therefore waste over 99.9% of all the photons emitted by the patient. That is the price one pays for using a collimator to determine what direction the photons came from. PET can get the same information—how many photons were emitted and what direction they came from—without a collimator, potentially making PET far more sensitive than SPECT. How is this done? Consider Fig. 1.4a, showing a ring of detectors surrounding the patient. Only four of the hundreds of detectors are shown (and those four are shown greatly enlarged for clarity). Imagine that a 511 keV photon has just struck detector 3, as in Fig. 1.4a. If this were the only piece of information that the PET scanner had, it would not be of any use. We would know that an annihilation had occurred, but we would not know from which

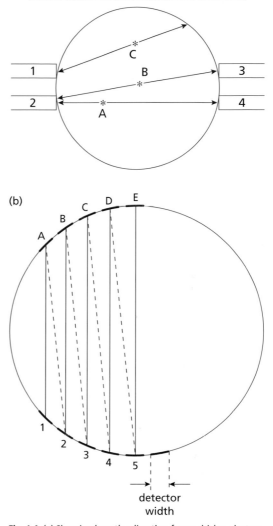

(a)   PET doesn't need a collimator
COLLIMATION BY COINCIDENCE DETECTION

(b)

Fig. 1.4 (a) Showing how the direction from which a photon came can be determined in PET by use of coincidence detection. When detectors 2 and 3 both detect a photon at the same time, the computer deduces that the pair of photons must have come from an annihilation along the line connecting detectors 2 and 3, as shown. (b) Showing how groups of detector pairs can form a projection image at a particular angle. Two projection angles are shown—the solid line shows the anterior-posterior projection, while the dashed lines show a projection about 10 degrees shifted.

direction it had come. It could have come from almost any direction. However, recall that for annihilation photons, there is always another photon traveling in the opposite direction. Therefore,

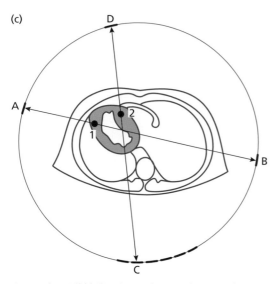

Fig. 1.4 *(cont'd)* (c) Showing a schematic diagram of coincidence detection among the crystals of one ring of detectors.

if a 511 keV photon struck detector 3 and simultaneously (i.e. in "coincidence") another 511 keV photon struck detector 2, then the computer would realize that this pair of photons must come from a positron that annihilated somewhere along the line B connecting the two detectors (see Fig. 1.4a). This is useful information—we know an annihilation occurred and we know from which direction the two photons came. This method of determining where the photons came from, without a collimator, is called "coincidence imaging" [7]. In reality the two photons may not be detected truly simultaneously. For example, the annihilation may occur closer to one of the detectors than the other, and so may reach that detector first (although the difference in time is usually on the order of a billionth of a second). One therefore usually accepts any pair of photons that occur within a narrow time interval as being in "coincidence". This window is called the "coincidence window" or "timing window" or the "resolving time" of the scanner, usually designated by the symbol τ. It is typically 5–20 nsec wide, depending on the scanner.

The pairs of detectors in Fig. 1.4b connected by solid lines (A-1, B-2, etc.) provide one "view" of the object at a given angle. Coincidences between A-2, B-3, C-4, etc. (dashed lines on Fig. 1.4b), provide another view of the object, at a slightly different angle. The PET camera has electronic circuits that can distinguish coincidences from every possible pair of detectors in the field of view of the camera.

In Fig. 1.4b, the solid lines comprising one "view" or projection are spaced rather far apart. To allow the PET scanner to distinguish small objects from one another, it is desirable that these lines be as close together as possible. This is accomplished by making the width of each detector small and placing the detectors as close together as possible. This decreases the spacing between lines and increases the number of possible angles (and therefore the number of views). Of course, increasing the total number of possible coincidences in this way increases the number of crystals, coincidence circuits, and other electronic components required, making the PET scanner more costly.

A factor that limits the number of crystals employed in a PET scanner is the number of photomultiplier tubes required. When a detector "detects" a gamma ray, it produces a small flash of light that is converted to an electronic pulse by a photomultiplier tube. Ideally each crystal would be attached to one photomultiplier tube, but the tubes cannot be made arbitrarily small and are quite expensive. Thus, manufacturers have devised schemes to allow one photomultiplier tube to share many crystals. A schematic diagram of coincidence detection among the crystals of one ring of detectors is shown in Fig. 1.4c.

Most scanners for cardiac imaging use several rings of detectors, often separated by lead shielding called "septa", to acquire data for multiple slices. When a PET scanner is operated with septa between rings it is said to be operating in "2D" mode. This is a bit of a misnomer, since of course such a scanner still acquires three dimensional data. As will be discussed later, some scanners operate without the septa. Those scanners are said to be operating in "3D" mode [8–11]. To increase the number of slices, coincidences are often recorded between one detector in one ring, and an opposing detector in an adjacent ring. Such a slice would be called a "cross" slice. With three rings of detectors (numbered I, II, and III) five slices could be produced. The first would consist of all coincident events from opposing pairs of detectors in ring I (a direct slice); the second would be a cross slice consisting of all coincident events between one detector in ring I and an opposing detector in ring II (or vice versa); the third would be formed from events only in ring II, and so on. Some PET scanners have completely separate rings of detectors. With this design, what constitutes a cross slice and what constitutes a direct slice is obvious. Other scanners have crystals so close together in the Z axis that the concept of physically separate rings no longer applies. What is important in any case is the final spatial resolution obtained (in all three directions) and the number of, and spacing between, slices.

Cardiac PET scanners reconstruct transaxial slices. The number and spacing of the slices is usually such that at least a 15 cm axial distance is encompassed by the slices—a quite adequate size for cardiac imaging—large enough to include the entire left ventricle in nearly all subjects. Depending on the scanner anywhere between 30–50 slices or more cover this ~15 cm axial field of view. It is often desirable to include some of the left atrium in the image also (even though it is not usually visualized well) to allow arterial blood concentrations of tracer to be measured. Some scanners permit a slight rotation and tilt of the gantry, but no scanner presently available can be positioned to yield true cardiac short-axis slices directly. Rather, one reformats the transaxial slices into short or long axis views.

It is important to understand the quantity being measured in the reconstructed image obtained from a PET scan. Each of the projections described previously measures simply the total number of coincidences seen by each detector pair at a given angle during a specific time period (the scan time). For example, in Fig. 1.4b, one projection is formed by the solid lines A-1, B-2, etc. The quantity measured by each detector pair in this projection is the number of coincidences per second seen along the line, for example that formed by A-1. This "line" is not an infinitesimally thin line, but has a width, because the detector pair A and 1 both have finite width. The number of coincidences seen by the pair A and 1 are those produced by all the radioactive material lying in the volume between them. The units of the measurement are therefore "coincidences per second per volume". These projection data are reconstructed to determine the number of coincidences arising from each point in the final reconstructed image. Since each point in the image

also represents a small volume in the object being imaged, the units are again coincidences per second per volume. Finally, it is assumed that the number of coincidences per second measured in a volume is directly proportional to the amount of radioactive material (usually measured in Bq (Bequerels) or Ci (Curies)) in that same volume. Providing all the corrections described below are made, this assumption is correct. The units of the PET scan can therefore be any of the following: Coincidences/s/cc, Bq (or nCi)/cc, or grams of radiolabeled material/cc. Use of the last unit is possible because Bq can be easily converted to number of atoms or grams as long as the half-life is known.

Accidental coincidences

Unfortunately, it is possible for two photons that did not come from the same annihilation event to be erroneously identified, quite by accident, as having occurred "simultaneously", that is, within the resolving time τ of the PET scanner.

Fig. 1.5 illustrates such a case. Only one of the photons from annihilation A has reached a detector; the other missed the ring. At nearly the same time atom B decayed. Only one of its photons was detected, the other also missing the ring. If these two separate events happen to occur at nearly the same time within the resolving time of the PET scanner, they will be considered to be in coincidence. The PET scanner then will falsely treat the detection of the two photons as if they resulted from a single annihilation that took place along the line between the two detectors (the dashed line in Fig. 1.5). Such false coincidence is called an accidental, or random coincidence. Random coincidences produce background activity in the reconstructed image that varies slowly in magnitude at different positions over the image, depending on the radioisotope distribution.

Accidental coincidences between unrelated photons must be distinguished from "true" coincidences between pairs of annihilation photons. The probability that an accidental coincidence will occur depends on the duration of the resolving time interval, τ: If it is very long, it becomes much more likely for two unrelated photons to be accidentally in coincidence. The resolving time of a PET scanner is therefore an important parameter,

RANDOMS

- Two single, unrelated photons are <u>accidentally</u> detected at same time
- # Randoms α (Activity)^2

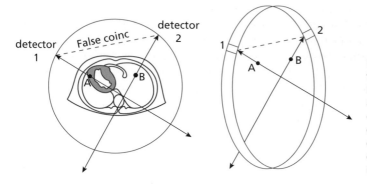

Fig. 1.5 Illustrating how if by accident, two separate annihilation events (A and B) are detected at nearly the same time a false or "accidental" coincidence can occur. This accidental (or "random") coincidence causes the PET camera to erroneously think the annihilation occurred along the dashed line indicated.

defining how well the scanner will distinguish true coincidences from accidental ones.

A second factor influencing the number of accidental events recorded is the amount and location of activity detected by the PET scanner. If the activity within the patient is doubled, the number of true coincidences will of course double also. The number of accidental coincidences, however, will increase by a factor of 4, i.e. as the square of activity. This has important ramifications. At sufficiently high levels of activity (e.g. for ^{82}Rb scans [9, 11, 12], the number of accidental coincidences may equal or even exceed true coincidences. With administration of excessive amounts of tracer, the patient may, therefore, be exposed to a higher radiation risk without a comparable increase in the amount of useful information obtained. The amount of activity constituting an excess varies with the machine used; it may be only a few millicuries in the field of view or as much as 50 or more mCi.

The reason that accidental events increase as the square of activity can be discerned from consideration of Fig. 1.5. Suppose that detector one measures S1 (S refers to "singles") counts per second, independent of whether these counts were in coincidence with any other detector. The count rate observed by a single detector, as opposed to a coincident pair of detectors, is called the singles count rate of that detector. Suppose also that detector 2 measures a singles rate of S2 per second. Consider that one photon has just struck detector 1. If an unrelated photon were to hit detector 2 within the

next τ s or has already hit detector 2 within the previous τ s, it will be in accidental coincidence with the event recognized by detector 1. Because there are S2 events detected by detector 2 each second, the number of these that will occur during the τ s before or the τ s after the event in S1 is S2 * 2 * τ. For every photon that strikes detector 1, there are therefore 2 * τ * S2 accidental coincidences per second. However, there are S1 photons striking detector 1 every second. Therefore the total number of accidental coincidences per second is:

Accidental coincidences/s = 2 * τ * S1 * S2

If the activity in the patient is doubled, the singles rate for every detector is also doubled, so both S1 and S2 double, giving a factor of 4 increase in accidental coincidences.

Consideration of the above equation suggests a way to correct for accidental coincidences. If the singles rate is measured at every detector, the number of accidental coincidences can be computed for every detector pair, and this number can be subtracted from the measured true events. Although measured singles rates include some counts from true coincidences, singles rates usually greatly exceed true coincidence rates. Thus, the error introduced by such a correction scheme is usually quite small.

Another approach to correction for random coincidences is the delayed coincidence method. Consider a single pair of opposing detectors in Fig. 1.5. The output of detector s is split. One of the signals goes to the coincidence circuitry as usual.

The other goes to a special circuit (or even a long length of wire) that causes a prolongation of travel time for the signal, perhaps of several 100 nsec. This second wire is connected to the usual circuit, which determines whether the two pulses (one from the delayed signal from the second wire of one detector, and the second from the undelayed, first wire of the opposing detector) occurred within time τ of each other. If a true coincidence event occurs, the delayed signal traveling down the second wire will not register as a coincidence with the undelayed signal of the opposing detector. The signal traveling down the long wire would reach the coincidence electronics much later than the undelayed signal from the opposing detector. Any coincidences measured by this long wire would, therefore, only be accidental coincidences, and not true coincidences. They could, therefore, be subtracted from the total number of coincidences measured with the undelayed standard short wires of both detectors to yield the number of true coincidences. The delayed coincidence method is quite accurate. However, it is limited by low signal-to-noise ratios because the number of randoms measured by the second delayed wire is often quite small, which may introduce additional noise into the final corrected image. On the other hand, use of the singles method discussed previously adds little noise to the image because the number of singles recorded by each detector is so high. However, the singles method requires measurement of τ, which is subject to inaccuracies.

Attenuation correction

If 511 keV annihilation gamma rays were made to travel through a substance with a very high atomic number, such as a lead brick, only a few of the photons would pass completely through the brick unaltered [13]. Most of the photons would interact with the atoms of lead. Of those that interacted, some would do so by a process called the photoelectric effect, which involves both an atomic electron and the nucleus of the lead atom. In this process, the photon completely disappears. It is totally absorbed or "stopped" by the lead, its energy transferred to the nucleus and a fast-moving atomic electron. Other gamma rays passing through the lead brick would interact by a process called scattering (or more prop-

erly Compton scattering, after A H Compton, its discoverer). In this process, the photon strikes one of the atomic electrons surrounding the atom, the gamma ray is deflected from its original direction and continues in a new direction with reduced energy. The bigger the angle of deflection, the more energy the gamma ray will have lost. A photon undergoing such a collision is said to have scattered. In lead, the two processes—complete absorption or stopping, and scattering—are both likely. In soft tissue, complete absorption almost never occurs. Instead, essentially all interactions result in the photon scattering. Even in bone, 511 keV photons are absorbed only rarely. Instead they simply scatter.

Now consider photons emitted by a small region of myocardium. Some small fraction of the annihilation photons will be headed in a direction such that both photons would strike a detector in the ring. As these photons travel toward the detector, they must pass through the tissue of the body. If either of the photons scatters, it will no longer be headed toward the detector. In all probability it will miss the ring entirely, or on those occasions that it does not, its energy may be too reduced to be detected. A coincident event that would have occurred in the absence of intervening tissue, now does not occur. The photons emanating from this small section of the myocardium are said to have been attenuated, and the loss of detected events due to interactions with atoms of the intervening tissue is called attenuation. The number of photons that make it through unscathed decreases exponentially with the thickness (d) of interposed tissue:

(No. of photons reaching the detector) = (No. of photons headed for detector) * $e^{-\mu^{*}d}$

The constant μ is the attenuation coefficient, and has a value of ~0.096 cm −1 for 511 keV photons in soft tissue. As can be seen by applying the equation above, only half of the photons will make it through 7.2 cm of tissue. Lower energy protons such as those emitted by ^{99m}Tc (140 keV) are attenuated more easily, because μ is higher at lower energies. It takes only 4.6 cm of tissue to stop half the photons of ^{99m}Tc from reaching their original destination. It would, therefore, seem that attenuation would be much more significant for SPECT scans than for PET scans, because the lower energy ^{99m}Tc photons used for SPECT scintigraphy are so much more easily attenuated. This presumption is, however, incorrect. In a PET scan, both photons in a pair must reach their respective detectors. As illustrated in Fig. 1.6a, a photon headed toward detector D1, must travel through a thickness of tissue X1 without interaction, and the photon going in the opposite direction must travel through thickness X2 to reach detector D2. The total attenuation is then:

coincidences = (# headed for D1 and D2) * (probability photons gets to D1) * (probability photon gets to D2)

= (# headed for D1 and D2) * $e^{-u(X1)}$ * $e^{-u(X2)}$

= (# headed for D1 and D2) * $e^{-u(X1+X2)}$

= (# headed for D1 and D2) * e^{-uD}

Where D is the total distance, X1 + X2, through the body.

Therefore the attenuation of the pair of photons depends only on D, the total amount of tissue the pair of photons has to traverse. It does not depend on where in the body the annihilation occurred. One does not need to know X1 and X2, only the attenuation resulting from its sum, D. This is not the situation for SPECT, in which only one photon is detected. In the SPECT case one needs to know what depth (e.g. X1) the photon came from. This is a piece of information that is usually unknown and unmeasurable.

For typical chest thicknesses up to ~90 per cent of the photons will be attenuated. Only ~10% will make it through the body. Photons traveling in other directions toward other detectors and those originating from other sections of the myocardium may be more or less extensively attenuated. In a 70 kg subject, attenuation by factors of 10–20 is common. Attenuation can be even greater in obese subjects. Obviously, attenuation has significant effects on the results of cardiac PET scans. Although this problem is serious with PET because both photons in a pair must survive intact, accurate attenuation correction is possible. In contrast, with methods such as single-photon emission computed tomography (SPECT) in which only one photon is involved, such correction is not possible because the attenuation correction factor, e − u(X1), depends on measurement of the depth at which the isotope is located in tissue. This measurement cannot be made before imaging. The value necessary for attenuation correction of PET images, however,

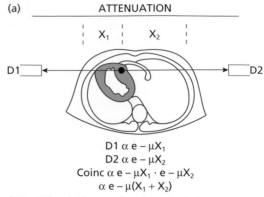

(a)   ATTENUATION

$D1 \propto e - \mu X_1$
$D2 \propto e - \mu X_2$
$Coinc \propto e - \mu X_1 \cdot e - \mu X_2$
$\propto e - \mu (X_1 + X_2)$

(X1 + X2) = thickness of patient. So it doesn't matter how deep the tracer is in body!

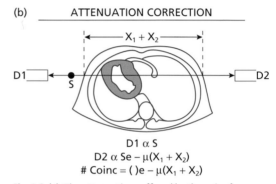

(b)   ATTENUATION CORRECTION

$D1 \propto S$
$D2 \propto Se - \mu (X_1 + X_2)$
Coinc = ( )e − μ(X₁ + X₂)

Fig. 1.6 (a) The attenuation suffered by the pair of photons does not depend on where in the body that pair of photons originated. No matter where they originate, together they have to traverse a thickness X1 + X2 of tissue. (b) Because of this, the same attenuation is experienced by a radioactive source placed outside the body, permitting the attenuation to be measured. One simply measures the number of pairs of photons detected without the patient and compares this to the number detected when the patient is present.

is (X1 + X2). This quantity is independent of how deep the isotope is located in the body and depends only upon the attenuation through the total body thickness, which can be measured accurately. The most common method for making this measurement involves performance of a "blank" scan and an "attenuation" scan (often called a transmission scan). Fig. 1.6b illustrates this approach for one detector pair [7, 14]. Before the patient to be imaged is placed in the ring, a small positron-emitting source is placed at one side (as in Fig. 1.6b) and the number of photons detected is recorded (just as in

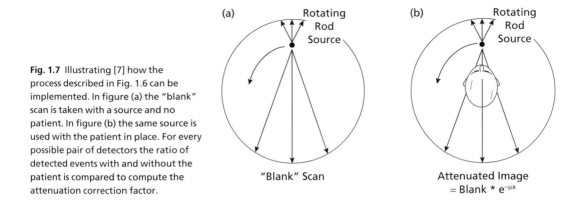

Fig. 1.7 Illustrating [7] how the process described in Fig. 1.6 can be implemented. In figure (a) the "blank" scan is taken with a source and no patient. In figure (b) the same source is used with the patient in place. For every possible pair of detectors the ratio of detected events with and without the patient is compared to compute the attenuation correction factor.

Fig. 1.6b but without the patient). The position of the source is maintained, and the patient is positioned in the ring (before injection of the isotope) as in Fig. 1.6b. Again, the number of photons are recorded. The difference in the counts detected in the blank and transmission scans is of course caused by attenuation through the patient. For example, if S coincident counts were recorded by the detector pair shown in Fig. 1.6b before the patient was in place, then $S * e^{-\mu*D}$ counts would be recorded by the same detector pair when the patient was interposed. The ratio of the counts without the patient (called the "blank" scan counts) to the counts with the patient in place (called the "transmission" scan counts) gives the factor $e^{+\mu*D}$, which is the factor needed to correct for attenuation for this particular detector pair. Making the same measurement for all detector pairs permits complete attenuation correction.

In order to make the measurement of attenuation for all detector pairs, often a rod of activity is used with its long dimension oriented along the Z axis (Fig. 1.7). Such a rod is attached to a mechanism that rotates it at a fixed speed around the gantry. The rod is usually filled with a relatively long lived positron emitter (^{68}Ge which decays to ^{68}Ga). The rod is first made to rotate without the patient, giving the "blank" scan counts (Fig. 1.7a). Then the patient is positioned and the measurement repeated (Fig. 1.7b) giving the transmission scan. The ratio of the counts in the blank to the counts in the transmission for every detector pair gives the attenuation correction factor for that detector pair.

As the rod rotates, only those detectors that lie on the line formed by the detector, the rod, and the opposing detector can possibly be in coincidence. By turning on only the appropriate detectors as the rod rotates around the gantry, most accidental and scatter coincidences can be eliminated. With proper correction software, this also permits the transmission measurement to be made even after activity has been injected [15, 16]. Some manufacturers use instead an isotope which emits only a single photon (e.g. ^{137}Cs). This makes it more difficult to remove scattered events, but in general both methods have been shown to work satisfactorily. Many modern PET scanners have been combined with a CT scanner, and in this case the CT scan (after suitable processing) can be used to perform attenuation correction. This will be discussed further later in this chapter.

A typical scanning sequence is: (1) obtain a blank scan (usually only done once per day, or week); (2) for static FDG imaging, inject the patient, wait for uptake (typically one hour) then position the patient in the gantry and obtain a transmission scan either immediately prior or immediately following, the emission scan. This minimizes motion between the transmission and emission scan. For dynamic scanning, the transmission scan must be taken prior to injection (or it can be done following the scan). As mentioned above, to perform the transmission scan after injection requires that hardware and software be available for correcting for emission activity present during the transmission scan. This is fairly straightforward when positron emitters (and coincidence detection) are used for the transmission source. It is often more difficult

SCATTER

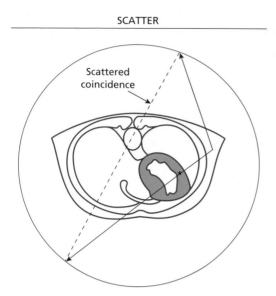

Fig. 1.8 Illustrating the effect of scattered radiation. If one of the pair of photons originating in the heart (shown as an asterisk in the free wall of the myocardium) scatters and is detected (as shown at about the 1pm position in the detector ring), the PET scanner will erroneously think the positron was emitted along the dotted line. A "scattered coincidence" will have occurred.

when single photon emitters are used for the transmission source. No matter what scheme is used, it is important to prevent patient motion between the transmission and emission scans. Such motion can produce appreciable errors in the uptake image [17].

Scatter

As described above, when annihilation photons pass through tissue, they frequently collide with electrons and scatter. The photon is deflected from its original direction and loses some fraction of its energy. The higher the angle of deflection, the greater the energy loss. The great majority of scattered photons never reach a detector, as illustrated in Fig. 1.8. A small percentage of scattered photons, however, may still hit a detector in the ring and register coincidences, as shown in Fig. 1.8. When this occurs, the PET camera erroneously computes the position of the radioactive atom (dotted line in Fig. 1.8). Such mispositioning of events can cause false counts to appear in cold areas of an image when a hot region is nearby. In general, the phenomenon slightly blurs sources of radioactivity from hot regions into cold regions (even those a

few cm away). This is of particular importance in cardiac imaging, since the observer is frequently trying to detect defects of uptake in segments of myocardium adjacent to normal regions (and perhaps adjacent to a hot liver).

Most PET scanners are designed to reduce the effects of scattered photons by rejecting those photons whose energy is below a certain threshold value. In most older, and some newer generation, scanners bismuth germinate (BGO) crystals are used. The energy resolution of these detectors is not very good, making it more difficult to reject scatter. Other crystal types (Lutetium oxyorthosilicate (LSO) or Gadolinium oxyorthosilicate (GSO)) in theory have better energy resolution, but in practice have yet to achieve much better scatter energy rejection than the new generation BGO scanners. In PET scanners with septa (2D scanners), scatter is usually fairly small anyway. However, as will be seen later, scanners without septa (3D mode) have several times higher scatter, and so the problem is more severe. If a scanner operates with an energy threshold of 360 keV, it can reject all photons that have been scattered by more than about 57°, but not those scattered less than this. Because photons are more likely to scatter at small angles, a large number of scattered photons will still be detected. Attempts to raise the energy threshold to, for example, 400 keV (as is being done in some of the scanners with LSO, or especially GSO crystals) would result in the rejection of photons that had scattered by more than about 44°, but of course the higher one raises the threshold, the larger the fraction of unscattered photons that are rejected as well. Energy rejection can, therefore, be used to reduce large-angle scattering, but can only eliminate smaller angle scattering at the expense of eliminating unscattered photons as well. This situation will improve if the energy resolution of the scanner can be improved. Meanwhile, more empirical methods must be applied to correct for the remaining scatter. Most modern scanners have relatively sophisticated algorithms for correcting for this residual scatter [18]. However, especially for cardiac imaging (with its mixture of lungs and adjacent soft tissue) the algorithms are not perfect. The situation for septa-out (3D) imaging is problematic, and as of this writing, further tests are necessary to determine how well such algorithms work for cardiac imaging [10, 11].

Deadtime

Quantitatively accurate PET studies require that the number of true coincidences be directly proportional to the concentration of radioactivity. In addition to physical phenomena such as scatter and accidental coincidences, a significant electronic effect in PET cameras can alter this relationship. Every time a photon produces a scintillation in a detector, a complex series of electronic events must occur: The light must be converted into an electronic pulse; the exact time of occurrence of the electronic pulse must be determined for use in timing coincidence, and the magnitude of the pulse must be computed to allow rejection of scattered events, etc. All of this takes time. If a second photon should arrive before the processing of the previous pulse is complete, the second pulse may be lost. There is, therefore, a time interval after a photon has interacted with a crystal during which the PET scanner electronics may be unable to process further pulses. Pulses that occur during this interval, termed the "deadtime", are lost. The higher the count rate, the larger will be the fraction of lost pulses. The number of coincidences per second at first increases linearly with activity, but at high activities it deviates from linearity due to this deadtime. Successive increases in activity produce successively smaller increases in coincidence rate. Manufacturers will frequently specify the activity concentration (e.g. MBq/cc in a 20 cm phantom) at which 50 per cent of the counts will be lost due to deadtime.

The principal source of deadtime is often not the number of coincident events the machine must process per se, but rather the rate at which the system must process single photons (each one of which must be analyzed to see if it meets the energy requirements and to see if it is in temporal "coincidence" with another photon, etc). The singles rate recorded by a detector is often one or more orders of magnitude greater than the coincident rate. Often the deadtime loss of a detector can be predicted quite accurately as a function of the singles rate measured by the detector. This relationship is the basis for one effective method for correcting for deadtime. The corrections can be quite large, especially with imaging techniques that require bolus injections of isotope (e.g. [82]Rb). It is probably best to limit the amount of activity injected so that the required deadtime correction during imaging will be less than a factor of 2. Activity levels greater than this will result in increased radiation exposure to the patient without a comparable increase in true coincidences. In addition, the accuracy of larger correction factors may be suspect.

In many circumstances cardiac PET studies are especially susceptible to the effects of deadtime. This is particularly true with dynamic cardiac studies that attempt to measure the wash-in or wash-out of activity from the myocardium, or to measure arterial activity as a function of time by monitoring the activity in the atrial or ventricular cavities. During a bolus injection or even during a one minute infusion of isotope, the PET camera field of view may contain a large fraction of the entire injected dose. This is in marked contrast to the 60 min postinjection static cardiac scans in which only a small percentage of the injected dose is in the field of view. The PET camera's deadtime characteristics (as well as random coincidences) may sometimes limit the amount of activity that can be administered. Again, the problem is far more severe when operating PET scanners in septa-out (3D) mode, than in septa-in (2D) mode.

Resolution

The term "resolution" is one of many parameters used to characterize PET scanners. The term requires

(a)

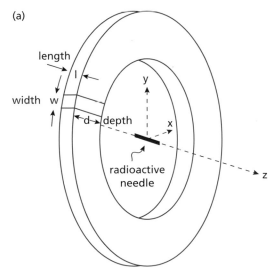

Fig. 1.9 (a) Showing placement of rod source to measure in-plane resolution [7].

(b)

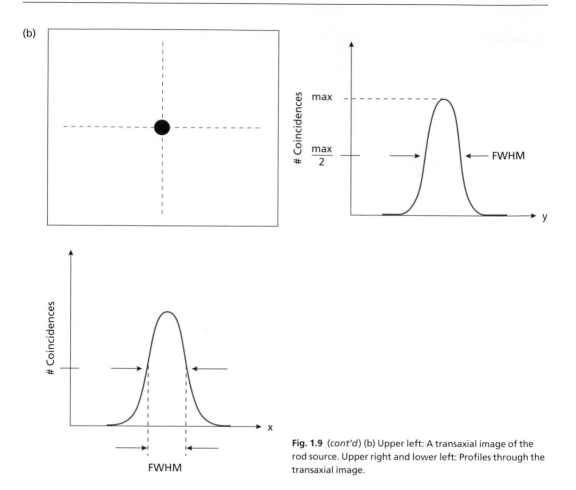

Fig. 1.9 (*cont'd*) (b) Upper left: A transaxial image of the rod source. Upper right and lower left: Profiles through the transaxial image.

more careful definition. The spatial resolution of a PET scanner is a measure of how well the scanner can distinguish two small objects placed closely together. Certain standard measurements of resolution have been adopted. With one, a very small spot of radioactivity is placed in the scanner's field of view and is imaged. If the range of the positron is very small (e.g. that of a positron from an isotope such as ^{18}F embedded in plastic or aluminum), then comparison of the apparent size of the object in the image and the actual size of the object allows calculation of the scanner's resolution. However, very small point sources of radioactive material are hard to construct. Instead, a thin rod of radioactive material, for example a long thin needle or capillary tube filled with ^{18}F, may be used. Steel prevents the positrons from leaving the needle. The needle or rod is placed in the scanner, with its long axis perpendicular to the plane of the ring as shown in Fig. 1.9a. Data are acquired and the image is reconstructed as shown in Fig. 1.9b. The top right of the figure shows a plot of the number of coincident events as a function of distance across the image. Typically such a plot follows a bell-shaped, approximately Gaussian curve. By convention, the width of this curve at half its maximum height (full width at half maximum, or FWHM) is used as a measure of spatial resolution. Since the initial measurement is obtained within one slice, or plane, it is called the "in-plane" resolution of the scanner. The in-plane resolution will usually be somewhat larger (perhaps a few millimeters or so, depending on the scanner) when the measurement is made at the edge of the field of view, rather than at the center. Because the free wall or apex of the myocardium may be 10 cm or more from the center of the field in a cardiac PET study, it is useful to know the PET scanner's resolution not just at the center, but also 10 or 15 cm from the center. In addition, at a given distance from the center of the scanner's field of view, the resolution in the anterior-posterior or Y direction may not be the same as that in the lateral, or X direction.

The scanner shown in Fig. 1.9a is made up of crystals with a width, W length, L, in the axial or Z direction, and a depth, D. As pointed out previously the width, W, of the detectors influences the in-plane resolution. Similarly the length, L, of the detector in the Z direction determines, in part, the resolution of the scanner in the axial direction. To measure the resolution in this direction, a small "dot" of radioactive material, placed on the bed of the gantry, might be used. An image could be made of this dot of activity, the source could be moved through the gantry by 1 or 2 mm, and a second image made. Progressively moving the source of activity through the scanner in 1 or 2 mm steps, making an image at each location, would result in a series of images as a function of the Z axis position of the source. Plotting the number of coincident events in each image as a function of the Z axis position (clinically, the bed position), would produce a plot similar to those in Fig. 1.9b. The FWHM resolution in the Z axis direction is sometimes called the "slice thickness" because it is a measure of how far into the Z axis the slice extends. A PET scanner, then, has at least two (possibly very different) spatial resolutions: The in-plane resolution (made up of the resolution in the anterior-posterior direction and the lateral directions, which are usually about the same) and the Z axis, or axial resolution.

The axial resolution, or slice thickness, should not be confused with the separation between slices. The spacing between slices may be greater or less than the "thickness" (i.e. FWHM in the axial direction) of each slice. If the spacing between slices is less than the thickness of the slice, then the slices may be considered to partially overlap. Even if the spacing between slices is greater than the slice thickness, some overlap will be present because the "edges" of a slice are not sharp but are Gaussian shaped.

The resolution of a PET image is determined by: The design of the machine (including crystal size and spacing, ring diameter, among other factors); physical factors such as the finite range of positrons

in tissue and the deviation of annihilation photons from exact co-linearity, and processing, including whatever smoothing is performed during or after reconstruction [19]. The effects of image processing are to some extent controllable. Positron range is of course a function of the isotope used. Its effects can be estimated as follows. If the number of positrons detected is plotted as a function of distance in tissue from the source, the number decreases almost exponentially with distance [20]. Some of the positrons therefore travel relatively far, altering the resolution curve from its usual Gaussian shape. The resolution curve produced by radioisotopes emitting very energetic positrons is a combination of the typical Gaussian curve illustrated in Fig. 1.9b and the approximately exponential curve associated with positron penetration [21]. Therefore, the curve is roughly Gaussian in shape near the center, but exhibits a long, nearly exponential tail. The amount of degradation in resolution that would occur with use of a positron with a relatively long range in tissue, such as ^{82}Rb, can be estimated as follows:

$$\text{Final resolution} = (R^2 + 1.89 * (2 * D)^2)^{0.5}$$

where R is the resolution of the scanner (including any smoothing) measured with a nearly zero-range positron source (e.g. when ^{18}F in a thin steel needle is used) and D is the average distance the positron travels, as shown in Table 1.1.

For example, with a scanner having 7 mm useable resolution as measured with ^{18}F, the resolution expected with the use of ^{82}Rb is based on the average distance an ^{82}Rb positron travels (D), 2.3 mm. The resolution of ^{82}Rb scan can be calculated from the equation above to yield a final resolution of approximately 9.4 mm FWHM—a significant increase compared with that of a lower energy positron emitter. The factor of 1.89 is entered into equation 1 in consideration of the fact that the number of positrons decreases with distance in an exponential rather than a Gaussian manner. Because the resolution curve is not Gaussian with an isotope such as ^{82}Rb, specifying the FWHM does not tell the full story. The number of positrons decreases exponentially with distance from the source, so many positrons will travel much farther than the average. Some ^{82}Rb positrons will travel more than a centimeter before annihilating. This produces an exponential tail on the resolution curve, in turn causing a small fraction of the counts in one part of an image to blur into other, distant parts of the image. To describe this effect, the full width at tenth maximum (FWTM) is measured in addition to FWHM.

To reduce the point-to-point random statistical fluctuations (called "noise") that are invariably present in a PET image, an image is often "smoothed" by averaging adjacent picture element (pixel) values together. Although this reduces image noise, it degrades resolution.

Various filters can be used at the time of reconstruction to facilitate smoothing. "Filtering" is the name given to the process of averaging neighboring pixels together [22] by replacing a pixel value with a weighted average of itself and its neighbors. For example, one commonly used filter replaces a pixel value with one-half times its own value plus one-eighth times each of its four nearest neighbors' values, so that the weighting factors for this filter would be 1/2 and 1/8. Such a filter will produce a less noisy image, but one with poorer spatial resolution. Filters are often given names (e.g. the "Hanning" and "Butterworth" filters). Despite their specialized names, all filters do nothing more than average neighboring pixels together; they differ only in their weighting factors, which may be positive or negative.

In addition to filters that reduce noise but worsen resolution, filters exist that improve resolution and exaggerate noise. Unfortunately, it is a consequence of the basic laws of physics that it is impossible to simultaneously reduce noise and improve resolution, and because of statistical fluctuations caused by the limited numbers of coincident events, PET images almost always must be filtered with a smoothing, rather than a resolution-improving, filter. Available PET scanner software usually gives the investigator a choice of which smoothing filter to use at the time of image reconstruction. It should be noted that iterative reconstruction techniques also have inherent "smoothing" (noise reduction combined with resolution worsening) built into them. In general, the more iterations (or iterations*subsets) the better the resolution and the worse the noise. In addition, some filtering is often applied postreconstruction. It is important for the user of a PET scanner to be able to estimate the resolution of the final image, given the reconstruction parameters selected. Comparing two images reconstructed with different parameters can result in misleading clinical conclusions.

It is important to clarify the difference between resolution and the distance between pixels. Imagine a PET scanner with 7 mm in-plane resolution (i.e. 7 mm FWHM) and a 41 cm field of view. The reconstructed image could be stored in an array (i.e. a digitized image) of 256×256 pixels. Each pixel would be 41 cm/256 or 1.6 mm apart. The 7 mm FWHM would therefore correspond to about 4.4 pixels. If instead the reconstructed image were stored in a 512×512 matrix, each pixel would comprise 41 cm/512 or 0.8 mm. The resolution would remain 7 mm FWHM which, with this matrix size, would be represented by 8.8 pixels. Resolution is a function of the scanner and the reconstruction and filtering processes; it cannot be improved by increasing the number of pixels in the image matrix. Below a certain number of pixels per centimeter, however, the image will no longer be able to reflect the resolution inherent in the scanner. In general, with PET images acquired *in vivo*, at least three pixels should be available for every FWHM [3]. So for example, if the final resolution of the image is to be 9 mm, then the pixel size must be 3 mm or smaller.

Pixels are spaced a fixed distance apart in the x and y direction and so occupy an area. Nearly all scanners are of course multislice machines. A pixel, then, can also be thought of as occupying a volume in space, in which case it is referred to as a voxel.

The partial volume effect

Quantitative data are usually extracted from PET images with the aid of regions of interest (ROIs) drawn on the images. Analysis of the data contained in such regions yields either the total number of events per second occurring within the region (proportional to the total activity in the region), or the mean number of events per second per voxel (proportional to the average concentration of activity in the region). Sometimes the maximum value within the ROI is also used. The resolution of the PET scanner, the size and placement of the region of interest, and the true anatomic size of the structure imaged all influence the accuracy of such measurements. Collectively, such influences are often described by a parameter called the partial volume effect [23].

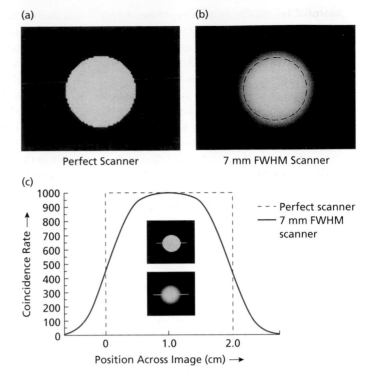

(a)   (b)

Perfect Scanner   7 mm FWHM Scanner

(c)

Fig. 1.10 (a) A transaxial image of a 20 cm diameter uniform cylinder, taken with a "perfect" PET camera. (b) The same image taken with a real PET scanner, with 7 mm FWHM resolution. Note blurry edges. (c) Line profile through the ideal image (dashed line) and through the real image (solid line). A region of interest (as shown in (b)) would recover only a portion of the activity in the image—the remaining activity would have blurred outside the region. The y axis is a relative scale proportional to the counts/sec at each pixel in the profile.

To better understand what the partial volume effect is, assume that a "perfect" PET scanner exists, and it is used to image a 2 cm diameter cylinder of radioactivity. Assume further that after imaging for 100 s, 100,000 coincident events would be detected (therefore 1000 events/s) in a transaxial slice of the cylinder. The perfect scanner would produce an image like the one shown in Fig. 1.10a. All pixels within the cylinder would have nearly the same value (apart from small statistical fluctuations which we will ignore), and all pixels outside it would have the value zero. Placing a 2 cm diameter region of interest around the image of the cylindrical object would give the total number of coincidences per second coming from the object (i.e. 1000 co-incidences/s). All of the coincidences that were detected would occur within the region of interest.

If the same 2 cm diameter cylinder of radioactivity was imaged with an imperfect PET scanner (e.g. one with 7 mm FWHM resolution), the same 100,000 coincidences (or 1000/s) would be detected, but some of the coincidences would be blurred or spread outside the true dimensions of the cylinder (Fig. 1.10b). Those from pixels near the center of the cylinder would not be affected as much because

just as many counts would be blurred out as blurred into them from neighboring pixels, whereas pixels near the edge would be particularly affected. The same 2 cm diameter region of interest (shown as a dashed circle in Fig. 1.10b) would now produce a value of only 785 events/s, the other 215 coincident events/s being spread out over pixels outside of the region of interest. The percentage of the counts retained in the region of interest is termed the "recovery coefficient": 785 of 1000 or 78.5% in this case.

The term "partial volume effect" describes this effect [23]. The poorer the resolution, the more blurred the data will be and the smaller the fraction of counts "recovered" within a given region of interest will be. As can be seen in Fig. 1.10, a larger fraction of the total events can be recovered by enlarging the region of interest to more than the true 2 cm object size. If the region of interest were increased to 2.4 cm, 914 of the original total 1000 events/s would be recovered. If the region were sufficiently large, all the original events would be recovered. Unfortunately, in patients, the size of the region drawn may be limited by the presence of substantial amounts of activity in structures close to the organ being imaged.

In the discussion so far, it has been tacitly assumed that the only quantity of interest is the total activity in the region, or the total number of events per second occurring in the "organ" (in this case, the cylinder). More commonly, the average concentration of activity within a region is sought and so the counts per second per number of pixels in the ROI is measured. This is in fact the unit most commonly produced by PET scanners (usually converted to MBq/cc).

We must now reconsider what impact the partial volume effect will have on accuracy of measurements of average concentrations of activity within an ROI. Drawing "too large" a region in an effort to recover all the counts will actually have the opposite effect on mean activity concentration measurements. It will reduce the measured counts per second per pixel by increasing the total number of pixels. Again, consider the 2 cm diameter cylinder shown in Fig. 1.10b. The "ideal" PET scanner might, for example, yield 1000 events/sec total within the 2 cm diameter. Let us also suppose that this value could be converted to a concentration of activity of perhaps 5 nCi/ml. The ideal PET scanner would, therefore, yield a value of 5 nCi/ml at every pixel within the 2 cm diameter, and zero outside. The mean value within any region of interest of 2.0 cm diameter or smaller would give the same value of 5 nCi/ml. If the region were enlarged to more than the true size of the object, however, the measured nanocuries per milliliter would fall because the region of interest would begin to include some pixels with 0 nCi/ml. For the 7 mm FWHM PET scanner producing the image in Fig. 1.10b, the 2.0 cm region of interest would yield too low a value for concentration of activity because events near the edge of the object would smear out to pixels outside the region. For the situation depicted in Fig. 1.10, the drop would be from 5–3.9 nCi/ml, again with a recovery coefficient of 78.5%. If the region of interest were decreased in size, however, it would no longer include pixels near the edge and the concentration of activity would approximate the correct value of 5 nCi/ml. If the region of interest were 1.8 cm in diameter, the average counts per second per pixel would correspond to 4.3 nCi/ml (85% recovery), and if the region of interest were decreased still further to 1.6 cm, the value would be 4.5 nCi/ml (90% recovery). For measurements in nanocuries per

milliliter or counts per second per pixel then, as the region of interest gets smaller, the average value within the region approaches the correct value.

Unfortunately, as the region of interest gets smaller, so does the total number of events contained in it, causing statistical fluctuations (the standard deviation) to increase. Conversely, if the region of interest is too large (larger than the object being imaged), the mean "nCi/ml" value drops. A rule of thumb is that if the edge of the region of interest is more than 2 FWHM interior to the object's anatomic borders, the influence of the partial volume effect will be small. Unfortunately, myocardial walls are typically no thicker than 1 to 2 cm (except in certain disease states), whereas FWHMs are typically no less than 0.7 cm. It will often be impossible to draw a region that is even one FWHM from both epi and endocardial borders. Accordingly, myocardial PET images are significantly influenced by partial volume effects. In general, recovery coefficients are significantly less than 100%. Even worse, since the myocardial wall varies in thickness around the heart, the thinner regions will artifactually appear to have lower activity than thick regions, even when the true underlying concentration is homogeneous.

In summary: (1) To measure only the total activity within an organ, the region of interest should be drawn very generously around the whole organ being imaged. This can only be done if there are no nearby structures containing activity. Ideally, edges of the region of interest should be at least two FWHM larger than the true organ borders. This will lead to recovery of nearly all events that have "blurred out" of the organ; (2) To measure radioactive concentrations within an organ rather than simply total activity: (a) the edges of the region should ideally be interior to the edges of the organ by two FWHM (this is of course often impossible); otherwise, recovery will be flawed, and (b) thin myocardial walls will in general give lower recovery than thick walls. The above discussion was focused on drawing regions within a slice. However, it should be remembered that partial volume effects occur in all three directions. The same considerations mentioned above for the x and y directions, also apply to the z direction.

It has been assumed that the activity concentration is uniform within the region of interest. If this is not the case, results should be interpreted with care because the mean value within a region of interest will depend on the position of the region within the heterogeneous structure.

It is possible to correct for the partial volume effect. If the true anatomic dimensions of the object being imaged and the resolution of the PET scanner (and reconstruction process) producing the image are known, it is possible to calculate the recovery coefficients and use them to correct the data. Unfortunately, the effects of cardiac wall motion also come into play. Sections of myocardium may move into and out of a region of interest as the ventricle contracts. Wall motion therefore produces its own "blurring" which influences the partial volume effect in exactly the same was as does the "real" blurring (i.e. the resolution) of the scanner itself.

2D vs 3D PET scanners

The PET scanners described above consist of separate rings of detectors, each of which is separated by a thin strip of lead, called the septum, Fig. 1.11a. The septa act as a sort of coarse collimator. The purpose of the lead septa between rings is to reduce the number of scattered photons seen by the detector, as shown in Fig. 1.11a, line "D". In addition, the septa reduce the number of photons from out of the field of view (e.g. from the bladder) which can hit the detectors, Fig. 1.11a, line "A". With the septa in place, only coincidences from crystals in the same ring (or a few adjacent rings) of detectors will be admitted. So the pair of annihilation photons "B" do not make it through the septa, while the annihilation pair of photons "C" do. As mentioned above, this mode of operation, with the septa in place, is called "2D" mode, or "septa-in" mode. The name "2D" is slightly misleading, since the data from a multislice PET scanner operating in 2D mode, is of course three dimensional. The nomenclature refers to the fact that the lead septa attempt to keep out any photons not originating from within a single detector ring (or a few adjacent rings). Together, the septa, combined with the limited energy discrimination, is able to reduce scatter in heart scans to about 10–15%—a quite clinically acceptable number. This remaining small scatter is easily, albeit approximately, corrected for by using software algorithms [24].

The interslice septa not only reduce scatter, but also reduce sensitivity. By restricting the coincidences to within a single ring or pair of adjacent rings, one has eliminated not only scattered photons, but also many of the photons that might have given valid coincidences between non-neighboring rings, for example line b in Fig. 1.11a. Typically, by using the scatter reducing septa, sensitivity for coincident photons is reduced by about a factor of 3–7 (depending on scanner design) compared to the situation if the septa had not been present. This is not nearly as big a reduction as incurred in SPECT by using a collimator (typically a SPECT collimator might reduce sensitivity by a factor of 1000 or more). Therefore even with the lead septa between rings, PET is still very much more sensitive

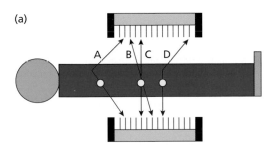

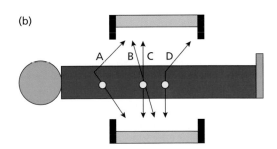

Fig. 1.11 (a) Illustrating a multislice PET camera with septa (misleadingly called a "2D" scanner). The septa stop scattered photons, like (D), out of field photons like (A) as well as valid photons that happen not to produce coincidences within the crystals in a single ring (or nearby rings). Only photon pair (C), shown in black, is detected. (b) The same scanner operating in "3D" mode—i.e. without the septa. Now both valid photons (B) and (C) are detected, increasing the sensitivity. However, this is at the expense of detecting lots of non-valid photons such as the scattered pair (D) and the out of field photon (A). (Figure re-drawn from: Reference 8, Bacharach SL. The new generation PET/CT scanners: Implications for cardiac imaging. In: Zaret BL & Beller GA, eds. *Clinical Nuclear Cardiology: State of the Art and Future Directions.* Mosby, Philadelphia, 2005: 141–152.

than SPECT. This is because SPECT requires a honeycomb of lead holes as its collimator, since the function of the SPECT collimator is to permit determination of the direction of the incident photons. PET uses coincidence detection to determine the location of the gamma rays, in principle requiring no collimator.

PET scanners with septa (i.e. 2D mode) actually work quite well for cardiac imaging. The sensitivity, despite the septa, is sufficient to obtain good quality images using 10–15 mCi FDG injections with 15 min of acquisition time. The septa keep random events and deadtime at acceptable levels, even for high dose studies, such as 40–50 mCi ^{82}Rb injections (imaging 90 s postinjection), or 20 mCi ^{13}N-ammonia injections. This is true even for relatively slow crystals such as BGO. The septa are able to accomplish this because random events (and deadtime) are greatly affected by the number of "singles" events/s. That is random events are determined by the count rate for individual detectors, rather than by the coincident count rate. The presence of the septa greatly limits the number of singles events per second, making 2D imaging advantageous for high activity studies. The use of septa, then, greatly reduces scatter, as well as random and deadtime corrections.

Despite the good performance of current generation 2D scanners for cardiac imaging, the need to perform whole body oncology scans made manufacturers look for ways to increase sensitivity. Cardiac imaging would also benefit from a sensitivity increase, provided it could be accomplished without sacrificing other machine characteristics important to cardiac imaging. A gain in sensitivity would permit either shorter imaging time (less of an issue for cardiac imaging than for whole body imaging), or increased total counts (useful for producing gated images), or better dosimetry, or some compromise between these factors.

Most new generation scanners have attempted to increase sensitivity by removing the septa, and operating in "3D" mode [8, 25–27], Fig. 1.11b. However, removing the septa greatly increases scatter, increases the effect of out of field activity, greatly increases randoms, and greatly increases the potential for deadtime. Comparing Fig. 1.11a and Fig. 1.11b illustrates why this is so. In 2D mode (Figure 1.11a) only one of the four photon pairs

(the black one) was detected. In Fig. 1.11b all four were detected. Only two of them (B and C) actually carry valuable information.

Typically, removal of the septa increases scatter in cardiac imaging to 50% or more for large subjects. Software to correct for scatter is available, but the accuracy of the correction is not nearly as good in 3D mode as in 2D mode for thoracic imaging, and of course the magnitude of the necessary correction is many times bigger for 3D mode than 2D. Scatter is especially important when imaging cold areas near hot regions, such as a defect surrounded by normal uptake tissue. In such situations, scatter artifactually increases the counts in the defect region. If the scatter correction algorithm is not perfect, the defect size and extent can be significantly biased. Scatter correction is thought to be slightly less important for hot spot tumor imaging, but of course even in this situation, scatter can result in inaccurate quantitation, or even artifacts. It was hoped that the better energy resolution of the newer crystal types (e.g. LSO and GSO) might greatly reduce the additional scatter caused by removing the septa. While these detectors have slightly improved the scatter problem, they have not yet proven to be the panacea originally hoped for. On the other hand, the faster response time of these new crystals was successful in reducing random events by roughly a factor of 1.5–2.

Despite the difficulties, the removal of the septa seems to have been clinically acceptable for oncology imaging—the reduced scan time compensating for a greater difficulty in quantifying uptake. For cardiac imaging much work is still being done to determine under what circumstances 3D imaging might be acceptable. Certainly it will be useful when dosimetry considerations dictate a low injected dose (e.g. for multiple sequential studies), or if only limited amount of the tracer was available (e.g. for some hard to produce radiopharmaceuticals). For static FDG imaging it may well prove perfectly acceptable (providing scatter can be adequately corrected). For dynamic imaging (e.g. bolus injections of ^{82}Rb or ^{13}N-ammonia) 3D imaging is more problematic. Much work is needed to determine the optimum activity levels that will be acceptable for 3D scanners, and whether 2D or 3D imaging is better in such circumstances. This is very important work, because many new generation scanners can only function in 3D mode (i.e. the septa can not be inserted or retracted at will).

An additional problem with removing the septa is that the axial sensitivity rapidly decreases from a maximum at the center of the axial field of view, to the end slices. This is because in 3D coincidences are allowed between many rings of detectors, as in Fig. 1.11b. This is fine in the center of the field, but as one approaches the edge of the field of view, there are fewer and fewer adjacent rings, causing the sensitivity to drop. This loss of sensitivity at the edges means that the effective overall sensitivity is not as high as one might predict. For oncology studies it means that significant overlap must occur between the axial fields of view at each imaging location. For cardiac studies it simply means that the noise will increase rapidly for slices further from the center of the axial field of view.

Use of PET/CT in cardiology

The vast majority of new PET scanners being sold today are combined with a CT scanner. The CT scan can be used to replace the much slower rotating ^{68}Ge rod source transmission scan thereby reducing scan time by 3–6 min per field of view. In addition the rotating rod transmission source, due to limited counts, introduced noise into the corrected PET images. The CT images are by comparison nearly noise free. The two scanners are physically located in the same gantry, but do not perform scans simultaneously. Instead one usually first acquires (for oncology) a rapid spiral CT scan (perhaps 20 s for a head to thigh scan) and then the much slower PET scan (several minutes per bed position). With the rotating rod source method scans of 4–6 minutes per bed position were commonly used. This resulted in 24–36 min of extra scan time for a six bed position oncology whole body scan. With CT this is reduced to ~20 s. In addition it soon became clear that much valuable clinical information was present in the fused CT and PET images.

Transmission scan time is much less an issue with single level cardiac scans. The reduced attenuation correction noise would, however, be beneficial. In addition, it is possible that combining CT cardiac data with PET metabolic or perfusion data, as obtained from PET/CT machines, will be of clinical value. There have been several reports in the past of the clinical utility of fusing coronary angiograms with SPECT perfusion data. Recently 16 slice helical CT scanners have begun to be marketed with PET scanners. Many of these scanners are fast enough to permit CT cardiac gating, and will even operate with commercially available CT coronary vessel software. To date, there has been no literature as to how these high speed scanners might best be used with PET data. Many of the cardiac CT procedures (other than angiography) that come to mind often still involve contrast media. For example, even with very low concentrations of contrast media in the blood, it is reasonably easy to identify the endo and epicardial borders using gated CT images. Thus one could correct the PET data for any partial volume effects, for example caused by thinning of one part of the myocardium compared to another. In addition, while gated FDG PET is adequate for global measures of ventricular function [28–34], the gated CT would also allow measurement of myocardial thickening—a very useful adjunct to PET physiologic (metabolic or perfusion) imaging.

Unfortunately, there are at present some unresolved issues associated with using a high speed CT scan for attenuation correction of cardiac images. A few of these are discussed briefly below.

Use of CT images for attenuation correction

As described above, when using a PET scanner, transmission related noise can be nearly eliminated by using the CT data to perform the attenuation correction. The physics of the process has been described in detail previously [35–38]. In short, a CT scan is taken of the patient immediately prior to the PET scan. Usually a quick scout acquisition is first taken, and from this scan, one can accurately position both the axial CT scan, and the subsequent PET imaging, over the cardiac chambers. Typical images are shown in Fig. 1.12. The CT scan is assumed to be aligned with the subsequent PET scan, just as the conventional transmission scan obtained with a ^{68}Ge rod source is assumed to be aligned. The CT scan, even at relatively low exposure settings (e.g. 140 kVp, 80 mA, 1.5 pitch, 0.8 s rotation speed) has far less noise than does the typical ^{68}Ge rod source transmission scan

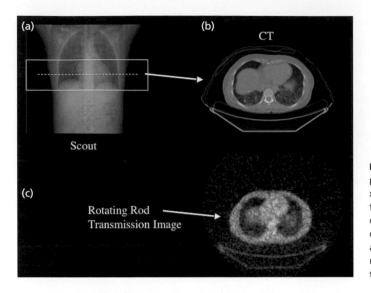

Fig. 1.12 (a) Scout view (single planar projection) taken with the stationary x-ray tube of a CT scanner. A single PET field of view (the box) is selected in order to produce CT tomographic slices, one of which is shown in (b). (c) shows a transmission image taken with a rotating ^{68}Ge rod source. Obviously the CT slice has much better statistics.

(Fig. 1.12). The CT scan is resampled to the same size as the PET data, is suitably blurred, and scaled [22] so as to convert the pixel values from Hounsfield units to the attenuation coefficients which would be obtained at 511 keV. The scaled, resampled CT data is then used to correct the PET data prior to reconstruction.

This procedure works reasonably well for oncology whole body imaging, although there are some difficulties. Some of these difficulties are potentially exacerbated when the process is applied to cardiac imaging. There is a small but growing body of literature concerning the accuracy and reliability of the CT attenuation correction for tumor imaging [35, 39, 40]. There is very little corresponding data validating the method for cardiac imaging [37, 41].

The two principal areas of concern for CT attenuation correction in cardiac PET are listed below:

I Scaling the CT Hounsfield units to 511 keV attenuation coefficients.

The x-ray beam from the CT scanner is of much lower energy than the 511 keV photons being imaged. In addition, the x-ray beam produces a continuous spectrum of energies all the way up to the peak (kVp). The attenuation of these lower energy CT photons is therefore much greater than the attenuation experienced by the 511 keV annihilation photons. To correct for this the attenuation values produced by the CT scanner have to be converted to 511 keV attenuation values. This aspect of PET/CT has been

well validated in oncology imaging, and has been shown to work quite well in general [35, 39, 40], with only a few caveats. The only potential difficulties that might occur during cardiac imaging are if contrast media has been used during or prior to the CT scan [40, 42–46], or if metallic objects (e.g. clips, shoulder or arm prostheses, etc) are in the plane of the cardiac images. When arms are not up (i.e. arms at the side), some artifacts and noise can be introduced into the CT scan. There may also be some small concern caused by the proximity of the myocardium to the ribs.

II Misalignment between CT and emission data

Misalignment between the CT data and the PET data is a potential problem when using CT data to perform attenuation correction for PET. The misalignment can be inadvertent (i.e. patient motion between the time of the CT and emission acquisitions) or "effective" misalignment due to patient respiration and myocardial motion during the cardiac cycle. We assume here that the PET and CT portions of the machine itself have been previously determined to be in accurate mechanical alignment.

The effects of a misalignment between the attenuation scan and the emission scan has already been investigated for PET [17]. Prior to PET/CT the only cause of this misalignment was whatever inadvertent patient motion might have occurred between the two scans. Relatively small misalignments can cause a myocardium with uniform uptake to appear

(a) 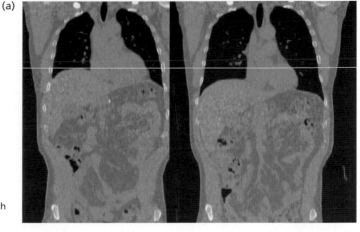 (b)

Fig. 1.13 Two coronal CT views at exactly the same level. (a) taken at normal end-expiration, (b) at normal end-inspiration. Note movement of both the dome of the liver and the heart.

non-uniform. In PET/CT the misalignment comes not only from inadvertent patient motion, but also from the motion of the internal organs caused by respiration. The CT scan is usually acquired quite rapidly, perhaps taking less than one second per slice. The CT therefore captures the chest at one phase of the respiratory cycle. The PET emission data, on the other hand, is acquired over many minutes, and so is an average over many respiratory cycles. The two data sets therefore do not overlay each other. The problem is most severe at the boundaries between low and high attenuation regions. For oncology studies this is usually at the dome of the liver. For heart studies it is all regions of the myocardium surrounded by lungs. In addition, not only does the heart itself appear to move with respiration, so too does the liver. As the liver moves into or out of the cardiac slices, the attenuation for those slices can change substantially. Fig. 1.13 illustrates the effect, showing a CT slice captured at normal tidal end-inspiration and normal tidal end-expiration.

Several studies have examined the effects of respiratory motion on PET/CT in oncology [47–51] and it is useful to consider how those findings might apply to cardiac imaging. In oncology applications, one of the most notable effects is at the dome of the liver, where respiratory motion is large and there is an air-tissue interface. In one study [51], nearly all (84%) subjects exhibited a cold artifact at the top of the liver, with 16% of the subjects having a defect categorized as moderate. The source of the defect was thought to be the incorrect attenuation correction,

due to inconsistencies at the lung/liver interface in the CT compared to the emission PET. It is quite possible similar effects would occur with the free wall of the heart. A tissue/lung interface exists, and there is indeed respiratory motion (as well as cardiac motion, depending on the speed of the CT scanner). The magnitude of such effects in the heart is not yet known [42], although previous data discussing misalignment between attenuation and emission data may be relevant [17]. Much work remains to be done in using CT images to correct for attenuation. One solution would be to slow down the CT scan (using very slow rotations and low mA) so as to average a few respiratory cycles together. While this may lengthen the scan unacceptably for multilevel oncology imaging, it might be quite practical for cardiac imaging. Another solution would be to use respiratory gating, but this of course adds considerable complexity to the acquisition, and potential noise to the data.

It should be noted that many CT scanners routinely scan fast enough to capture only a portion of the cardiac cycle itself. Again, problems similar to those described above may occur. Here, however, the motion (and so potential misalignment) is presumably much smaller. In addition only a minimal reduction in CT scan speed would average several cardiac cycles together.

In summary, combining CT with PET imaging may well prove even more valuable for cardiac imaging than for oncology imaging. The additional information associated with overlaying physiologic data (metabolism, blood flow, etc) with CT angiographic data, coupled with wall thickness and thickening measurements would seem to portend significant advances in the field of cardiac imaging. However, the problems associated with respiratory motion are likely to be much worse for cardiac imaging than for oncology imaging. Considerable work therefore needs to be done before cardiac PET/CT can achieve to its full potential.

References

1. ICRP. *Radionuclide Transformations*. Pergamon Press, New York, 1983.

2. Dilsizian V. *Myocardial Viability: A Clinical and Scientific Treatise*. Futura, Armonk, NY, 2000.

3. Bacharach SL, Bax JJ, Case J *et al.* PET myocardial glucose metabolism and perfusion imaging: Part I—guidelines for patient preparation and data acquisition. *J Nucl Cardiol* 2003; **10**: 545–556.

4. Lederer CM, Shirley VS. *Table of Isotopes*, 7th edn. Wiley, New York, 1978.

5. Parker J. *Image Reconstruction in Radiology*. CRC Press, Boca Raton, 1990.

6. Maass RE, Bacharach SL. Imaging instrumentation. In: Iskandrian AE & Verani MS, eds. *Nuclear Cardiac Imaging: Principles and Applications*. Oxford Press, New York, 2003: 28–50.

7. Bacharach SL. The physics of positron emission tomography. In Bergmann SR & Sobel BE, eds. *Positron Emission Tomography of the Heart*. Futura Publishing Co, Mount Kisco, NY, 1992: 13–44.

8. Bacharach SL. The new generation PET/CT Scanners: Implications for cardiac imaging. In: Zaret BL & Beller GA, eds. *Clinical Nuclear Cardiology: State of the Art and Future Directions*. Mosby, Philadelphia, 2005: 141–152.

9. Knesaurek K, Machac J, Krynckyi *et al.* Comparison of 2-dimensional and 3-dimensional Rb-82 myocardial perfusion PET imaging. *J Nucl Med* 2003; **44**: 1350–1356.

10. Knesaurek K, Machac J, Krynckyi *et al.* Comparison of 2D and 3D myocardial PET imaging. *J Nucl Med* 2001; **42**: 170.

11. Machac J, Chen H, Almeida OD *et al.* Comparison of 2D and high dose and low dose 3D gated myocardial Rb-82 PET imaging. *J Nucl Med* 2002; **43**: 777.

12. Votaw JR, White M. Comparison of 2-dimensional and 3-dimensional cardiac Rb-82 PET studies. *J Nucl Med* 2001; **42**: 701–706.

13. Murphy PH. Radiation physics and radiation safety. In: Iskandrian AE & Verani MS, eds. *Nuclear Cardiac Imaging: Principles and Applications*. Oxford University Press, New York, 2003: 7–27.

14. Bacharach SL. Attenuation correction: Practical considerations. In: Schwaiger M, ed. *Cardiac Positron Emission Tomography*. Kluwer Academic Publishers, Boston, 1996: 49–64.

15. Carson RE, Daubewitherspoon ME, Green MV. A method for postinjection pet transmission measurements with a rotating source. *J Nucl Med* 1988; **29**: 1558–1567.

16. Thompson CJ, Ranger NT, Evans AC. Simultaneous transmission and emission scans in positron emission tomography. *Ieee Trans Nucl Sci* 1989; **36**: 1011–1016.

17. McCord ME, Bacharach SL, Bonow RO *et al.* Misalignment between Pet transmission and emission scans—its effect on myocardial imaging. *J Nucl Med* 1992; **33**: 1209–1214.

18. Bendriem B, Soussaline F, Campagnolo *et al.* A technique for the correction of scattered radiation in a PET system using time-of-flight information. *J Comput Assist Tomogr* 1986; **10**: 287–295.

19. Hoffman EJ, Phelps ME. Resolution limit for positron-imaging devices—reply. *J Nucl Med* 1977; **18**: 491–492.

20. Evans R. *The Atomic Nucleus*. McGraw-Hill, New York, 1995: 625–629.

21. Phelps ME, Hoffman EJ, Huang SC *et al.* Effect of positron range on spatial-resolution. *J Nucl Med* 1975; **16**: 649–652.

22. Bacharach SL. Image analysis. In: Wagner HN, Buchanan SZ & Buchanan JW, eds. *Principles of Nuclear Medicine*. W B Saunders, Philadelphia, 1995: 393–404.

23. Hoffman EJ, Huang SC, Phelps ME. Quantitation in positron emission computed tomography: Effect of object size. *J Comput Assist Tomogr* 1979; **3**: 299–308.

24. Bergstrom M, Eriksson L, Bohm C *et al.* Correction for scattered radiation in a ring detector positron camera by integral transformation of the projections. *J Comput Assist Tomogr* 1983; **7**: 42–50.

25. Muehllehner G, Karp JS, Surti S. Design considerations for PET scanners. *Q J Nucl Med* 2002; **46**: 16–23.

26. Alessio AM, Kinahan PE, Cheng PM *et al.* PET/CT scanner instrumentation, challenges, and solutions. *Radiol Clin North Am* 2004; **42**: 1017–1032.

27. Surti S, Karp JS, Kinahan PE. PET instrumentation. *Radiol Clin North Am* 2004; **42**: 1003–1012.

28. Schaefer WM, Lipke CSA, Nowak B *et al.* Validation of an evaluation routine for left ventricular volumes, ejection fraction and wall motion from gated cardiac FDG PET: A comparison with cardiac magnetic resonance imaging. *Eur J Nucl Med Mol Imaging* 2003; **30**: 545–553.

29. Rajappan K, Livieratos L, Camici PG *et al.* Measurement of ventricular volumes and function: A comparison of gated PET and cardiovascular magnetic resonance. *J Nucl Med* 2002; **43**: 806–810.

30. Machac J, Mosci K, Almeida OD, *et al.* Gated Rubidium-82 cardiac PET imaging: Evaluation of left ventricular wall motion. *J Am Coll Cardiol* 2002; **39**: 393A–393A.

31. Khorsand A, Graf S, Pirich C *et al.* Gated cardiac PET for assessment of LV volume and ejection fraction. *J Nucl Med* 2001; **42**: 741.

32. Block S, Schaefer W, Nowak B *et al.* Comparison of left ventricular ejection fraction calculated by EGG-gated PET and contrast left ventriculography. *J Nucl Med* 2001; **42**: 734.

33. Willemsen AT, Siebelink HJ, Blanksma PK *et al.* Left ventricle ejection fraction determination with gated (18)FDG-PET. *J Nucl Med* 1999; **40**: 166P.

34. Cooke CD, Folks RD, Oshinski JN *et al.* Determination of ejection fraction and myocardial volumes from gated FDG PET studies: A preliminary validation with gated MR. *J Nucl Med* 1997; **38**: 198–198.

35. Burger C, Goerres G, Schoenes S *et al.* PET attenuation coefficients from CT images: Experimental evaluation of the transformation of CT into PET 511 keV attenuation coefficients. *Eur J Nucl Med Mol Imaging* 2002; **29**: 922–927.

36. Koepfli P, Wyss CA, Hany TF *et al.* Evaluation of CT-transmission for attenuation correction in quantitative myocardial perfusion measurement using a combined PET-CT scanner: A pilot dose-finding study for different CT energies. *Circulation* 2001; **104**: 2778.

37. Koepfli P, Hany TF, Wyss CA *et al.* CT attenuation correction for myocardial perfusion quantification using a PET/CT hybrid scanner. *J Nucl Med* 2004; **45**: 537–542.

38. Kinahan PE, Hasegawa BH, Beyer T. X-ray-based attenuation correction for positron emission tomography/computed tomography scanners. *Semin Nucl Med* 2003; **33**: 166–179.

39. Nakamoto Y, Osman M, Cohade C *et al.* PET/CT: Comparison of quantitative tracer uptake between germanium and CT transmission attenuation-corrected images. *J Nucl Med* 2002; **43**: 1137–1143.

40. Visvikis D, Costa DC, Croasdale I *et al.* CT-based attenuation correction in the calculation of semi-quantitative indices of F-18 FDG uptake in PET. *Eur J Nucl Med Mol Imaging* 2003; **30**: 344–353.

41. Vass M, Sasaki K, Pan T. Investigation of heart motion with multi-slice cardiac CT for attenuation correction of PET emission data. *Radiology* 2002; **225**: 520.

42. Dizendorf E, Hany TF, Buck A *et al.* Cause and magnitude of the error induced by oral CT contrast agent in CT-based attenuation correction of PET emission studies. *J Nucl Med* 2003; **44**: 732–738.

43. Nakamoto Y, Chin BB, Kraitchman DL *et al.* Effects of non-ionic intravenous contrast agents at PET/CT imaging: Phantom and canine studies. *Radiology* 2003; **227**: 817–824.

44. Cohade C, Osman M, Nakamoto Y *et al.* Initial experience with oral contrast in PET/CT: Phantom and clinical studies. *J Nucl Med* 2003; **44**: 412–416.

45. Burger CN, Dizendorf EV, Hany TF *et al.* Impact of transient oral contrast agent on CT-based attenuation correction in combined PET/CT studies. *Radiology* 2002; **225**: 409.

46. Antoch G, Jentzen W, Stattaus J *et al.* Effect of oral contrast agents on CT-based PET attenuation correction in dual-modality PET/CT tomography. *Radiology* 2002; **225**: 423–424.

47. Beyer T, Antoch G, Blodgett T *et al.* Dual-modality PET/CT imaging: The effect of respiratory motion on combined image quality in clinical oncology. *Eur J Nucl Med Mol Imaging* 2003; **30**: 588–596.

48. Goerres GW, Buehler TC, Burger C *et al.* CT based attenuation correction using a combined PET/CT scanner: Influence of the respiration level on measured FDG concentration in normal tissues. *J Nucl Med* 2002; **43**: 887.

49. Goerres GW, Burger C, Kamel E *et al.* Respiration-induced attenuation artifact at PET/CT: Technical considerations. *Radiology* 2003; **226**: 906–910.

50. Goerres GW, Kamel E, Heidelberg TNH *et al.* PET-CT image co-registration in the thorax: Influence of respiration. *Eur J Nucl Med Mol Imaging* 2002; **29**: 351–360.

51. Osman MM, Cohade C, Nakamoto Y *et al.* Respiratory motion artifacts on PET emission images obtained using CT attenuation correction on PET-CT. *Eur J Nucl Med Mol Imaging* 2003; **30**: 603–606.

CHAPTER 2

Cardiovascular magnetic resonance: Basic principles, methods and techniques

Joseph B. Selvanayagam, Matthew D. Robson,
Jane M. Francis & Stefan Neubauer

Introduction

Unlike the physics of x-ray imaging (attenuation of x-ray beam by tissue) or the physics of ultrasound imaging (reflection of ultrasound by tissue), the physics underlying magnetic resonance imaging (MRI) is substantially more complex. This technique has evolved over the past half-century through a number of landmark discoveries and investigations. In 1946, Bloch [1] and Purcell [2] independently discovered the phenomenon of *Nuclear Magnetic Resonance*, or NMR (later shortened, although physically incorrect, to *Magnetic Resonance*, or MR), and both later shared the Nobel Price in Physics for this discovery. In 1973, Lauterbur [3] and Mansfield independently proposed that the spatial distribution of nuclear spins may be determined through local variation of field strength, i.e. by use of a magnetic field gradient; both received the 2003 Nobel prize in Medicine for this discovery. In 1976, again working independently, Radda's [4] and Jacobus's [5] groups were the first to record an MR signal from the heart, in the form of a ^{31}P-MR spectrum. Cardiac MR spectroscopy (MRS) thus substantially preceded the development of cardiac MRI (CMR). In 1977, Damadian's group [6] reported whole-body MRI, and soon thereafter, MRI of the brain and of other non-moving or easily immobilized organs became ready for clinical prime time. The heart has long escaped high-resolution

detection by MRI, because it is a constantly moving structure, posing a number of additional technical challenges to its detection by MR. CMR has come to fruition only since the mid 1990s, mainly because of major advances in hardware design (high-field, highly homogeneous magnets), coil design (cardiac phased array etc), sequence development (TrueFISP etc.) and computing power. The latter has been instrumental in speeding up image reconstruction and postprocessing, a previously critical bottleneck in CMR. In coming years, further major technical breakthroughs in CMR development are anticipated, e.g. in perfusion, coronary, and atherosclerosis imaging and in MRS. It is conceivable that, because of its unique versatility and non-invasive nature, CMR may become the primary diagnostic modality in cardiovascular medicine.

Physical principles underlying MRI

Magnetic resonance imaging views the water and fat in the human body by observing the hydrogen nuclei in these molecules. Magnetic resonance is sensitive to any nucleus that possesses a net "spin". Nuclear spin is a fundamental property of atomic nuclei that depends on the numbers of neutrons and protons it contains, and so nuclei either have it (e.g. hydrogen (^{1}H), phosphorus (^{31}P), sodium (^{23}Na)) or they do not (e.g. helium (^{4}He), carbon (^{12}C), oxygen (^{16}O), see Table 2.1). Certain common

Table 2.1 Myocardial tissue concentrations and MR sensitivity of elements important for MR imaging/spectroscopy.

Nucleus	Natural abundance	Relative MR sensitivity	Myocardial tissue concentrations
^{1}H	99.98%	100%	H_2O 110 M; up to ~90 mM (CH_3 -^{1}H of creatine)
^{13}C	1.1%	1.6%	labeled compounds, several mM
^{23}Na	100%	9.3%	10 mM (intracellular); 140 mM (extracellular)
^{31}P	100%	6.6%	up to ~18 mM (PCr)

elements occur as a mixture of different isotopes, and in this case only a fraction may be visible (i.e. ^{3}He is visible but ^{4}He is not). The high concentration of hydrogen (^{1}H) nuclei in the human body (up to 110 mol/L) coupled with its high "relative MR sensitivity", make it the nucleus most suitable for high-resolution MRI.

Nuclei possessing net spin will behave as tiny radiofrequency receivers and transmitters when placed in a strong magnetic field. Both the frequency and the strength of the transmitter increase with increasing magnetic field strength. Typical clinical MRI systems possess fields of 1.5 Tesla (the Tesla (T) is the unit of magnetic field strength, or more accurately magnetic flux density). Even at these high magnetic field strengths the signals obtained from biological tissues are still very small, and the size of this signal can limit the quality of the images resulting in noise (graininess) obscuring the structures of interest. The nuclear magnetic resonance (NMR) phenomenon on which MRI is based involves transmitting radiofrequency pulses to the nuclei, which elevates them to a different energy level, from which they subsequently re-emit a radiofrequency signal. We can receive and acquire this re-emitted signal, and by manipulating this basic process we can perform MR imaging.

General physics of MR

One feature of MR is that the frequency at which signals are received and re-emitted (known as the resonant frequency) is exquisitely sensitive to the exact magnetic field, for example hydrogen nuclei (lone protons) resonate at 42.575 Hz/Tesla. So, if we have two regions where the magnetic field is different by a small amount (e.g. at 1.000 Tesla and 1.001 Tesla), then the protons in one region will transmit at 42.575 MHz (the Larmor frequency for

protons), and the protons from the other region will transmit at 42.575+0.042 MHz. If we sample this transmitted signal it is possible to determine these two different frequencies in the same way that a musician can distinguish between two tones at different audible frequencies. Numerically this transformation from a sampled signal to the component frequencies is known as a Fourier transform (Fig. 2.1).

Instead of using two discrete regions, in MRI we generally apply a linearly increasing magnetic field (lower at one side of the magnet and higher at the other side). As a result, each point in the body will have a discrete resonance frequency and hence the amplitude of the signal at a specific frequency will represent the number of protons at that specific location. Using a magnetic field gradient while the data are sampled allows the patient to be "imaged" in a single dimension, and comprises part of standard imaging methods. The direction of this gradient is described as the "read-out" direction in the MR image. To extend acquisition to two or more dimensions, additional switched magnetic field gradients (generally known simply as "gradients") need to be applied in the directions perpendicular to the "read-out" direction. For two-dimensional imaging, the above process is repeated a large (typically 256) number of times with different "gradients" applied in the second dimension for short intervals prior to acquisition, and the position is encoded in the phase of the signal. Each of these steps is known as a "phase encode" step and the number of these is generally[a] equal to the number of pixels in the phase-encode direction. The time

---

[a] This generalization is broken by partial Fourier, and by the parallel acquisition approaches (iPAT, SENSE, SMASH etc.).

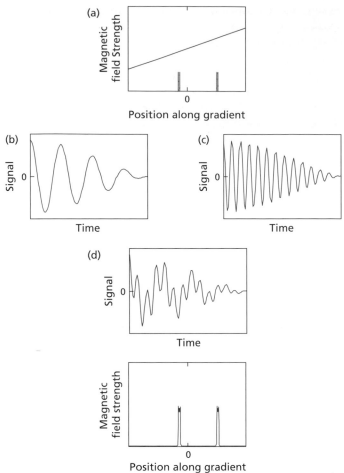

Fig. 2.1 (a) Two regions of protons are shown within a field gradient. The signals from each of the two regions are shown ((b) and (c)), but in reality it is only the sum of these two signals that we can sample (d). By Fourier transforming the signal we can examine the sample.

required for each phase-encode step is known as the repetition time and signified as TR.

As we are interested in slices through the sample that are thin, rather than projections of the sample (as in an x-ray) we also use a process known as slice selection. This involves using a radiofrequency (RF) excitation pulse that only contains a narrow range of frequencies. By playing out such a pulse whilst a field gradient is applied we only excite nuclei within a narrow slice. By applying the above three mechanisms we can obtain a two-dimensional image from a discrete slice of the sample. By modifying the frequency of the RF pulse, and by playing out the gradient pulses on more than one axis simultaneously we can move the slice of interest freely. We are not limited to axial planes, and can acquire data with oblique or doubly oblique axes with complete flexibility.

Basic imaging sequences

The term "pulse sequence" or "imaging sequence" describes the way in which the scanner plays out RF pulse and gradient fields and how it acquires and reconstructs the resultant data to form an image. Different orders of these pulses have defined names (e.g. FLASH, True-FISP, FSE) to describe them. The details of the sequence required for its application will also need to include the exact timings (i.e. TR), the amplitude, duration, and shapes of the gradient and RF pulses; the resolution parameters, and for cardiovascular applications these details will also include information on the cardiac gating strategy. This set of additional parameters is labeled the "protocol". Varying the protocol provides enormous flexibility for each imaging sequence.

In CMR we usually obtain 2D data acquired from a slice (e.g. 5 mm thick). Images can either be acquired in real time or over a series of heart beats. In the first case the spatial and temporal resolution will be limited by the available imaging time. In the second case we require that the breath is held[b] and so assume that the heart is perfectly periodic and that a fraction of the phase-encoding steps of the image is acquired at the same relative phase of the cardiac cycle. The latter approach results in improved spatial and temporal resolution. If the assumption of periodicity is broken (e.g. in the case of arrhythmia, or failure to hold breath for long enough) then image artifacts[c] will result.

The basic imaging sequences used in cardiac MR are:

- FLASH (Fast Low Angle SHot). This plays out a small excitation RF pulse which is followed by a rapid read-out and then spoiling (or removing) of the residual signal to prevent it appearing as an artifact in subsequent acquisitions. The process is repeated yielding a single phase-encode line per acquisition.
- TrueFISP (aka Balanced FFE (Balanced Fast Field Echo)). This sequence is similar to FLASH but instead of spoiling the magnetization at the end of each acquisition it re-uses that signal. Compared to FLASH the benefit of this approach is that the images are of higher signal-to-noise, the disadvantages being increased sensitivity to artifacts, increased RF power deposition, and contrast that is more complex to interpret.
- FSE (Fast Spin Echo, TSE (Turbo Spin Echo)). This sequence acquires a number of phase-encode lines per acquisition by playing out a series of refocusing pulses after the initial excitation pulse. These refocusing pulses are a phenomenon of MR (not described here), which allow us to hold onto the signal created by the excitation pulse for longer so that we can sample it multiple times. The optimum excitation pulse can be used, which

maximises the available signal, and it is possible with this sequence to obtain T_2 contrast without the undesirable effects of T_2^* (see below). It is possible to acquire all the phase encodes in FSE in a single acquisition (this variant is known as HASTE, EXPRESS, and Single-Shot FSE), which has some advantages, although this is likely to result in low temporal resolution.

Additional modules can be included with the above sequences to modify the image contrast, for example:

- Black-blood pulses can be applied which effectively remove all the signal from material that moves quickly (i.e. blood). This is usually performed using double inversion, which requires a delay prior to acquisition so is most compatible with FSE-based sequences.
- Inversion recovery is a prepulse method that allows us to introduce T_1 contrast into an image. We can choose an inversion time that completely removes the signal from materials with a certain T_1. In practice this is often used when we want to see small changes in T_1 in late enhancement type sequences (see section on viability).
- Fat suppression (or water suppression) can be used to remove all the signal from either of these tissues, which may improve the delineation of the structures of interest.

The above acquisition approaches represent no more than the "tip of the iceberg" regarding all possible MRI acquisition strategies, but will include 95% of all practical CMR applications.

Image contrast

If all the nuclei behaved identically, then the above imaging methods would provide a map of the patient whereby the intensity at a pixel would depend purely on the concentration of that nucleus at that location in the body. However, several additional mechanisms affect this simple picture, which make MRI a considerably more powerful technique.

- Spin-lattice relaxation (T_1) relates to the time it takes for the signal to recover after an excitation pulse. This can simply be thought of as the time needed for the proton system to become active again, and so if we acquire separate phase-encodes rapidly (i.e. short TR), then tissues with a long T_1 will not recover quickly enough and will be darkened in the image (this effect is known as

---

[b] Breath-holding provides the most simple and robust method for cardiac imaging. Alternative approaches do exist that involve determining the phase of breathing either using external devices, or using MRI based measurements, and dynamically modifying the scan accordingly, therefore eliminating the requirement for breath-holding. The MRI based (or navigator) methods allow for long scans where breath-holding is impossible.

[c] An artifact is an imperfection in the image that is not due purely to noise. Noise appears as a speckling of the image.

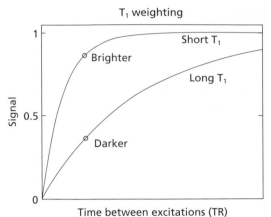

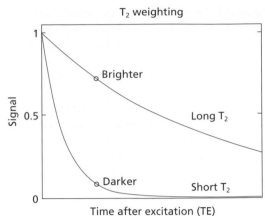

Fig. 2.2 This oversimplified figure shows that the magnetization recovers quickly for tissues with a short T_1 but more slowly for tissues with a long T_1. By manipulating the repetition time (in this figure, but also the "flip angle") we can convert this difference in longitudinal magnetization into transverse magnetization and hence image intensity.

Fig. 2.3 The transverse magnetization from the tissue with short T_2 decays rapidly after excitation, whereas this magnetization persists for the long T_2 species. These two tissues can be distinguished in an image by using a long echo time (as shown by the markers).

"saturation"), whereas tissues with a short T_1 will recover more quickly and so will be brighter in the image (Fig. 2.2). T_1 contrast can also be manipulated by changing the size of the excitation pulse (this parameter is known as the "flip angle"), as the spins will require more time to recover from the application of large flip angle than from a small one. Consequently, decreasing TR and increasing the flip angle will both increase the amount of T_1 weighting, whereas decreasing TR and the flip angle will decrease the amount of T_1 weighting.

- The spin-spin relaxation time (T_2) relates to the time that the signal is available for sampling after excitation. To benefit from this method we can excite the nucleus, and then wait a short period (e.g. 50 ms) before acquiring data. Tissues with a short T_2 (i.e. fast decay rate) will be darkened almost completely in the image, whereas tissue with a long T_2 (i.e. slow decay rate) will be darkened much less in the image (Fig. 2.3). T_2 is used to refer specifically to the relaxation rate in fast-spin-echo type sequences (i.e. the family of FSE sequences described above), and a different parameter T_2^* is used to describe the equivalent time for a gradient echo type sequence (i.e. FLASH). This is useful, for example to look at iron overload where the T_2^* is shortened [7]. The echo time (TE) is the time between excitation and

acquisition and determines the amount that the image is affected by the T_2^* and T_2 (known as the degree of T_2-weighting).

- In-flow. In the cardiovascular system the motion or flow of the protons will affect the image contrast in a similar way as the T_1. In this case spins may move out of the imaging slice, where they are not affected by the flip angle, to a location where they become visible in our image. In this case the in-flowing spins will have additional brightness as they will not be subject to the signal attenuation because of the effect of T_1 saturation (described above). MR angiography utilizes this in-flow to make blood in vessels (i.e. moving blood) bright, while suppressing the stationary signals (Fig. 2.4) Alternative methods exist to quantitatively examine flow velocities. These methods use the field gradients to encode the position of the blood and then decode this position at a later time. Stationary signal is unaffected by this encoding and decoding, but moving tissues accumulate a change in the phase of their signal which provides quantitative information on flow rates. This method is known as "phase-velocity", as the velocity is encoded in the phase of the signal [8].

Contrast agents

Up until this point we have only been concerned with the indigenous contrast in the sample that

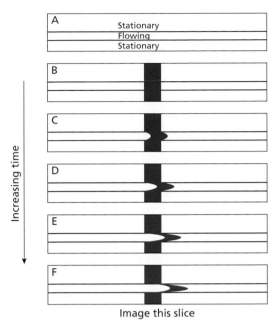

Image this slice

Fig. 2.4 The above figures show the sample evolving with time. Initially (A) none of the sample is saturated. With the application of a slice selective saturation pulse a slab of signal is saturated (B). As time progresses unsaturated blood flows into the region that was previously saturated. If we select our slice thickness and imaging time correctly we can obtain an image that shows the blood without the stationary tissues.

is due to the molecular environment of the water and fat. Addition of even small amounts of certain molecules, called MR contrast agents, can massively change relaxation rates (i.e. T_1, T_2 and T_2^*) within the patient, which results in major changes in the appearance of an MR image. Fundamentally, there are two types of contrast agents:

- T_1 contrast agents, which by interaction with the nuclear spins, shorten the T_1 of the sample. For this to operate there needs to be intimate contact between the agent and the protons.
- T_2 and T_2^* contrast agents. In this case the contrast agents will shorten the T_2 and T_2^* of the sample. These effects do not need close interactions between the nuclei and the agent as they occur over much larger distances.

In each case the contrast agents are based upon molecules or ions that are magnetically active. Paramagnetic moieties (typically, Fe, Dy, Gd but also O_2) are used because these demonstrate the greatest effects. The most commonly used nucleus

is Gd (gadolinium), and this is chelated (with diethylenetriaminepentaacetate, DTPA) so as to render it non-toxic and safe for injection. Gd compounds act predominantly as T_1 contrast agents in the blood and myocardium, although where the contrast cannot freely mix with the observed water (i.e. in the brain because of the blood-brain barrier), their small T_2 and T_2^* effects can also be observed. Gd-based contrast agents are approved for clinical use, but for historic reasons at the time of writing these are not yet approved for cardiac application in the US, although this will most likely be rectified in the near future. Iron-oxide particles predominantly affect the T_2 and T_2^* of the sample. In MR images the regions where these particles accumulate will decrease the signals in T_2-weighted images. For both types of contrast agent the effects are regionally specific, i.e. compounds affect the contrast at the site of the contrast agent and by an amount that increases with contrast agent concentration. This can be used, for example when looking at myocardial infarction when contrast agent remains within infarcted tissue at higher concentration than in surrounding normal tissue ~10–20 min after administration of an appropriate agent (see viability imaging). By adding MR contrast agents to compounds that can adhere to specific molecules (e.g. Fibrin) we can create "targeted contrast agents". This type of molecular imaging provides a promising approach for the future.

Contrast agents can be produced that remain within the vascular system, and are thus termed "intravascular". With an agent that decreases the T_1 it is possible to boost the signal in angiographic examinations, and hence improve the image quality. Presently Gd-DPTA is used in such angiographic examinations, but as it is not an "intravascular" agent the acquisition needs to occur when the Gd-DTPA is undergoing its first pass through the vascular tree. "Intravascular" contrast agents would remove this restriction, enabling longer, and hence higher quality, imaging. Presently no agents of this kind are approved for clinical use.

The CMR scanner—how we use the physics

The physics and engineering of MRI are immensely complex, but much like a modern motor car it is not essential to understand all the details to be able to use the machine.

To minimize the effects of electrical interference from the outside world (e.g. radiotransmitters, electronic devices etc.) the MRI system is placed within an electrically shielded "box" (a Faraday cage), which is normally hidden in the walls of the scanning room. CMR scanners are a subset of MRI scanners, but with specific characteristics. Here MRI systems are described with special note as to what is required for CMR.

The most important feature of the CMR scanner is the magnet. A strong homogeneous magnetic field can be obtained by building a solenoidal electromagnet from superconducting wires carrying large electrical currents at very low temperatures. These magnets are kept permanently at magnetic field. Some clinical systems operate at 0.5, 1.0T and some new systems are available at 3.0T, but the majority of MR systems operate at 1.5T. Cardiac imaging at fields outside this range is more difficult, although scientific results have been demonstrated. The field of the magnet is highest in the centre of the bore[d] of the magnet and this is where the organs of interest (i.e. the heart and vascular system) need to be positioned. The magnetic field also extends out from the magnet. Modern systems use "active shielding" which minimizes this effect, but even with this technology the "fringe" field will extend to approximately 3–5 m (10–16 ft) or so in each direction around the magnet (including the floors above and below).

The equipment for transmitting RF pulses into the patient (the RF transmit coil), and for creating the linear magnetic field gradients (the gradient coil) are enclosed within the bore of the magnet and are not visible during operation. The gradient system on CMR machines needs to be particularly powerful because this component relates directly to the rate at which images can be acquired. The rapidly switching currents in the gradient coil interact with the magnetic field of the magnet, which results in forces being exerted on the gradient coil. The gradient coil is strongly built so as to resist these forces, but these small motions and distortions of the coil act like a speaker, producing large amounts of audible noise when running fast imaging sequences.

Additional RF reception coils are placed onto the patient, and may also be built into the patient bed, and these are used to receive the signals that are re-emitted by the nuclei. Smaller coils provide a higher signal-to-noise ratio than large coils, but also have a smaller region of sensitivity. RF coil manufacturers tailor their designs for specific parts of the body to optimise this trade off, and frequently will use multiple coils within a single structure to maximise the signal, while also maximising the region of sensitivity. These complex coil combinations are known as "phased array" coils and are standard for cardiac imaging.

The other visible component of an MRI system is the patient bed. This is required to position the patient accurately at the center of the MRI system. The MRI system is operated away from the magnet itself via a computer, which allows the operator to acquire and display images. An additional room is required to house the electronics, cooling and other control hardware associated with the MRI system; this equipment is generally hidden. Fig. 2.5 shows a typical layout of these components for a cardiovascular imaging system.

CMR imaging techniques

General overview of the CMR examination

Careful preparation of the patient is necessary in order to maximize diagnostic information from the CMR scan. This includes screening of the patient to exclude any contraindication to the MR examination (see section on safety), checking that the patient is not wearing any clothes with metallic fastenings, and adequate preparation of the chest prior to electrode positioning for ECG gating. To ensure good contact it may be necessary to shave the chest to remove any excess hair, and/or use an abrasive skin preparation to remove any dead skin cells and moisture. It is possible to double the amplitude of the signal with correct preparation and a simple, important rule is: "No trigger, no scan". If repeated breath-hold images are to be taken then it may be worthwhile training the patient outside the magnet about the breathing commands to be used.

Fig. 2.6 demonstrates the use of a four-lead ECG configuration and electrode positioning placed both anteriorly and posteriorly. The benefits of

---

[d] The term "bore" is used to describe the hole through the middle of the magnet.

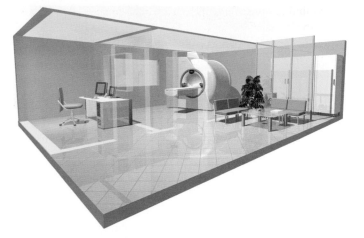

Fig. 2.5 Computer generated diagram of an MR scanning suite. The internal walls are displayed semi-opaque so each part of the system is visible. Note the operator console, magnet, and control hardware (image supplied courtesy of Siemens Medical Solutions).

Fig. 2.6 Suitable sites on the anterior (A, B) or posterior (C) chest wall for optimal ECG detection. (D) demonstrates the correct positioning of the body flex array coil for CMR examination. (Image supplied courtesy of Siemens Medical Solutions).

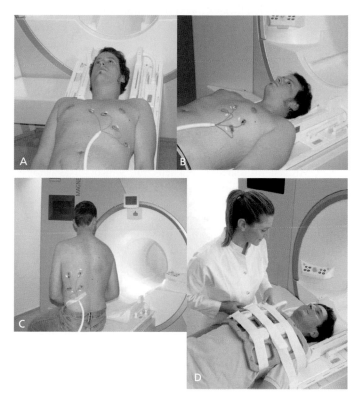

anterior lead placement are larger amplitude and ease of repositioning, but there may be respiration-induced artifacts. Posterior lead placement can help counteract this at the expense of signal amplitude. Once the patient is ready then he/she is placed supine on the scanner table and an RF receiver coil is placed over the anterior chest wall. This is used in combination with elements of the spine array coil

to ensure good signal from both the anterior and posterior chest wall.

ECG gating and physiological monitoring

Gating is described simply as the detection of the R-wave by the MR system and is used to "trigger" or synchronize the acquisition to the patient's heart rate. Correct gating relies on good R wave detection

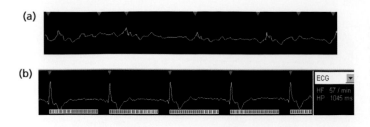

Fig. 2.7 (a) An example of poor R wave recognition in a patient positioned within the magnet bore. In contrast (b), there is accurate R wave detection during this prospectively gated cine acquisition. Cine frames are indicated by the green squares below the trace.

and a regular R-R interval. Deterrents to successful CMR imaging include poor R wave detection (Fig. 2.7), an inadequate ECG, and the presence of tachyarrhythmias and/or ventricular ectopic beats. When using prospective cardiac gating, the MR system detects the R-wave and then begins the imaging sequence. However, as this method only uses 80–90% of the R-R interval, data are not acquired during end-diastole.

Retrospectively gated sequences are now widely available, whereby the sequence is continuously repeated, the R-R interval monitored and the data retrospectively fitted, allowing acquisition of the entire cardiac cycle. This method has the added benefit of compensating for some variation in the R-R interval during acquisition. A new feature of some CMR systems is arrhythmia detection, which allows the R-R interval that is used for acquisition to be fixed by the operator, thus eliminating data obtained during ectopic beats. This approach may particularly aid data acquisition in patients with atrial fibrillation.

One important consideration is the effect of the magnetic field on the ECG waveform. Blood flow, particularly in the aorta, causes an additional electrical signal detected by the ECG, leading to a magnetohydrodynamic effect. This is generally superimposed on the T wave and can make the analysis of the ECG within the magnetic field very difficult. The only diagnostic feature of the ECG that is reliable while a patient is inside the bore is the heart rate (provided QRS detection is good), whereas it is difficult to comment on changes in the P wave, the ST segment and the T wave. The development of techniques such as the vector ECG, which uses 3D collection of ECG data and separates artifact from the true ECG signal, have helped to overcome some of the ECG problems associated with CMR and to improve image quality and scan efficiency [9]. Another novel method of ECG

synchronization is the self gating approach where information regarding cardiac motion is extracted from the image data [10]. This method does not require an ECG to be obtained.

The other main cause of image degradation in CMR is respiration-artifact. Most patients are able to hold their breath during image acquisition, particularly with the recent introduction of parallel imaging techniques such as iPAT and SENSE which reduce breath-hold times considerably. However, especially in instances where the patients cannot hold their breath (e.g. older subjects, significant cardiac/respiratory disease), and/or in cases where longer acquisition times are unavoidable (e.g. coronary artery imaging), respiratory gating with MR navigators is essential for artifact free images. Navigator echo techniques are used for respiratory compensation, in conjunction with ECG gating. The navigator echo is combined with the imaging sequence and enables movement to be tracked throughout the respiratory cycle. It consists of a signal from a column perpendicular to the direction of movement. The usual placement for CMR is on the dome of the diaphragm, and the sequence only acquires when the diaphragm is in a predefined position with a small tolerance window. Although this might reduce scan efficiency and hence prolong imaging time, it does allow acquisition to take place with the patient breathing freely (Fig. 2.8). Fig. 2.9 shows some common artifacts encountered during CMR imaging.

Cardiac anatomy

Cardiac anatomy can easily be demonstrated using MR imaging techniques, which are not confined to the three orthogonal planes (transverse, coronal and sagittal) as in conventional imaging. The multiplanar capabilities of CMR can be used to define the conventional imaging planes of the heart, such as the horizontal and vertical long axes, and the

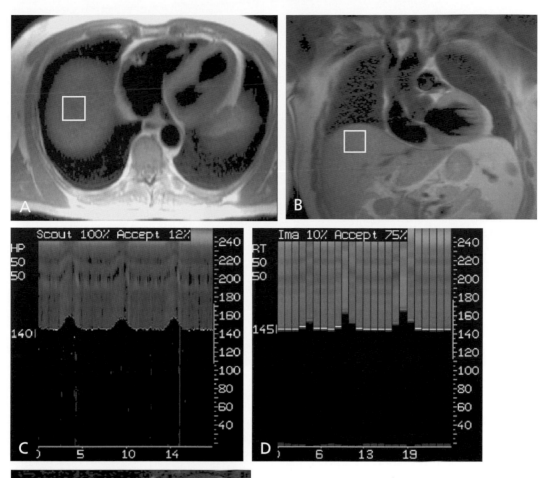

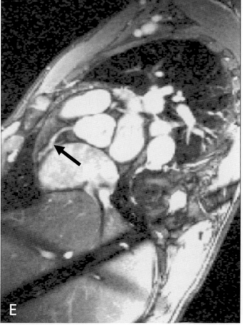

Fig. 2.8 Placement of a navigator (white square) on the right hemi-diaphragm in the transverse (A) and coronal (B) planes. (C)—diaphragm position during the respiratory cycle (y axis) against time (x axis). (D)—navigator trace during image acquisition set at 145 mm +/− 8 mm. Acquisition takes place as indicated by white "bar". (E)—resulting short axis view showing the right coronary artery—black arrow.

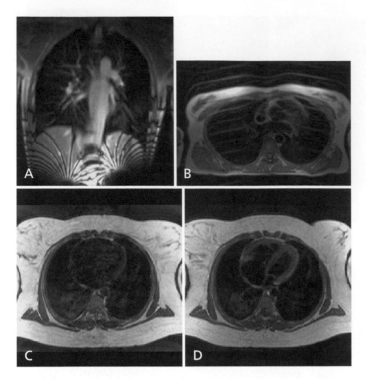

Fig. 2.9 Common artifacts seen during CMR imaging: (A) Metal artifact from a small clip in the patient's trousers, highlighting the importance of removing all clothing with metal fastenings. (B) Respiration artifact during a spin echo anatomical imaging sequence. (C) Poor definition of cardiac structures with spin echo sequence because of incorrect positioning of ECG electrodes. (D) Significant improvement seen after repositioning of the ECG electrodes.

short axis, as well as to prescribe any imaging plane specific to a particular pathology. This is particularly useful in cases of congenital heart disease. The three orthogonal planes (see Fig. 2.10) remain important for diagnosis and these can be easily and quickly acquired using the newer single shot techniques such as HASTE, where a stack of images can be obtained in a single breath-hold.

The transverse plane is useful for a good overview of size, shape and position of the cardiac chambers and great vessels and should be inclusive from the top of the aortic arch (including the great vessels) to the inferior wall of the right ventricle, typically covering 20–24 slices. The coronal plane is useful for an assessment of the descending aorta, IVC (inferior vena cava) SVC (superior vena cava), both ventricles, left atrium and pulmonary veins, and the LVOT (left ventricular outflow tract). The slices should reach from the descending aorta posteriorly to the right ventricle anteriorly. The sagittal plane is useful for visualizing the descending aorta, IVC (inferior vena cava), SVC (superior vena cava), and the right ventricle. In addition, the oblique sagittal view, which is planned from the

transverse multislice series can be a useful addition when assessing the aorta and gives the familiar "hockey stick" view of the whole of the aorta.

Cardiac function

CMR has rapidly become the imaging method of choice and the gold standard in the assessment of cardiac function of both normal and abnormal ventricles [11–14]. Given its 3D nature and order of magnitude greater signal-to-noise ratio, CMR is highly superior to 2D echocardiography for the measurement of global left ventricular function [11]. This has allowed reductions of study sizes of 80–97% to achieve the same statistical power

Fig. 2.10 (*opposite*) Anatomical images obtained with a turbo spin echo sequence showing the heart and great vessels in a transverse (A-D), coronal (E-H) and sagittal (I-K) planes. (L) shows an oblique sagittal view of the ascending and descending aorta, the so called "hockey stick" view. LV denotes left ventricle; RV denotes right ventricle; MPA, main pulmonary artery; RVOT, right ventricular outflow tract; AA, proximal ascending aorta; DA, descending aorta; LA, left atrium; RA, right atrium; SVC, superior vena cava; PDA, proximal descending aorta.

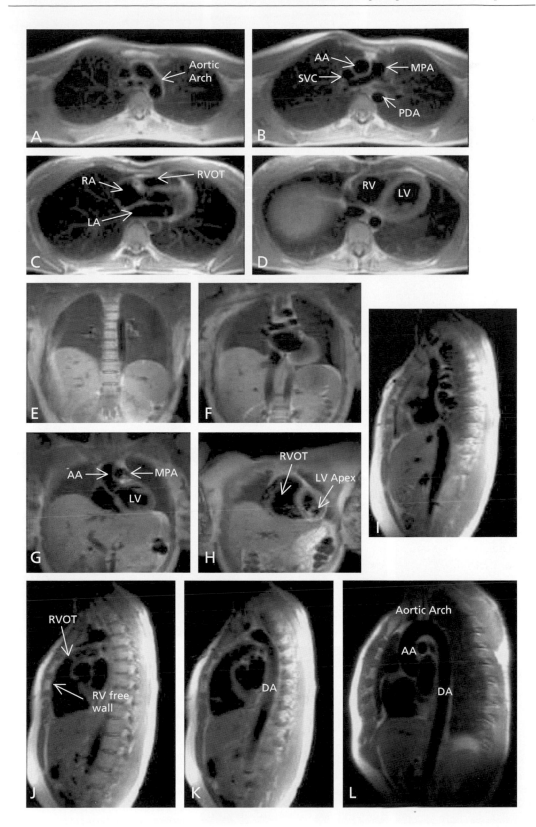

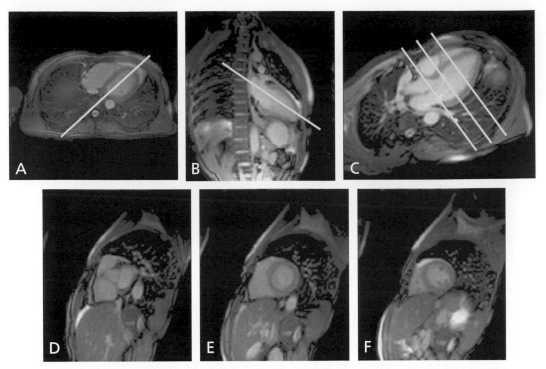

Fig. 2.11 Sequence of images (A-F) demonstrating the correct acquisition of the long axis and short axis planes for cine imaging. Initially, multiplanar localizer images are performed in a single breath-hold (A). Using the transverse localizer (A), in the plane indicated by the solid line in (A), pilot images are then performed in the vertical long axis (VLA) plane (B). The resultant VLA pilot is used to prescribe (as indicated by the solid line in (B)) the horizontal long axis (HLA) pilot (C). Using the HLA and VLA pilots, three short axis (SA) slices (D-F) are next acquired with the basal slice parallel to the atrioventricular (AV) groove (indicated by three solid lines in (C)).

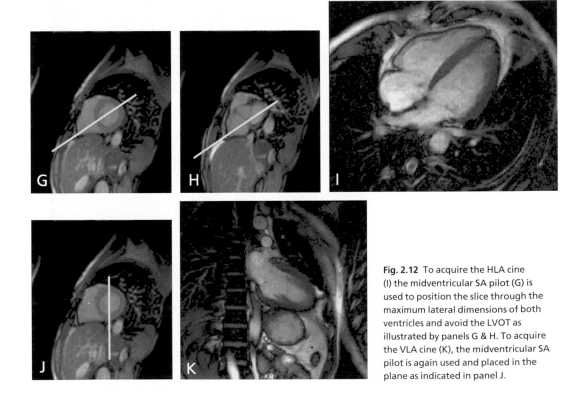

Fig. 2.12 To acquire the HLA cine (I) the midventricular SA pilot (G) is used to position the slice through the maximum lateral dimensions of both ventricles and avoid the LVOT as illustrated by panels G & H. To acquire the VLA cine (K), the midventricular SA pilot is again used and placed in the plane as indicated in panel J.

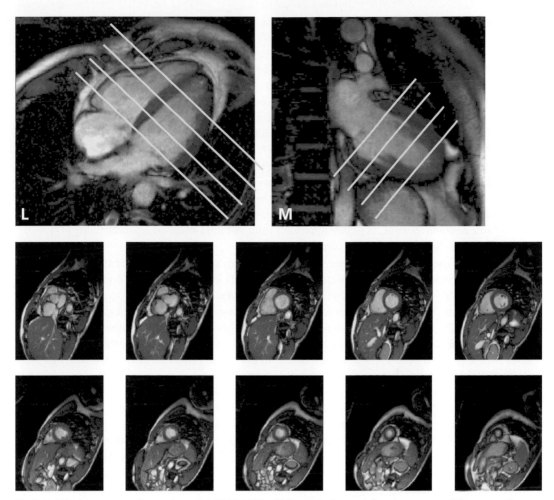

Fig. 2.13 This demonstrates the resultant HLA (L), VLA (M) and short axis cine stack from base to apex (bottom panel). Placement of only 4 short axis slices shown for image clarity.

for demonstrating given changes of left ventricular volumes, ejection fraction, or cardiac mass [11]. It can be performed quickly and easily, and can be incorporated into a comprehensive CMR examination.

The following method is employed at the authors' institution, and is a widely accepted approach to quantify left ventricular volumes, mass and function (Fig. 2.11, Fig. 2.12 and Fig. 2.13). The methods described may not be possible from all manufacturers, and variations from the described protocol may be necessary. After careful preparation of the patient and explanation of the importance of consistent breath-hold technique, multislice, multiplanar localizer images are performed in a single breath-hold. Prescribing a plane from the transverse plane using the mitral valve and the apex of the left

ventricle as anatomical markers, localizer ("pilot") images are obtained in the vertical long axis (VLA). The resultant VLA pilot is then used to prescribe the horizontal long axis (HLA) pilot using the same anatomical landmarks.

It is important to accurately define the base of the heart when using this or a similar piloting method. As illustrated in Fig. 2.11, using the HLA and VLA pilots, three short axis (SA) slices are acquired with the basal slice parallel to the atrioventricular (AV) groove. The distance between the slices is chosen such that they encompass the basal, mid and apical regions of the left ventricle. These "scout" images can then be used to plan cine images in two long-axis (HLA, VLA), and left ventricular outflow tract (LVOT) views.

When acquiring the short axis volume stack

from the two long axis cines, the position of the basal slice is critical. Most errors in volume calculation are introduced here if this stage is not carefully planned. Using the end-diastolic frames from the VLA and HLA cines, the first slice is placed in the atrioventricular (AV) groove. Subsequent slices are placed parallel to this, covering the entire left ventricle. Typically slice thickness is 7–8 mm with a 3 or 2 mm interslice gap. Imaging is usually performed in expiration as this generally produces a more consistent, reproducible breath-hold position.

Volume and mass data are calculated by drawing epicardial and endocardial regions of interest (ROI) at end-systole and end-diastole. Papillary muscles and trabeculae should be included in mass calculation and excluded from ventricular volumes. Various programmes are available to aid calculation of these values, e.g. ARGUS ® (Siemens Medical Solutions), and MASS ®, (Medis, Netherlands). Normal, gender specific values for left and right ventricular volumes and mass in adults have been defined [14]. Earlier studies used a gradient echo approach, such as a turboFLASH sequence, which has inferior blood/myocardial contrast definition when compared to newer steady state acquisition techniques such as TrueFISP. Recent studies have provided normal volume and mass ranges using steady state free precession (SSFP) sequences [13]. These show that SSFP sequences produce larger ventricular volumes and smaller ventricular mass measurements (when compared to gradient echo sequences) in the same reference population due to the improved definition of the blood-endocardial border.

CMR is also considered to be the most accurate imaging method for the evaluation of right ventricular (RV) volumes. CMR measurement of RV volumes has been validated with close correlation between RV and LV stroke volumes, and between RV stroke volumes and tricuspid flow measurements [15]. The inherent 3D nature of CMR makes it particularly well suited to studying the RV, given its complex and variable (even in normal volunteers) morphology [16]. CMR measurements of the RV volumes can either be acquired in a transverse (axial) orientation or in an axis aligned along the LV short axis. Both methods have their advantages and limitations. Using the LV short axis plane, only one data set is required for both LV and RV measurements. In addition, in the images acquired using the axial orientation, the partial volume effect of blood and myocardium on the inferior wall of the RV can make it difficult to identify the blood/myocardial boundary. However, assessment of the RV in the LV short axis orientation also has important limitations: The position of the pulmonary and tricuspid valves cannot be clearly identified and therefore, the basal boundary of the RV can be difficult to define. This can result in significant error because the basal slice has a large area. In a recent study that compared the two methods for RV volume measurements, Alfakih *et al.* found that there were systematic differences between them, and that the axial orientation resulted in better inter and intra-observer reproducibility [17].

Dynamic measures of left ventricular function

Given its ability to visualize myocardial segments accurately, CMR can be used to define ventricular function during pharmacological stress, principally with dobutamine (DSMR). Although DSMR imaging has been performed since 1992 [18], early studies to document inducible myocardial ischemia were limited by an inability to image the entire cardiac cycle during peak stress, and concerns about patient safety. Recent software and hardware advances have enabled the investigators to overcome some of these limitations. Shorter repetition times, phase encoding grouping and phased array surface coils allow for acquisition of images with high temporal resolution and with spatial resolution sufficient to delineate the endocardial border during peak stress [19]. Earlier concerns about patient safety have been alleviated by the introduction of hemodynamic monitoring and wall motion display software that allows the physician to safely monitor patients during stress testing.

Practical Aspects of DSMR Imaging

In preparation for a DSMR study patients are instructed to refrain from taking any ß-blockers and nitrates 24 hours prior to the examination. Short acting ß-blocker (e.g. Esmolol 0.5 mg/kg) is used as an antidote and should be easily accessible during scanning. Table 2.2 details the monitoring requirements needed for stress MR imaging. As with its use in other cardiac imaging, severe arterial hypertension (>220/120 mmHg); recent acute coronary syndrome; significant aortic stenosis; complex cardiac arrhythmias, and significant hypertrophic obstructive cardiomyopathy are some of the contraindications to the use of dobutamine stress testing.

Table 2.2 Monitoring requirements needed for stress MR imaging.

Heart rate and rhythm	Continuously
Blood pressure	Every minute
Pulse oximetry	Continuously
Symptoms	Continuously
Wall motion abnormalities	Every dose increment

Scan protocol: All 17 segments of the heart can be covered by a combination of three SA and two long axis views (HLA, VLA). The three SA and two long axis cines are performed at rest and are also repeated during stress at each dobutamine dose. Scans are terminated when the submaximal heart rate is reached; systolic blood pressure decreases >20 mmHg below baseline; blood pressure increases >240/120 mmHg; intractable symptoms, and new or worsening wall motion abnormalities occur in at least two adjacent left ventricular segments, or in the presence of complex cardiac arrhythmias.

Image interpretation: Multiple cine loop display is recommended, showing at least four different stress levels for each slice simultaneously. The ventricle is analyzed by 17 segments per stress level [20]. Analysis is carried out visually according to the standards suggested by the American Society of Echocardiography. Segmental wall motion is classified as normokinetic, hypokinetic, akinetic or dyskinetic and assigned one to four points, respectively. The sum of points is divided by the number of analyzed segments and yields the wall motion score. Normal contraction results in a wall motion score of one, a higher score is indicative of wall motion abnormalities. During dobutamine stress with increasing doses, a lack of increase in either wall motion or systolic wall thickening, a reduction of both, or significant changes in the rotational pattern of left ventricular myocardium ("tethering") are indicative of pathological findings. Nagel *et al.* compared DSMR imaging to dobutamine stress echocardiography (DSE) in patients referred for diagnostic coronary angiography [21]. They showed that DSMR imaging provided superior specificity (86% vs 70%) and sensitivity (89% vs 74%) in detecting coronary stenosis >50%, principally because the number of myocardial segments visualized as "good" or "very good" image quality was far greater with DSMR than with DSE. Among patients with regional wall motion defects at rest, DSMR has been shown to have a sensitivity of 89% and specificity of 85% for identifying coronary artery stenosis greater than 50% [22].

Tissue contractility

Beyond analysis of global and segmental function, MR offers techniques for assessment of regional and tissue contractility.

MR tagging: This method was first developed by Zerhouni and colleagues [23]. A radiofrequency tag is a region within the imaged tissue where the net magnetization has been altered with radiofrequency pulses. Each tag or "saturation grid" is created as a 3D plane that extends through the tissue, and it is seen as a tag line when imaged in an orthogonal view (Fig. 2.14). Typical tagging schemes include stacks of parallel lines [24], grids [25], and radial stripes [26]. By tracking material points as a function of

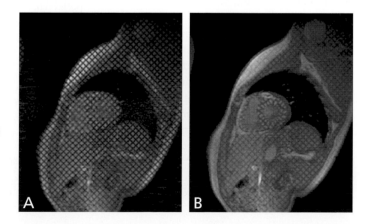

Fig. 2.14 Cardiac tagging short axis images obtained in a normal heart using a complementary spatial modulation of magnetization (CSPAMM) technique. The initial rectangular tagging grid at diastole (A) is distorted by cardiac contraction, as seen in the end-systolic image (B).

time, it is possible to compute the description of motion around a given point in the tissue as it traverses through time and space. Although the concept of radiofrequency tagging was proposed over a decade ago, automated software to analyze the images has only recently become available, [27, 28] and the clinical use of the method remains to be determined.

Tissue phase mapping and DENSE: The tissue phase mapping technique allows the determination of three-dimensional velocity tensors over the cardiac cycle, i.e. for rotation, radial and longitudinal movement, with a pixel-by-pixel spatial resolution nearing that of "conventional" cine MRI [29]. This is currently being investigated in clinical studies. Displacement encoded imaging using stimulated echoes (DENSE) can also provide information on myocardial displacement, velocity and strain [30].

Assessment of myocardial viability

Viability assessment can be defined practically as detecting myocardium that shows severe dysfunction at rest, but which will improve function, either spontaneously with time (stunned) or following revascularization (hibernating). The identification of residual myocardial viability is critical to the management of patients with ischemic heart disease. Contrast-enhanced MRI (ceMRI) with gadolinium-DTPA was described in 1984 in a canine model of acute MI [31]. Injured myocardium demonstrates significantly greater T1 shortening after contrast. These initial studies were hampered, however, by insufficient image contrast between normal and injured myocardium due to technical (e.g. gradients, phased array etc.) and sequence limitations.

Delayed enhancement MRI

In recent years, a number of studies have demonstrated the effectiveness of a segmented inversion recovery fast gradient echo (seg IR-GE) sequence for differentiating irreversible injured from normal myocardium with signal intensity differences of nearly 500% [32]. This technique of delayed enhancement imaging (DE-MRI), pioneered by Simonetti, Kim and Judd, has been shown in animal and human studies, to identify the presence, location, and extent of acute and chronic myocardial irreversible injury [33–36]. Delayed enhancement MRI (DE-MRI), allows assessment of the trans-

mural extent of irreversible injury, and is superior to SPECT for the identification of subendocardial myocardial infarction [37–39]. Furthermore, it permits quantification of even small areas of myocardial necrosis, both due to native coronary disease and, after percutaneous and surgical revascularization [40–42].

Practical aspects of delayed enhancement image acquisition

Delayed enhancement imaging can be performed in a single brief examination, requiring only a peripheral intravenous line. It does not require pharmacological or physiological stress. Initially cine images are obtained (as described above) to provide a matched assessment of left ventricular morphology and contractile function. A bolus of 0.10–0.20 mmol/kg intravenous gadolinium is then given by hand injection. After a 10–15 min delay (see below), high spatial resolution delayed-enhancement images of the heart are obtained at the same imaging planes as the cine images using the segmented IR-FGE pulse sequence. Each delayed-enhancement image is acquired during a 10–14 s breath-hold, and the imaging time for the entire examination (including cine imaging) is generally 30–40 min. Fig. 2.15 demonstrates two patient examples.

Segmented inversion recovery fast gradient echo sequence (IR-GE)

The timing diagram for the segmented IR-GE pulse sequence is shown in Fig. 2.16. Immediately after the onset of the R wave trigger, there is a delay period before a non-selective 180° inversion pulse is applied. Following this inversion pulse, a second variable wait period (usually referred to as the inversion time or TI), occurs corresponding to the time between the inversion pulse and the centre of acquisition of k-space lines. The flip angle used for radiofrequency excitation for each k-space line is shallow (20°–30°) to retain regional differences in magnetization that result from the inversion pulse and TI delay.

The following factors need to be considered when performing DE-MRI:

Dose: The dose of gadolinium given is usually 0.1–0.2 mmol/kg. Early validation studies used doses as high as 0.3 mmol/kg in animal models [34] and

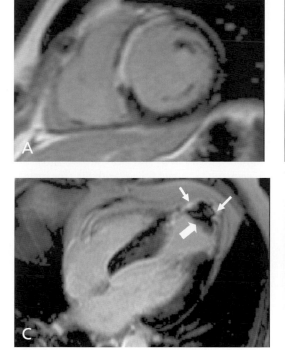

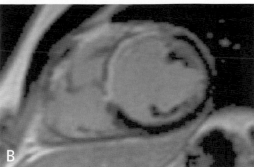

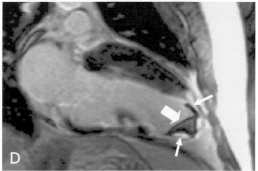

Fig. 2.15 Two patient examples of delayed hyperenhancement (DHE) imaged with a segmented inversion recovery gradient echo sequence at 10 min postGd-DTPA injection (0.1 mmol/kg). Panels A–B, demonstrate anteroseptal DHE in a patient presenting with two-week-old anterior myocardial infarction and proximal left anterior descending artery (LAD) occlusion. C–D are from a patient with history of apical myocardial infarction 12 months prior and midLAD occlusion, showing thinned apical wall with fully transmural DHE (small arrows). Co-existent apical thrombus is also seen in this patient (large arrows).

Fig. 2.16 Timing diagram of two-dimensional segmented inversion-recovery fast gradient echo pulse sequence. ECG = electrocardiogram, TI = inversion time delay, α = shallow flip angle excitation. See text for further details. (Figure re-drawn from: Reference 32, Simonetti OP, Kim RJ, Fieno DS *et al.* An improved MR imaging technique for the visualization of myocardial infarction. *Radiology* 2001; **218**: 215–223. Re-drawn with permission of publishers.)

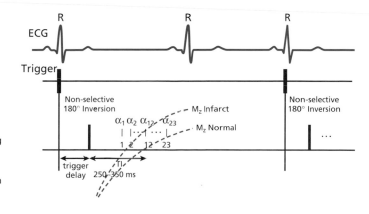

0.2 mmol/kg in patients [43]. More recent studies have found that using 0.1–0.15 mmol/kg still provides excellent image contrast between injured and normal myocardium with the added advantage that the time required to wait after contrast administration is reduced [41, 44]. It is necessary to allow the blood pool signal in the LV cavity to decline and provide discernment between LV cavity and hyperenhanced myocardium. This is particularly important in imaging small subendocardial infarcts, and when using a higher dose (i.e. 0.2 mmol/kg).

Gating factor: Image contrast is also optimized by applying the inversion pulse every other heart beat in order to allow for adequate longitudinal relaxation between successive 180° inversion pulses. If there are limitations related to breath-hold duration and/or bradycardia, every heart beat imaging may have to be performed. In this situation there may be incomplete relaxation of normal myocardium. Incomplete relaxation will result in not only an artificially shorter "effective" TI needed to null normal myocardium, but may also lead to a reduction in the image intensity differences between infarcted and normal myocardium.

Inversion time (TI): This is defined as the time between the 180° pulse and the center of acquisition of the k-space lines. Selecting the appropriate TI is probably the most important element in obtaining accurate imaging results. The TI is chosen to "null" normal myocardium, the time at which the magnetization of normal myocardium reaches the zero crossing (Fig. 2.16). This is when the image intensity difference between infarcted and normal myocardium is maximized. If the TI is too short, normal myocardium will be below the zero crossing and will have a negative magnetization vector at the time of k-space data acquisition. Since the image intensity corresponds to the magnitude of the magnetization vector, the image intensity of normal myocardium will increase as the TI becomes shorter and shorter, whereas the image intensity of infarcted myocardium will decrease until it reaches its own zero crossing.

At the other extreme, if the TI is set too long, the magnetization of normal myocardium will be above zero and will appear gray. Although areas of infarction will have high image intensity, the relative contrast between infarcted and normal myocardium will be reduced. Usually only one or two "test" images need to be acquired as with experience one can estimate the optimal TI based on the amount of contrast agent that is administered and the time after contrast agent administration. As the gadolinium concentration within normal myocardium gradually washes out with time the TI will need to be adjusted upwards (e.g. 10 ms every 3–4 images) to provide optimal image quality with multiple time-point imaging. Recently available automated TI finding sequences can also help in establishing the optimal inversion time.

Postprocessing

For routine clinical reporting, the 17-segment model recommended by the American Heart Association can be used [20]. The extent of hyperenhanced tissue within each segment is graded visually using a 5-point scale in which a score of 0 indicates no hyperenhancement; 1, hyperenhancement of 1–25% of the segment; 2, hyperenhancement of 26–50% of the segment; 3, hyperenhancement of 51–75% of the segment, and 4, hyperenhancement of 76–100% of the segment. It is advisable to interpret the delayed-enhancement images with the cine images immediately adjacent which provide a reference for the diastolic wall thickness of each region.

Assessment of myocardial perfusion

Contrast agents based on paramagnetism (e.g. gadolinium) or superparamagnetism (e.g. Fe^{2+}) can be tracked as they traverse the myocardium after intravenous injection to assess myocardial perfusion at rest and with a vasodilator (e.g. adenosine). Quantitative results have been achieved in animal studies with an intravascular agent such as a macromolecular blood pool marker, although such compounds are not yet licensed for use in humans. At the same time, semiquantitative/quantitative approaches are feasible in humans with a conventional extracellular MR contrast agent (Gd-DTPA).

First pass imaging

In first pass imaging a bolus of contrast agent is injected directly into a peripheral vein and a sequence of images is then obtained to show the dynamic passage of the tracer through the heart (Fig. 2.17).

MR sequences and contrast agents

The most significant parameter that a perfusion sequence must optimize is the temporal resolution, because the contrast agent only spends a relatively short period of time passing through the myocardium. During this time the required data must be obtained at a sufficient rate so that the reconstructed images provide a measure of the change in contrast agent concentration over time. For a complete perfusion study, up to three to five separate short axis slices need to be simultaneously obtained to achieve sufficient coverage of the myocardium. The most commonly used perfusion sequences are turboFLASH, SSFP, multishot echo planar (EPI)

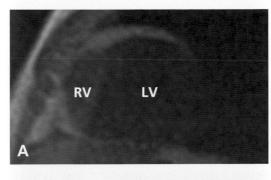
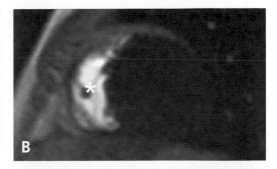
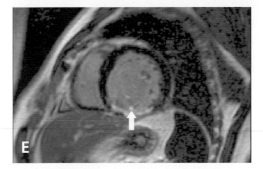
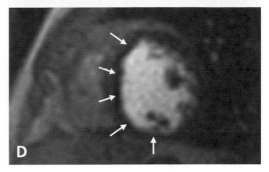
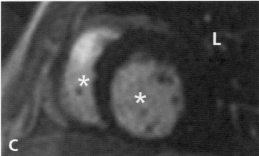

Fig. 2.17 Example of CMR perfusion images obtained with a turboFLASH sequence during first pass rapid injection of an extracellular contrast agent (Gd-DTPA). Images were acquired in a basal short axis view, and show: (A)—before contrast injection, (B)—contrast agent first in the right ventricle, (C)—contrast agent then in the lungs and left ventricle and (D)—agent in the left ventricle cavity and myocardium. Perfusion defect is seen in the anteroseptum, inferoseptum and inferior wall (arrows). Corresponding "delayed enhancement" image (E) is shown at the same slice position, demonstrating inferior wall delayed hyperenhancement (block arrow). Patient had evidence of significant left anterior descending artery and right coronary artery disease. RV = right ventricle, LV = left ventricle, L = lungs, * = contrast agent.

and hybrid EPI-gradient echo (GRE) sequences. Fast T_1 weighted imaging sequences such as spoiled gradient-echo imaging with TRs as short as 2 ms and a magnetization preparation (either inversion recovery or saturation recovery) for T_1 weighting are applied to image the contrast enhancement during the first pass of contrast agent.

The most common compound bolus used is an extracellular MR contrast agent such as Gd-DTPA.

Rapid contrast injection is crucial as this improves the sensitivity for detecting changes in myocardial perfusion [45]. The goal is to assure that the primary bottleneck to the rate of contrast enhancement is the rate of transport of the contrast through the myocardial tissue and not the rate at which the contrast agent is injected. The regional image intensity contrast enhancement should ideally be proportional to the contrast agent concentration.

Such an approximate linear relationship between regional signal intensity and contrast agent concentration is only observed at lower contrast agent dosages—typically, <0.05 mol/Kg of Gd-DTPA for fast IR-prepared gradient echo sequences (TR < 3 ms; TE < 2 ms) [46].

Vasodilator stress

A complete discussion of the effects of adenosine/dipyridamole is beyond the scope of this chapter. Briefly, vasodilation with dipyridamole or adenosine induces an increase of blood flow in myocardial areas supplied by normal coronary arteries ("coronary steal"), whereas no (or only minimal) change is found in areas supplied by stenotic coronary arteries. With adenosine a maximal coronary vasodilation can be achieved safely with an intravenous infusion at a rate of 140 µg/kg/min. For cardiac imaging 4–6 min of infusion is recommended. The vasodilatory effect of adenosine may result in a mild to moderate reduction in systolic, diastolic and mean arterial blood pressure (<10 mmHg) with a reflex increase in heart rate. Although some patients may complain about anginal chest pain or dyspnea, these effects respond promptly to discontinuation of the drug and usually do not require medical intervention. Studies in over 10,000 patients during thallium radionuclide imaging, echocardiography, SPECT and MRI have shown that pharmacological stress testing with adenosine presents a safe method of acquiring stress imaging data [47, 48]. However, adenosine should be used with caution in patients with pre-existing atrioventricular (AV) block or bundle branch block and should be avoided in patients with high-grade AV block, sinus node dysfunction or reversible airways obstruction (e.g. asthma).

Practical aspects of image acquisition

An intravenous line should be started before the examination for administration of the contrast agent. A16G or 18G peripheral needle is usually sufficient together with a power injector at a rate of 5–10 ml/s. Contrast administration needs to be followed without delay by an injection of physiologic saline solution to assure that the entire contrast agent dose is injected into the vein. Monitoring of the patient's blood pressure, heart rate, and, preferably, also the arterial oxygen saturation is recommended.

Practical tips that aid successful perfusion imaging:
1 The recommended contrast agent dose varies from 0.02 mmol/kg to 0.1 mmol/kg Gd-DTPA depending on the sequence used and the type of assessment needed (quantitative versus qualitative).
2 Double oblique slices that give a short axis view of the heart are recommended. For multislice acquisitions the interslice gap should be 30–50% of the chosen slice thickness. Slice positions are customarily chosen to cover the location of wall motion defects that are detected on the cine imaging, which is usually performed beforehand.
3 Minimize the field of view without causing aliasing ("wrap around") artifacts. It is our practice to perform a test image (without contrast) to determine any wrap artifact and to adjust the slice position accordingly. Choosing the read-out direction parallel to the chest wall often reduces the likelihood of aliasing and other artifacts.
4 Perform the scan with the patient holding their breath in inspiration. Begin the scan as soon as the patient starts the breath-hold; the contrast agent injection can be started after acquisition of three to five "baseline" images.

Qualitative analysis and visualization

Currently, only limited data is available regarding the accuracy of visual assessment, and experience is required to reach an acceptable standard. The main artifacts occurring during the initial passage of the contrast bolus are due to susceptibility at the endocardium blood-pool interface, sometimes making diagnosis of subendocardial perfusion deficits difficult. The trabeculae of the papillary muscles are especially prone to susceptibility artifacts and such findings should not be interpreted as evidence of a regional ischemic perfusion abnormality.

Semiquantitative analysis

Most publications in the literature have been based on semiquantitative analysis of regional myocardial perfusion. Here the endo- and epicardial contours of left ventricular myocardium are traced and corrected manually for changes of diaphragmatic position due to breathing or diaphragmatic drift. The myocardium is then divided into six to eight equiangular segments per slice, and an additional region of interest is placed within the cavity of the left ventricle, excluding the myocardial segments

(a)

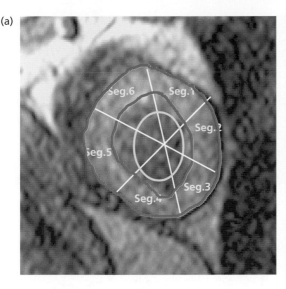

(b)

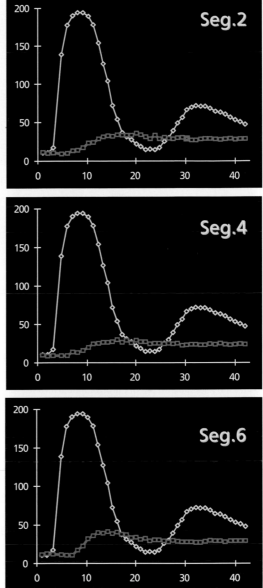

Fig. 2.18 (a) A T$_1$-weighted gradient-echo image in the short-axis view is shown with user-traced endo and epicardial contours, and region of interest in the center of the LV cavity. The LV wall was subdivided into six transmural myocardial segments that are arranged in circumferential order, starting at the anterior junction of the RV and LV, which serves here as an anatomical landmark. Signal intensity in each segment is compared with signal intensity curves of left ventricular cavity (b). Signal intensity is given in arbitrary units. (Figure modified from: Reference 49, Al-Saadi N, Nagel E, Gross M *et al.* Non-invasive detection of myocardial ischemia from perfusion reserve based on cardiovascular magnetic resonance. *Circulation* 2000; **101**: 1379–1383. Reproduced with permission of the publishers).

and the papillary muscles (Fig. 2.18 and Fig. 2.19). Images acquired after premature ventricular beats or insufficient cardiac triggering need to be excluded from the analysis to guarantee steady-state conditions. Signal intensity is determined for all dynamics and segments. The upslope of the resulting signal intensity time curve is determined by the use of a linear fit. To correct for possible differences of the input function, the results of the myocardial segments are corrected by dividing the upslope of

each myocardial segment by the upslope of the left ventricular signal intensity curve. Perfusion reserve index is calculated by dividing the results of stress imaging by the results obtained at rest.

Quantitative analysis

Quantification of myocardial blood flow and measurement of myocardial perfusion reserve is based both on the Fermi model of constrained deconvolution, as well as on other independent models

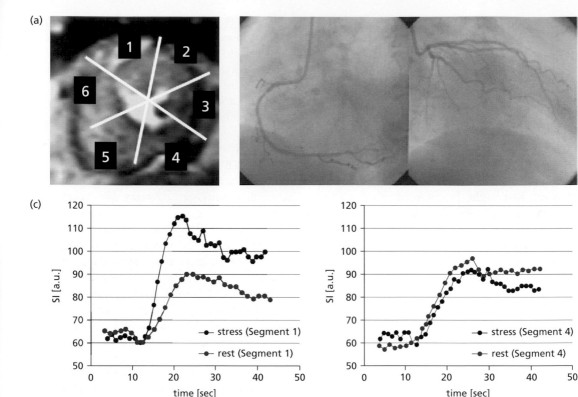

Fig. 2.19 (a) Segmentation of the myocardium into six equiangular segments per slice, starting clockwise from the anterior septal insertion point of the right ventricle. (b) Coronary angiogram of the patient showing critical right coronary artery stenosis. In the normally perfused anterior segment, there is a clear increase of the upslope after adenosine (●) when compared with rest (●), whereas in the inferior segment of the same slice there is no change of the upslope after vasodilation (c). (Figure re-drawn from: Reference 47, Nagel E, Klein C, Paetsch I *et al*. Magnetic resonance perfusion measurements for the non-invasive detection of coronary artery disease. *Circulation* 2003; **108**: 432–437. Re-drawn with permission of the publishers.)

[50–52]. Compared to the Fermi-model-based analysis, model-independent deconvolution provides an impulse response that is a more accurate representation of the true impulse response, albeit at the price of higher complexity in the implementation of the algorithms. The model-independent analysis works well for analyzing contrast enhancement with intravascular and extracellular contrast agents. For the extracellular contrast agents, the Fermi model requires that the fit to the measured data be limited to approximately the first pass, as the leakage of contrast agent from the vascular space into the interstitial space is not reproduced well by the Fermi impulse response model. The model-independent analysis overcomes this shortcoming of the Fermi model [53]. However, more experience, as well as standardization of the analysis method will be needed to determine the clinical value of absolute quantification of perfusion.

Future requirements: A general limitation to MR perfusion imaging using gadolinium contrast is the use of different technical approaches by different vendors and different centers, which discourages comparison of results and limits multicenter trials. A standardized approach is needed both for image acquisition (e.g. image sequences, contrast dose, number of slices etc) as well as postprocessing (e.g. color coded maps). This would then pave the way for long term, multicenter trials in larger heterogeneous patient groups, which are necessary to establish the prognostic value of this technique in coronary artery disease.

Non-contrast perfusion and BOLD Sequences

Spin labeling techniques exploit the labeling of the nuclear magnetization of water protons, either by direct preparation of inflowing spins or by specific preparation of the imaging slice. In both cases, water is used as a free diffusible contrast agent. Although easily repeatable, arterial spin labeling techniques applied at 1.5 Tesla yield only a relatively small signal difference between normal and underperfused myocardium (44% in a recent study by Wacker *et al.* [54]), but these techniques may become more practical when applied at higher field.

Blood oxygenation level-dependent (BOLD) MRI may overcome the tracer kinetic limitations of first pass perfusion imaging by observing changes in tissue oxygenation directly. BOLD utilizes the T_2^* effect, that is the incoherence in the phase behavior due to local inhomogenities in the magnetic field. Wacker and colleagues show that dipyridamole was associated with an increase of T_2^* in healthy volunteers but with a T_2^* decrease in patients with stenotic coronary arteries [55]. Although significant progress is being made [54, 56], BOLD imaging is not yet ready for clinical application to the heart as it is currently only possible to analyze single slices and the T_2^* signal differences remain small. The arrival of 3T systems hold much promise in this regard, as at 3 Tesla the blood T_2 is much more sensitive to its oxygenation level than it is at 1.5 Tesla, consequently intravascular contrast (a significant mechanism for BOLD in the myocardium) will be increased at 3 Tesla.

Measurement of blood flow

Velocity encoded cine (VENC) MR imaging allows accurate estimation of velocity profiles across a valve or any vascular structure, comparable to those provided by Doppler ultrasonography [57, 58]. In addition, MR imaging is able to quantify flow volumes and does not have the same limitations with respect to acoustic penetration of different portions of the heart and therefore is better able to demonstrate distribution and velocity of flow throughout the heart. On cine gradient-echo MR images, blood has bright signal intensity due to fresh inflowing blood that has not been saturated. Abnormal flow patterns encountered in valvular disease cause dephasing of the spins within a voxel and result in signal loss (flow void). This flow void is seen with either stenosis or regurgitation and is caused by high-velocity flow and turbulence [59]. Its appearance depends on technical factors including display parameters (window width and level), flip angle and TE [60]. With long-TE sequences (12 ms),

the flow void is well demonstrated, whereas with short-TE sequences (<7 ms), it tends to be smaller. These variables must be taken into account when evaluating flow anomalies.

Flow-sensitive imaging techniques permit the measurement of flow expressed as either velocity or volume per unit of time. Currently, the most popular flow-sensitive cine MR imaging technique is referred to as phase-contrast, phase-shift, or velocity encoded (VENC) MR imaging. As described in the section on image contrast, this is based on the principle that the phase of flowing spins relative to stationary spins along a magnetic field gradient changes in direct proportion to flow velocity. Magnitude images can be reconstructed to provide anatomical information, and phase images can provide flow velocity information. The phase shift is displayed as variations in pixel signal intensity on the phase map image. Stationary tissue appears gray on this image, whereas flow in a positive direction along the flow-encoding axis will appear bright, and flow in a negative direction will appear dark (Fig. 2.20). As a result, it is possible to differentiate antegrade from retrograde flow. Furthermore, as with Doppler ultrasonography, the phase map image can be color coded to reinforce the differentiation between antegrade and retrograde flow. Velocity can be encoded in planes that are perpendicular to the direction of flow by using section-selective direction (through-plane velocity measurement), in planes that are parallel to the direction of flow by using phase encoded or frequency encoded directions (in-plane velocity measurement), or, more recently, in 3D. However, VENC MR imaging also has certain limitations and potential sources of error [61]. Because of the cyclic nature of phase, aliasing may appear if more than one cycle of phase shift occurs. To avoid aliasing, which occurs when the chosen velocity range is lower than the predicted maximum velocity, the velocity threshold must be correctly selected prior to acquisition.

VENC MR imaging can be used to calculate absolute velocity at any given time during the cardiac cycle at specified locations in the plane of data acquisition. Velocity can be measured for each pixel within a region of interest encircling all or part of the cross-sectional vessel area or across a valve annulus. The product of cross-sectional area (as determined from the magnitude image) and spatial

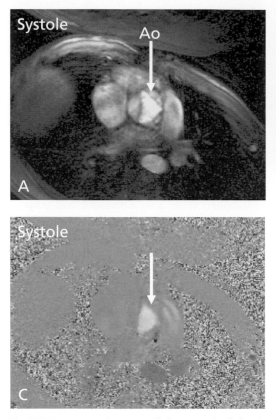

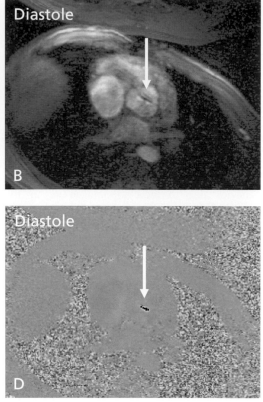

Fig. 2.20 Transverse velocity encoded MR magnitude (A, B) and phase (C, D) images centered on the aortic valve in a patient with severe aortic regurgitation. In systole (A, C), the leaflets are open and bright signal, indicating anterograde flow (arrows). In diastole (B, D) absence of coaptation is demonstrated, and dark signal indicates central retrograde flow. In (D), there is also adjoining lighter area due to aliasing effects.

mean velocity (i.e. the average velocity for all pixels in the cross-sectional area on the phase image) yields the instantaneous flow volume for each time frame during the cardiac cycle. Integration of all instantaneous flow volumes throughout the cardiac cycle yields the flow volume per heart beat. This technique has been evaluated *in vitro* as well as *in vivo* by several authors and allows accurate measurement of aortic and pulmonary arterial flow, which represent the stroke volumes of the left and right ventricles, respectively [62]. It has also been used to calculate the ratio of pulmonary to systemic flow, thereby allowing non-invasive quantification of left-to-right shunts [63] and separate measurement of right and left pulmonary flows [64]. Moreover, these measurements can be used in the evaluation and quantitative assessment of valvular regurgitation and stenosis.

MR angiographic techniques

In recent years there has been considerable interest in magnetic resonance angiography (MRA) in which images of blood vessels are produced without detail from surrounding stationary tissue. MRA techniques fall into three broad categories: Time of flight (TOF), phase contrast and contrast-enhanced MRA. These have applications in imaging various vessels, particularly the aorta, carotid, renal, and peripheral arteries.

Time of flight MRA (TOF MRA): Time of Flight MRA relies on the flow of fully relaxed material into the imaged volume for image contrast (see earlier section on image contrast). Fast gradient echo imaging is commonly used to perform 2D or 3D TOF MRA. In the former, thin slices are acquired one at a time, while in the latter, a volume is excited by the radiofrequency (RF) pulse.

Phase contrast MRA: Phase contrast MRA relies on changes in the phase of the transverse magnetization induced by the application of a bipolar, flow sensitized gradient, which generate a phase difference between the stationary tissues and the moving blood. Phase contrast angiography has effective background suppression and provides quantitative flow measurements, but the acquisition time is long and the technique is only sensitive to a certain range of blood velocities.

Contrast-enhanced MRA (CE-MRA): This has become an increasingly popular angiographic technique over recent years as it can be acquired during a single breath-hold, and hence has particular advantages in imaging areas of major respiratory motion such as the thorax and abdomen. The appropriate intravenous injection of Gd-DTPA leads to substantial local blood signal enhancement because of the shortening of the T_1 relaxation time of blood. Timing of the scan with respect to the intravenous bolus is critical for data collection. Consequently, it is good practice to administer a "test bolus" to estimate the contrast arrival time at the targeted vessel. Contrast-enhanced MRA is the preferred MRA technique for the evaluation of aortic aneurysms, pulmonary arterial disease, and peripheral arterial disease. Renal CE-MRA is indicated in patients with hypertension to exclude vascular causes, and in patients with worsening renal function to exclude bilateral renal artery stenosis.

Coronary and bypass graft imaging

The epicardial coronary arteries are small structures, demanding images of high spatial resolution. For such high resolution imaging the need for high signal-to-noise (SNR) and contrast-to-noise (CNR) ratios often means prolonged imaging time. However, longer imaging time makes the image vulnerable to motion-related blurring, artifact and image degradation. Hence, adequate cardiac and respiratory motion suppression (see earlier section) is imperative for artifact free coronary imaging.

The principal sequences used for coronary imaging (summarized below) utilize the "time of flight" angiography principle that was mentioned above. "Black blood" coronary MRA (CMRA) takes advantage of the negative contrast between flowing coronary blood and surrounding tissues. "Black blood"

methods may be particularly useful for patients with bypass grafts or intracoronary stents, as they are less sensitive to metallic implant susceptibility artifacts than gradient echo ("bright blood") imaging. Contrast-to-noise ratio can also be improved by the use of MR contrast agents. Gadolinium-based agents considerably reduce the T_1 relaxation time of blood, resulting in an improved differentiation between coronary blood and the adjoining myocardium. Imaging can be done using saturation recovery or inversion recovery prepulses. Extracellular agents appear best suited to first pass breath-hold approaches, whereas intravascular contrast agents may be best for longer navigator/free breathing CMRA.

Proximal coronary artery visualization has been the main aim of CMRA since initial studies were performed more than 10 years ago [65, 66]. This showed that visualization is possible of proximal segments in a majority of motivated volunteers and patients. Two of the most commonly used techniques for CMRA, which are performed at various CMR centres, are briefly described below (Fig. 2.21). A full discussion of all the available techniques is beyond the scope of this chapter, but is available elsewhere [68].

3D segmented k-space gradient echo CMRA: First described by Li [65] and Botnar [69], this technique takes advantage of superior SNR and postprocessing capabilities of 3D imaging and provides high spatial resolution. As the data acquisition period is long, exceeding standard breath-hold duration, navigators are needed for respiratory gating. The use of T_2 preparatory pulses are also needed to enhance CNR and facilitate better identification of the coronary arteries from underlying tissue.

3D segmented k-space echoplanar CMRA: With fast breath-hold or free breathing 3D EPI coronary MRA, two to four excitation pulses are followed by a short EPI read-out train [70, 71]. This takes advantage of the EPI speed while keeping the echo and acquisition time short to minimize blood flow and motion related artifacts.

Bypass grafts: Early CMR studies for bypass graft assessment used non-respiratory compensated, ECG-triggered 2D spin echo and gradient echo techniques. Current approaches (often used in

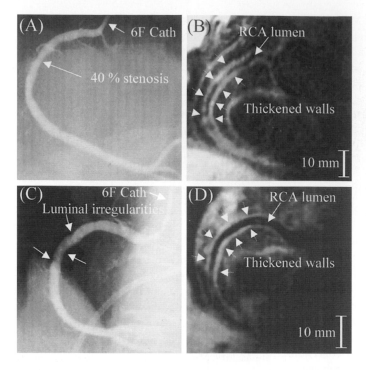

Fig. 2.21 Black-blood 3D CMR vessel wall scans (B, D) demonstrate an irregularly thickened RCA wall (>2 mm) indicative of an increased atherosclerotic plaque burden. The inner and outer RCA walls are indicated by the white dotted arrows. Comparison is made with the corresponding diagnostic x-ray angiographic images (A, C). (Figure reproduced from: Reference 67, Kim WY, Stuber M, Börnet P. Three-dimensional black-blood cardiac magnetic resonance coronary vessel wall imaging detects positive arterial remodelling in patients with non-significant coronary artery disease. (*Circulation* 2002; **106**: 296. Reproduced with permission of the publishers.)

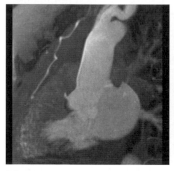
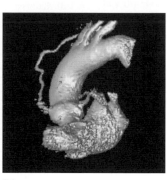
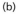

(a)   (b)

Fig. 2.22 Contrast enhanced MR angiogram of a patent LIMA graft six months post surgery. Acquisition of a 3D data set allows postprocessing with multiplanar reformation and maximum intensity projection (a). Surface rendered image is shown (b). (Images courtesy of Drs. O. Mohrs and T. Voigtlaender, Frankfurt/Main, Germany.)

combination) can be broadly divided into techniques that assess patency, such as turbo spin echo (e.g. HASTE) and MR angiography, and those that assess graft flow reserve, which can give information about graft stenosis. 3D MR angiography using rapid contrast injection (after initially performing a timing sequence to determine the onset of peak gadolinium-DTPA enhancement) is the preferred technique for assessing graft patency. Acquisition of a 3D data set allows postprocessing with multiplanar reformation and maximum intensity projection to identify grafts. Surface rendering of this 3D data set is also possible (see Fig. 2.22).

Despite recent advances in technique development, MR coronary angiography at 1.5 T produces (at best) in-plane resolution of around 0.7 mm, which is inferior to that obtained with invasive x-ray coronary angiography (around 0.3 mm). As such, currently, it cannot replace the latter for routine clinical use.

Atherosclerosis imaging

High-resolution magnetic resonance (MR) has emerged as the leading *in vivo* imaging modality for atherosclerotic plaque characterization, given the inherent advantages of non-invasiveness and high

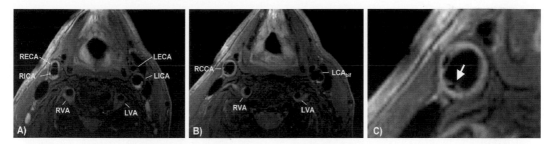

Fig. 2.23 Example of *in vivo* carotid plaque imaging in a 61-year-old smoker who presented with recent anterior circulation transient ischemic attack (TIA). (A) Magnetic resonance T$_2$-weighted turbo-spin-echo images in a transverse plane, showing increased wall thickness of the carotid and vertebral arteries. (B) Significantly thickened vessel wall in the left carotid bifurcation (LCA). Also shown are two arteriosclerotic lesions in the right common carotid artery (RCCA) with dark lipid core and thin fibrous cap (C). Close up of right common carotid artery suggestive of plaque rupture (arrow). (Figure reproduced from: Reference 77, Wiesmann F, Robson MD, Francis JM *et al.* Visualization of the ruptured plaque by magnetic resonance imaging. *Circulation* 2003; **108**: 2542. Reproduced with permission of the publishers.)

spatial resolution. MR differentiates plaque components on the basis of biophysical and biochemical parameters such as chemical composition and concentration, water content, physical state, molecular motion, or diffusion.

Since detected MR signals rely on the relaxation times T$_1$ and T$_2$ and on proton density, the MR images can be "weighted" to the T$_1$, T$_2$, or proton density values through adaptation of the imaging parameters (such as repetition time and echo time). For example, in a T$_1$-weighted (T$_{1w}$) image, tissues with lower T$_1$ values will produce pixels with high signal intensity. Conversely, tissues with a longer T$_2$ relaxation time will appear hyperintense in a T$_2$-weighted (T$_{2w}$) image. In a proton density-weighted (PD$_W$) image the contrast relies mainly on the differences in density of water and fat protons within the tissue. This contrast is also referred to as intermediate-weighted, as it represents a combination of T$_1$ and T$_2$ contrast. Applying these different "weightings", one can produce maps with varying contrast of the same object [72]. This makes the MR method uniquely suitable for the assessment of the vascular wall [73]. Improvements in MR technology, including the development of high-sensitivity coils and faster imaging protocols, have allowed the study of atherosclerotic plaques using multicontrast (T$_{1w}$, T$_{2w}$, and PD$_w$) MR imaging [74]. MR imaging has been used for the study of atherosclerotic plaque in the human aorta [75], carotid arteries (Fig. 2.23) [76, 77], and in peripheral arteries [78]. Successful MR imaging of the coronary artery wall has been performed

(Fig. 2.24) [80], but is technically demanding because of the small size and highly tortuous course of the coronaries. Additionally, to obtain artifact-free images, cardiac and respiratory motion must be reliably suppressed. Use of navigator echoes accounts for any cardiac or diaphragmatic motion and allows visualization of the coronary wall in a time-efficient way without the need for breath-holding [81].

Studies on human atherosclerosis

Carotid artery: In vivo images of advanced lesions in carotid arteries were initially performed in patients referred for endarterectomy [82]. As the carotid arteries are superficial and less mobile than the aorta and the coronary arteries they pose less of a technical challenge for imaging. Some of the MR studies of carotid arterial plaques include the imaging and characterization of normal and pathological arterial walls, the quantification of plaque size, and the detection of fibrous cap "integrity". Typically the images are acquired with resolution of 0.4 × 0.4 × 3 mm^3 using a carotid phased-array coil. Most of the *in vivo* MR plaque imaging and characterization have been performed using a multicontrast approach with high-resolution black-blood spin echo- and fast spin echo-based MR sequences. The signal from the blood flow is rendered black by the use of preparatory pulses (e.g. radiofrequency spatial saturation or inversion recovery pulses) to better visualize the adjacent vessel wall.

MR angiography (MRA) and high-resolution black-blood imaging of the vessel wall can be combined. MRA demonstrates the severity of stenotic

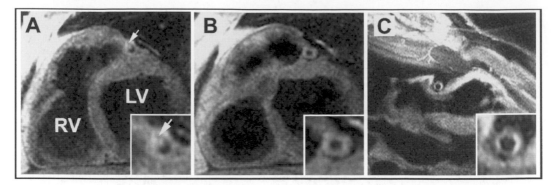

Fig. 2.24 Human *in vivo* MR black-blood cross-sectional images that demonstrate a plaque with (presumed) deposition of fat (arrow, A) and a concentric fibrotic lesion (B) in the left anterior descending artery, and an ectatic, but atherosclerotic, right coronary artery (C). (Figure reproduced from: Reference 79, Fayad Z, Fuster V, Nikolaou K *et al.* Computed tomography and magnetic resonance imaging for non-invasive coronary angiography and plaque imaging: Current and potential future concepts. *Circulation* 2002; **106**: 2026. Reproduced with permission of the publishers.)

lesions and their spatial distribution, whereas the high-resolution black-blood wall characterization technique may show the composition of the plaques and may facilitate the risk stratification and selection of the treatment modality. Improvements in spatial resolution (<250 μm) have been possible with the design of new phased-array coils tailored for carotid imaging [83] and new imaging sequences such as long echo train fast spin echo imaging with "velocity-selective" flow suppression or double-inversion recovery preparatory pulses (black-blood imaging).

Aorta: In vivo black-blood MR atherosclerotic plaque characterization of the human aorta has been reported recently. Fayad *et al.* [75] assessed thoracic aorta plaque composition and size using T_{1W}, T_{2W}, and PD_W images. The acquired images had a resolution of $0.8 \times 0.8 \times 5$ mm^3 using a torso phased-array coil. Rapid high-resolution imaging was performed with a fast spin echo sequence in conjunction with velocity-selective flow suppression preparatory pulses. Matched cross-sectional aortic imaging with MR and TEE showed a strong correlation for plaque composition and mean maximum plaque thickness.

Cardiac magnetic resonance spectroscopy

Cardiac MRI uses the ^{1}H nucleus in water and fat molecules as its only signal source. In contrast, cardiac MR spectroscopy (MRS) allows the study of many additional nuclei with a net nuclear spin, i.e. with an uneven number of protons, neutrons or both. Importantly, MRS is the only available method for the non-invasive study of cardiac metabolism without external radioactive tracers (as used, for example in positron emission tomography). Table 2.1 lists the nuclei most frequently used in cardiac MRS: ^{1}H (protons from metabolites other than water and fat), ^{13}C, ^{23}Na and ^{31}P. Cardiac MRS is a fascinating method but has one major limitation: Low spatial and temporal resolution. The nuclei studied with MRS have a much lower MR sensitivity than ^{1}H and are present in much lower concentrations than those of ^{1}H nuclei of water and fat (Table 2.1). Therefore, the resolution of MRS is several orders of magnitude lower than that of MRI.

Basic principles of MR spectroscopy

The most extensively studied nucleus in cardiac MRS is phosphorus (^{31}P), and the basic principles of MRS, relevant for all nuclei, are best derived from a ^{31}P-MRS study of the most widely used animal model, the isolated buffer-perfused rodent heart [84]. MRS is performed using an MR spectrometer, which consists of a high-field (up to 18 Tesla) superconducting magnet with a bore size ranging between ~5 cm and ~1 m. The magnet bore holds the nucleus-specific probe head with the radiofrequency (RF) coils, which are used for MR excitation and signal reception. The magnet is inter-

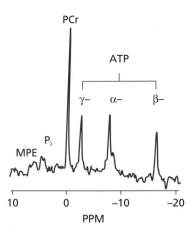

Fig. 2.25 ^{31}P-MR spectrum of an isolated, buffer-perfused rat heart obtained within 5 min at 7 Tesla.

faced with a control computer, a magnetic field gradient system, and an RF transmitter and receiver. The magnetic field requires homogenization with shim gradients, as MRS demands high magnetic field homogeneity. A radiofrequency impulse is sent into the RF coils for spin excitation. The resulting MR signal, the free induction decay (FID) is then recorded. The FID is subjected to Fourier transformation, which results in an MR spectrum.

A typical ^{31}P-MR spectrum from an isolated, beating rat heart, obtained in 5 min at 7 T is shown in Fig. 2.25. A ^{31}P-spectrum shows six resonances, corresponding to the three ^{31}P-atoms of Adenosine Tri-phosphate (ATP), phosphocreatine (PCr), inorganic phosphate (Pi) and monophosphate esters (MPE). Different metabolites resonate at distinct frequencies, and this is termed the chemical shift phenomenon (quantified relative to the B_0 field in ppm = parts per million): Different positions in the molecule lead to subtle differences in the local magnetic field strength, spreading the resonance frequencies of ^{31}P metabolites over a range of ~30 ppm. From the fully relaxed state, the area under each ^{31}P-resonance is proportional to the amount of each ^{31}P-nucleus in the sample, and metabolite resonances are quantified by measuring peak areas. Relative metabolite levels are calculated directly (such as the phosphocreatine/ATP ratio), and absolute metabolite concentrations are calculated by comparing tissue resonance areas to those of an external ^{31}P-reference standard (e.g. phenylphosphonate) [85–87]. ^{31}P-MRS has been used extensively to study the

relationships between cardiac function and energy metabolism in acute ischemia/reperfusion and in chronic heart failure models [84, 88–90]. These experimental studies suggest a crucial role of altered cardiac energetics in injured myocardium.

Because of the low sensitivity of MRS, many FIDs have to be signal averaged to obtain MR spectra with a sufficient signal-to-noise ratio. Typically, for a perfused rat heart experiment at 7–12 Tesla, 100–200 FIDs are acquired and signal averaged. In MRS, it is important to account for the effects of partial saturation when selecting pulse angles and TR: A full MR signal from a given nucleus can only be obtained when the nucleus is excited from a fully relaxed spin state, i.e. when a time of at least $5 \times T_1$ has passed since the previous excitation (for example, T_1 of phosphocreatine at 1.5 Tesla ~4.4 s requiring TR of 22 s); "fully relaxed" spectra can therefore only be obtained with long TRs, leading to prohibitively long acquisition times. In practice, shorter TRs are used, but these yield spectra where a part of the signal is lost due to saturation effects ("partially saturated"). Since the T_1s of ^{31}P-metabolites such as phosphocreatine and ATP are different (T_1 of phosphocreatine is ~ twice as long as T_1 of ATP), the extent of saturation also varies for different ^{31}P-resonances. Thus, when quantifying partially saturated spectra, "saturation factors" need to be used for correction. These factors are determined for each metabolite by comparing fully relaxed and saturated spectra.

^{1}H has the highest MR sensitivity of all MR-detectable nuclei and very high natural abundance (Table 2.1). Many metabolites can be detected by ^{1}H-MRS, such as creatine, lactate, carnitine, taurine and -CH$_3$ and -CH$_2$ resonances of lipids [91–93]. Particularly promising is the non-invasive measurement of total creatine [94, 95]. Furthermore, tissue oxygenation can be followed non-invasively by ^{1}H-MRS using the oxymyoglobin and deoxymyoglobin resonances [96]. However, ^{1}H-MRS is technically demanding, as we need to suppress the strong ^{1}H signal from water which is 1,000,000 times more intense than the metabolite signals. Furthermore, the complex ^{1}H spectra show overlapping resonances, many of which remain to be characterized. Cardiac ^{1}H-MRS is only in its infancy, but the technique has enormous potential for clinical application.

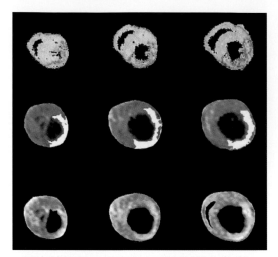

Fig. 2.26 Bottom row: Three adjacent slices of a 3D ^{23}Na-MRI dataset in an isolated rat heart four weeks post-MI after segmentation. Middle row: The region with signal elevation of double standard deviation over mean in the ^{23}Na image is delineated in white, and is chosen for infarct size measurement. Top row: Corresponding histological slices with stained infarcted area. The area of increased ^{23}Na signal intensity closely matches the histologic scar area (r = 0.91; p < 0.0001) (Figure reproduced from: Reference 88, Horn M, Weidensteiner C, Scheffer H et al. *Magn Reson Med* 2001; **45**: 756–764. Reproduced with permission from Wiley & Sons, New York.)

The ^{13}C nucleus has a low natural abundance (~1%), and for a ^{13}C-MRS experiment, the heart has to be loaded with ^{13}C-labeled compounds such as, e.g. 1-^{13}C-glucose. Typically, these are added to perfusion media or infused into a coronary artery during a defined study protocol. Substrate utilization by the heart [97, 98] may then be investigated, or the activities of key enzymes or entire metabolic pathways can be quantified, e.g. citric acid cycle flux, pyruvate dehydrogenase flux and beta-oxidation of fatty acids [99–101]. Clinical applications have yet to be reported for the heart, because MR sensitivity and concentrations of ^{13}C nuclei are too low for spatially resolved detection in human heart within an acceptable acquisition time.

^{23}Na-MRS is the only non-invasive method for evaluation of changes in intra and extracellular ^{23}Na during cardiac injury [102]. Maintenance of the sarcolemmal ^{23}Na concentration gradient (extracellular/intracellular concentration gradient ~14:1) is a requirement for normal cardiac function. A cardiac ^{23}Na spectrum yields a single peak representing all ^{23}Na in the heart (the total Na$^+$ signal), and for discrimination of intra and extracellular ^{23}Na pools paramagnetic shift reagents, e.g. [TmDOTP]$^{5-}$, have to be added to the perfusate. These high molecular weight chelate complexes are distributed in the extracellular space only, and ^{23}Na in the close vicinity of shift reagents undergoes a downfield chemical shift of its resonance frequency, so that extracellular and intracellular ^{23}Na peaks can be discriminated. This method is being used experimentally to examine the mechanisms of intracellular Na$^+$ accumulation in ischemia-reperfusion injury [103]. Unfortunately, ^{23}Na-MR shift reagents for clinical use are currently not yet available, so that only imaging of the total Na signal is feasible, as first demonstrated by DeLayre et al. [104]. However, even the total ^{23}Na signal holds biologically important information: In acute ischemia, the total myocardial ^{23}Na MRI signal increases because of breakdown of ion homeostasis and intra and extracellular edema formation [105]. Furthermore, the total Na signal remains significantly elevated during chronic scar formation, as we have demonstrated in an experimental model [106], because of the expansion of the extracellular space in scar (Fig. 2.26). In contrast, ^{23}Na content is not elevated in akinetic, but stunned or hibernating myocardium [88]. For these reasons, ^{23}Na MRI may allow detection of myocardial viability based on intrinsic tissue contrast.

Clinical cardiac MRS methods

Almost all human cardiac MRS studies have so far been confined to the ^{31}P nucleus. Clinical cardiac spectroscopy is a complex technique. There are hardware requirements that usually do not come with a standard CMR system: The RF generator has to be able to produce frequencies other than ^{1}H ("broadband capability"), and a specific ^{31}P-cardiac surface coil is needed, typically with a loop diameter of 10–15 cm. The low resolution of MRS cannot simply be offset by increasing imaging time, which, for practical reasons, is limited to 60–90 min. ECG gating is required, but, given the large voxel sizes and the already extended acquisition time, respiration gating is currently not employed. Field strength of clinical MRS systems is much lower than that of experimental systems, i.e. typically 1.5 Tesla, although 3 Tesla systems have recently become

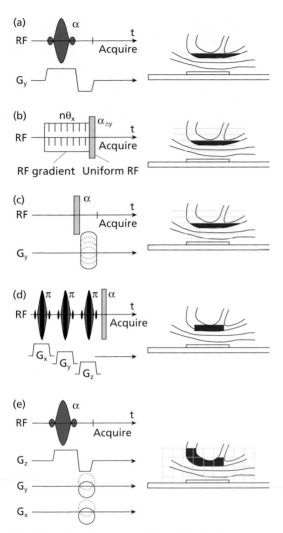

Fig. 2.27 Basic pulse sequences for localized cardiac spectroscopy with surface coils. (a) "depth-resolved surface coil spectroscopy". A single section parallel to the plane of the surface coil is selected by applying an MR imaging gradient G in the presence of a modulated radiofrequency excitation pulse of flip angle. (b) The "rotating frame" MR method uses the gradient inherent in a surface coil to simultaneously spatially encode spectra from multiple sections parallel to the surface coil by means of application of a flip angle pulse, which is stepped in subsequent applications of the sequence. (c) The "one-dimensional chemical shift imaging" method similarly encodes multiple sections but uses an MR imaging gradient whose amplitude is stepped. (d) The "image-selected *in vivo* spectroscopy" method localizes to a single volume with selective inversion pulses applied with G_x, G_y and G_z MR imaging gradients. All eight combinations of the three pulses must be applied and the resultant signals added and subtracted. (e) A section-selective "three-dimensional chemical shift imaging" sequence employs MR imaging section selection in one

available. The cardiac muscle lies behind the chest wall skeletal muscle, whose ^{31}P-signal requires suppression by means of spectroscopic localization techniques. Localization methods used for cardiac MRS include DRESS (depth-resolved surface coil spectroscopy); rotating frame; 1D-CSI (chemical shift imaging); ISIS (image-selected *in vivo* spectroscopy), and 3D-CSI. Some details are given in Fig. 2.27; for a full description of localization methods see the review by Bottomley [107]. Although less comfortable for the patient, it is currently recommended that MRS studies be performed in prone position rather than supine, as this reduces motion artifacts and brings the heart closer to the surface coil, thus improving sensitivity. [1]H scout images are first obtained to select the spectroscopic voxel(s), followed by ^{31}P-acquisition for 20–50 min. Given the low sensitivity, ^{31}P-MRS voxel sizes have been large, typically ~30 ml. A typical ^{31}P-MR spectrum of a healthy volunteer is shown in Fig. 2.28. Compared to the rat heart spectrum, two additional resonances are seen: 2,3-diphosphoglycerate (2,3-DPG), arising from the presence of blood (erythrocytes) in the voxel, and phosphodiesters (PDE), a signal due to membrane as well as serum phospholipids. The 2,3-diphosphoglycerate resonances overlap with the inorganic phosphate peak, which therefore cannot be detected in most human ^{31}P-MR spectra. For relative quantification of human ^{31}P-spectra, the phosphocreatine/ATP and phosphodiester/ATP peak area ratios are calculated. The phosphocreatine/ATP ratio is a powerful indicator of the energetic state of the heart. The meaning of the phosphodiester/ATP ratio remains poorly understood, and this ratio may not change with cardiac disease. Human ^{31}P-resonances require correction for the effects of partial saturation according to the principles described for experimental MRS. In addition, to account for saturation, either adiabatic pulses (creating identical flip angles across the entire sample volume) or B_1 field characterization (taking into account variations in flip angle) are

dimension and phase encoding in two dimensions. (Figure reproduced from: Reference 107, Bottomley PA. MR spectroscopy of the human heart: The status and the challenges. *Radiology* 1994; **191**; 593–612. Reproduced with permission from the Radiological Society of North America.)

(a)

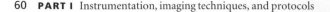

(b)

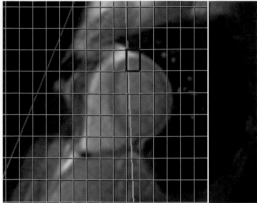

(c)

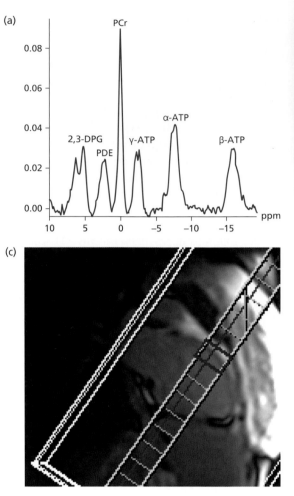

Fig. 2.28 ^{31}P-MR spectrum from a healthy human volunteer (a), 3D-CSI technique. Voxel size 25 × 27 × 30 mm (20 ml). 2,3-DPG = 2,3-Diphosphoglycerate; PDE = phosphodiesters, PCr = phosphocreatine, γ-, α-, β-ATP = the three phosphorus atoms of adenosinetriphosphate. The right panels show short axis (b) and the vertical long axis (c) proton scout images. The entire voxel grid of the 3D-CSI localization is shown in green, and the voxel corresponding to the ^{31}P spectrum is shown in blue.

required. ^{31}P-spectra should also be corrected for blood contamination: Blood contributes signal to the ATP-, 2,3-diphosphoglycerate- and phosphodiester-resonances of a cardiac ^{31}P-spectrum. As human blood spectra show an ATP/2,3-diphosphoglycerate area ratio of ~0.11 and a phosphodiester/2,3-diphosphoglycerate area ratio of ~0.19, for blood correction, the ATP resonance area of cardiac spectra is reduced by 11% of the 2,3-diphosphoglycerate resonance area, and the phosphodiester resonance area is reduced by 19% of the 2,3-diphosphoglycerate resonance area [106].

Absolute quantification of phosphocreatine and ATP is difficult, but is an essential step for further development of clinical cardiac MRS, as the phosphocreatine/ATP ratio cannot detect simultaneous decreases of phosphocreatine and ATP, which have

been demonstrated, for example, in the failing [108] or in the infarcted non-viable, myocardium [109]. Quantification of absolute ^{31}P-metabolite levels is possible by obtaining simultaneous signal from a ^{31}P-standard and estimates of myocardial mass based on MR imaging [110]. An alternative strategy [111] is to use simultaneous acquisition of a ^{1}H-spectrum and to calibrate the ^{31}P-signal to the tissue water proton content. Probably the most advanced technique in this respect is SLOOP (spectral localisation with optimum pointspread function), which allows interrogation of curved regions of interest matching the shape of the heart, and absolute quantification with high accuracy [112]. SLOOP requires a ^{31}P reference standard, flip angle calibration, B_1 field mapping, and measurement of myocardial mass.

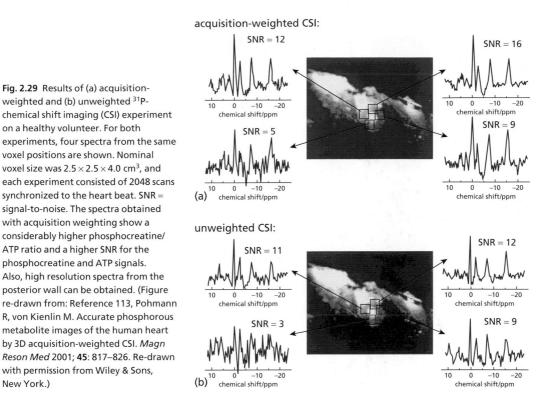

Fig. 2.29 Results of (a) acquisition-weighted and (b) unweighted ^{31}P-chemical shift imaging (CSI) experiment on a healthy volunteer. For both experiments, four spectra from the same voxel positions are shown. Nominal voxel size was $2.5 \times 2.5 \times 4.0$ cm^3, and each experiment consisted of 2048 scans synchronized to the heart beat. SNR = signal-to-noise. The spectra obtained with acquisition weighting show a considerably higher phosphocreatine/ATP ratio and a higher SNR for the phosphocreatine and ATP signals. Also, high resolution spectra from the posterior wall can be obtained. (Figure re-drawn from: Reference 113, Pohmann R, von Kienlin M. Accurate phosphorous metabolite images of the human heart by 3D acquisition-weighted CSI. *Magn Reson Med* 2001; **45**: 817–826. Re-drawn with permission from Wiley & Sons, New York.)

It has previously been impossible to interrogate the posterior wall of the human heart, because of its distance from the ^{31}P-surface coil. Pohmann and von Kienlin [113] have recently implemented acquisition-weighted ^{31}P-chemical shift imaging, which reduces the signal contamination between adjacent voxels, and, for the first time, ^{31}P-spectra from the posterior wall could be obtained. Acquisition-weighting should thus be implemented for all cardiac MRS protocols (Fig. 2.29). Clinical applications of ^{31}P-MRS are described in Chapter 7.

Methods for clinical ^{23}Na-MRI

Although methods for clinical ^{23}Na-MRI are considered in this spectroscopy section, ^{23}Na acquisition is strictly speaking an imaging technique, as there is a single frequency. Human sodium imaging requires specialist-built RF coils. Images are gated to the end-diastolic phase of the cardiac cycle but are acquired without respiratory gating due to the long duration of the scans (see Fig. 2.30). The sodium nucleus is a spin-3/2 system, which in practical terms means that the decay is bi-exponential,

giving rise to two T_2 values. To completely characterize the signal, both components need to be obtained, and as the short T_2 is around 1 ms, specialist acquisition approaches are required for this. A number of such approaches have been developed [114, 115]. One benefit arising from the properties of the sodium nucleus is that T_1 is very short and hence it is possible to use short repetition times, so that a large number of signal averages can be acquired to improve the SNR. The high concentration of sodium in the blood pool seriously hampers detection of endocardial infarction using present methods. Developments such as advanced coil designs, higher field strengths and the use of navigated acquisitions should improve the quality of human cardiac sodium imaging.

Perspective on MRS

Human cardiac MRS is feasible, but it is clear that a major technical development effort is still required to allow MRS to enter clinical practice. Major advances should be achievable in coil and sequence design, and through implementation of MRS at

Sodium (^{23}Na) images   Proton (^{1}H) images

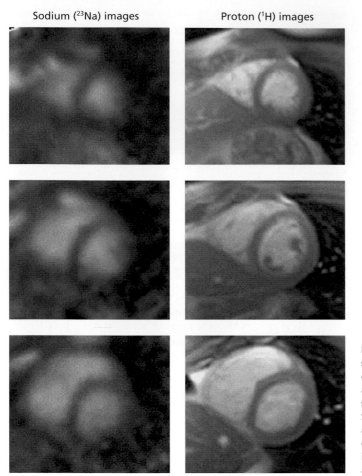

Fig. 2.30 Here three slices from a 3D sodium data set show the concentration of the long T$_2$ in the tissue. Proton slices acquired during the same imaging session are shown for comparison. Sodium acquisition was cardiac gated and required a 22 min acquisition using our ultra-short TE CSI approach. The image quality shown here is typical for all the acquisition methods at 1.5 T.

higher field strength [116]. Standardization of cardiac MRS approaches used at different centers is also an important issue. Until that time, MRS will remain a fascinating clinical research tool, allowing insight into cardiac metabolism in various forms of human heart disease.

Safety and contraindications

As an MR system consists of a large, static magnetic field in which RF energy is periodically released during imaging, possible hazards are associated with its use. In general, the potential hazard of implants or devices is dependent on such factors as their degree of ferromagnetism, geometry, location in the body, as well as the gradient and field strength of the imaging magnet.

In assessing whether a particular patient should be subjected to a CMR scan, the main rule, as with other investigations in medicine, is to determine the risk-benefit ratio to the patient of the proposed study. It is absolutely essential to carefully interview a patient prior to an MRI examination, and most centers would require a safety questionnaire to be completed. Whenever there is a concern about the safety of a patient with an implant, the CMR examination should be deferred until the device and the issues associated with it are clarified. Reference texts [117] and web based information (www.MRIsafety.com) on the safety of specific devices are available.

Older cerebral aneurysm clips are ferromagnetic and there are a number of reports of fatal cerebral hemorrhage after MR examinations in this setting. Although modern aneurysm clips are non-ferromagnetic, the type of clip should be established with certainty prior to performing the examination. Previous history of eye injury with metallic shards should also be sought and an x-ray performed of the orbit if there is doubt that the metallic fragment has not been removed. Electronic devices such as cochlear implants, nerve stimulation units and a number of modern implants can be damaged or malfunction as a result of being in a magnetic field and are best avoided. Sternal wires and vascular clips are not contraindicated, although they do produce artifacts.

Pacemakers and cardioverter defibrillators (ICDs): Despite early reports [118] and a recent large study [119] of non-pacemaker dependent patients being safely scanned in a high field system, a pacemaker-dependent patient is generally considered as an absolute contraindication to CMR scanning. Cardiac pacemakers and ICDs present potential problems for patients undergoing MR procedures from several mechanisms including: (1) movement of the device (e.g. the pulse generator and/or leads) because of the magnetic field of the MR system; (2) MR-related heating of leads by the time-varying magnetic fields; (3) inhibition or modification of the function of the device by the electromagnetic fields used for MR procedures, and (4) inappropriate or rapid pacing due to the pulsed gradient magnetic fields and/or pulsed radiofrequency (RF) fields (i.e. electromagnetic interference with the lead acting as an antenna) [120–122]. These problems may result in serious injuries or lethal consequences for patients, as well as device malfunctions or damage [122].

Stents: Every year approximately 457,000 metallic coronary artery stents are placed in the US alone [123]. In patients with coronary stents, MRI is believed to be safe once endothelialization [124] has occurred, presumably because this opposes possible dislodgement [117]. Therefore, manufacturers of stents and professional associations of cardiologists [123] have traditionally recommended postponing elective MRI examinations for four to eight weeks after stent placement. However, *in vitro* and animal studies [125–127] have shown that ferromagneticity and stent migration are absent or minimal with MRI of currently available stents. Early clinical studies on the outcome of patients who undergo MRI early after coronary stent placement also indicated that CMR at 1.5 T was safe in patients early after stent implantation [128, 129]. Recently, a retrospective review of 111 patients who underwent MRI at 1.5 T (39% head/neck, 27% spine, 9% chest) fewer than eight weeks after stent placement (and treated with aspirin and thienopyridine) showed that the risk of cardiac death, MI, or need for repeat revascularization because of associated stent thrombosis was very low [130]. Although the study did not have 30 day angiographic follow-up, the results are consistent with the 30-day cardiac event rates (0.5% to 1.9%) after coronary stent placement with contemporary anti-platelet therapy in patients not undergoing MRI [131]. These findings indicate that postponing CMR until after eight weeks following coronary stenting does not seem necessary.

Valvular prostheses: Heart valve prostheses are all safe for CMR. These most recent recommendations supersede earlier suggestions that pre-6000 series Starr-Edwards valves might cause problems during MR. Studies at 1.5 T to 2.35 T static magnetic fields have shown that there is no hazardous deflection during exposure of the magnetic field [117, 132].

Claustrophobia: Despite the development of shorter magnets, and more open designs, up to 10% of patients may experience varying degrees of claustrophobia. In our experience, the number is nearer to 5% [41], which can be reduced even further to about 2% of patients by the use of explanation, reassurance and, when necessary, light sedation [133].

Acknowledgements

The authors thank Drs Saul Myerson and Damian Tyler for critical review of various subsections of this chapter. We are also deeply grateful to the late Dr Frank Wiesmann, who played a crucial part in atherosclerosis imaging at our unit.

References

1. Bloch F. Nuclear induction. *Physical Review (Physics)* 1946; 460–473.
2. Purcell E, Torrey, H, Pound R. Resonance adsorption by nuclear masgnetic moments in a solid. *Physical Review (Physics)* 1946; 37–38.
3. Lauterbur P. Image formation by induced local

interactions: examples employing nuclear magnetic resonance. *Nature* 1973; **242**: 190–191.

4. Garlick PB, Radda GK, Seeley PJ. Phosphorus NMR studies on perfused heart. *Biochem Biophys Res Commun*. 1977; **74**: 1256–1262.

5. Jacobus WE, Taylor GJT, Hollis DP *et al*. Phosphorus nuclear magnetic resonance of perfused working rat hearts. *Nature* 1977; **265**: 756–758.

6. Goldsmith M, Koutcher JA, Damadian R. Nuclear magnetic resonance in cancer. Application of NMR malignancy index to human lung tumors. *Br J Cancer* 1977; **36**: 235–242.

7. Anderson LJ, Holden S, Davis B *et al*. Cardiovascular T_2-star (T_2^*) magnetic resonance for the early diagnosis of myocardial iron overload. *Eur Heart J*. 2001; **22**: 2171–2179.

8. Bryant DJ, Payne JA, Firmin DN *et al*. Measurement of flow with NMR imaging using a gradient pulse and phase difference technique. *J Comput Assist Tomogr* 1984; **8**: 588–593.

9. Chia JM, Fischer SE, Wickline SA *et al*. Performance of QRS detection for cardiac magnetic resonance imaging with a novel vectorcardiographic triggering method. *J Magn Reson Imaging* 2000; **12**: 678–688.

10. Larson AC, White RD, Laub G *et al*. Self-gated cardiac cine MRI. *Magn Reson Med* 2004; **51**: 93–102.

11. Bellenger NG, Davies LC, Francis JM *et al*. Reduction in sample size for studies of remodeling in heart failure by the use of cardiovascular magnetic resonance. *J Cardiovasc Magn Reson* 2000; **2**: 271–278.

12. Grothues F, Smith GC, Moon JC *et al*. Comparison of interstudy reproducibility of cardiovascular magnetic resonance with two-dimensional echocardiography in normal subjects and in patients with heart failure or left ventricular hypertrophy. *Am J Cardiol* 2002; **90**: 29–34.

13. Alfakih K, Plein S, Thiele H *et al*. Normal human left and right ventricular dimensions for MRI as assessed by turbo gradient echo and steady-state free precession imaging sequences. *J Magn Reson Imaging* 2003; **17**: 323–329.

14. Lorenz CH, Walker ES, Morgan VL *et al*. Normal human right and left ventricular mass, systolic function, and gender differences by cine magnetic resonance imaging. *J Cardiovasc Magn Reson* 1999; **1**: 7–21.

15. Helbing WA, Rebergen SA, Maliepaard C *et al*. Quantification of right ventricular function with magnetic resonance imaging in children with normal hearts and with congenital heart disease. *Am Heart J* 1995; **130**: 828–837.

16. Helbing WA, Bosch HG, Maliepaard C *et al*. Comparison of echocardiographic methods with magnetic resonance imaging for assessment of right ventricular function in children. *Am J Cardiol* 1995; **76**: 589–594.

17. Alfakih K, Plein S, Bloomer T *et al*. Comparison of right ventricular volume measurements between axial and short axis orientation using steady-state free precession magnetic resonance imaging. *J Magn Reson Imaging* 2003; **18**: 25–32.

18. Pennell DJ, Underwood SR, Manzara CC *et al*. Magnetic resonance imaging during dobutamine stress in coronary artery disease. *Am J Cardiol* 1992; **70**: 34–40.

19. Fayad ZA, Connick TJ, Axel L. An improved quadrature or phased-array coil for MR cardiac imaging. *Magn Reson Med* 1995; **34**: 186–193.

20. Cerqueira MD, Weissman NJ, Dilsizian VJ *et al*. Standardized myocardial segmentation and nomenclature for tomographic imaging of the heart. A statement for healthcare professionals from the Cardiac Imaging Committee of the Council on Clinical Cardiology of the American Heart Association. *Int J Cardiovasc Imaging* 2002; **18**: 539–542.

21. Nagel E, Lehmkuh HB, Bocksch W *et al*. Non-invasive diagnosis of ischemia-induced wall motion abnormalities with the use of high-dose dobutamine stress MRI: Comparison with dobutamine stress echocardiography. *Circulation* 1999; **99**: 763–770.

22. Wahl A, Roethemeyer S, Paetsch I *et al*. High Dose dobutamine stress MRI for follow-up after coronary revascularization procedures in patients with wall motion abnormalities at rest. *J Cardiovasc Magn Reson* 2002; **4**: 22–23.

23. Zerhouni EA, Parish DM, Rogers WJ *et al*. Human heart: Tagging with MR imaging—a method for non-invasive assessment of myocardial motion. *Radiology* 1988; **169**: 59–63.

24. Mosher TJ, Smith MB. A DANTE tagging sequence for the evaluation of translational sample motion. *Magn Reson Med* 1990; **15**: 334–339.

25. Axel L, Dougherty L. Heart wall motion: Improved method of spatial modulation of magnetization for MR imaging. *Radiology* 1989; **172**: 349–350.

26. Bolster BD Jr, McVeigh ER, Zerhouni EA. Myocardial tagging in polar coordinates with use of striped tags. *Radiology* 1990; **177**: 769–772.

27. Ryf S, Spiegel MA, Gerber M *et al*. Myocardial tagging with 3D-CSPAMM. *J Magn Reson Imaging* 2002; **16**: 320–325.

28. Croisille P, Guttman MA, Atalar E *et al*. Precision of myocardial contour estimation from tagged MR images with a "black-blood" technique. *Acad Radiol* 1998; **5**: 93–100.

29. Hennig J, Schneider B, Peschl S. Analysis of myocardial motion based on velocity measurements with a black-blood prepared segmented gradient-echo sequence: Methodology and applications to normal volunteers and patients. *J Magn Reson Imaging* 1998; **8**: 868–877.

30. Gilson WD, Yang Z, French BA *et al*. Measurement of myocardial mechanics in mice before and after infarction using multislice displacement-encoded MRI with

3D motion encoding. *Am J Physiol Heart Circ Physiol* 2004; **288**: H1491–1497.

31. Wesbey G, Higgins C, McNamara M *et al*. Effect of gadolinium-DTPA on the magnetic relaxation times of normal and infarcted myocardium. *Radiology* 1984; **153**: 165–169.

32. Simonetti OP, Kim RJ, Fieno DS *et al*. An improved MR imaging technique for the visualization of myocardial infarction. *Radiology* 2001; **218**: 215–223.

33. Sandstede JJ, Pabst T, Beer M *et al*. Assessment of myocardial infarction in humans with (23)Na MR imaging: Comparison with cine MR imaging and delayed contrast enhancement. *Radiology* 2001; **221**: 222–228.

34. Kim RJ, Fieno DS, Parrish TB *et al*. Relationship of MRI delayed contrast enhancement to irreversible injury, infarct age, and contractile function. *Circulation* 1999; **100**: 1992–2002.

35. Choi KM, Kim RJ, Gubernikoff G *et al*. Transmural extent of acute myocardial infarction predicts long-term improvement in contractile function. *Circulation* 2001; **104**: 1101–1107.

36. Selvanayagam JB, Kardos A, Francis JM *et al*. Value of delayed-enhancement cardiovascular magnetic resonance imaging in predicting myocardial viability after surgical revascularization. *Circulation* 2004; **110**: 1535–1541.

37. Wu E, Judd RM, Vargas JD *et al*. Visualisation of presence, location, and transmural extent of healed Q-wave and non-Q-wave myocardial infarction. *Lancet* 2001; **357**: 21–28.

38. Wagner A, Mahrholdt H, Holly TA *et al*. Contrast-enhanced MRI and routine single photon emission computed tomography (SPECT) perfusion imaging for detection of subendocardial myocardial infarcts: An imaging study. *Lancet* 2003; **361**: 374–379.

39. Wu KC, Zerhouni EA, Judd RM *et al*. Prognostic significance of microvascular obstruction by magnetic resonance imaging in patients with acute myocardial infarction. *Circulation* 1998; **97**: 765–772.

40. Wu KC, Kim RJ, Bluemke DA *et al*. Quantification and time course of microvascular obstruction by contrast-enhanced echocardiography and magnetic resonance imaging following acute myocardial infarction and reperfusion. *J Am Coll Cardiol* 1998; **32**: 1756–1764.

41. Selvanayagam JB, Petersen SE, Francis JM *et al*. Effects of off-pump versus on-pump coronary surgery on reversible and irreversible myocardial injury: A randomized trial using cardiovascular magnetic resonance imaging and biochemical markers. *Circulation* 2004; **109**: 345–350.

42. Selvanayagam JB, Porto I, Channon K *et al*. Troponin elevation following percutaneous coronary intervention directly represents the extent of irreversible myocardial injury: Insights from cardiovascular magnetic resonance imaging. *Circulation* 2005; **111**: 1027–1032.

43. Kim RJ, Wu E, Rafael A. The use of contrast-enhanced magnetic resonance imaging to identify reversible myocardial dysfunction. *N Engl J Med* 2000; **343**: 1445–1453.

44. Ricciardi MJ, Wu E, Davidson CJ *et al*. Visualization of discrete microinfarction after percutaneous coronary intervention associated with mild creatine kinase-MB elevation. *Circulation* 2001; **103**: 2780–2783.

45. Wilke N, Jerosch-Herold M, Stillman AE *et al*. Concepts of myocardial perfusion imaging in magnetic resonance imaging. *Magn Reson Q.* 1994; **10**: 249–286.

46. Jerosch-Herold M, Wilke N, Stillman AE. Magnetic resonance quantification of the myocardial perfusion reserve with a Fermi function model for constrained deconvolution. *Med Phys* 1998; **25**: 73–84.

47. Nagel E, Klein C, Paetsch I *et al*. Magnetic resonance perfusion measurements for the non-invasive detection of coronary artery disease. *Circulation* 2003; **108**: 432–437.

48. Cerqueira MD, Verani MS, Schwaiger M *et al*. Safety profile of adenosine stress perfusion imaging: Results from the Adenoscan Multicenter Trial Registry. *J Am Coll Cardiol* 1994; **23**: 384–389.

49. Al-Saadi N, Nagel E, Gross M *et al*. Non-invasive detection of myocardial ischemia from perfusion reserve based on cardiovascular magnetic resonance. *Circulation* 2000; **101**: 1379–1383.

50. Jerosch-Herold M, Wilke N. MR first pass imaging: Quantitative assessment of transmural perfusion and collateral flow. *Int J Card Imaging* 1997; **13**: 205–218.

51. Wilke N, Simm C, Zhang J *et al*. Contrast-enhanced first pass myocardial perfusion imaging: Correlation between myocardial blood flow in dogs at rest and during hyperemia. *Magn Reson Med* 1993; **29**: 485–497.

52. Larsson HB, Fritz-Hansen T, Rostrup E *et al*. Myocardial perfusion modeling using MRI. *Magn Reson Med* 1996; **35**: 716–726.

53. Jerosch-Herold M, Seethamraju RT, Swingen CM *et al*. Analysis of myocardial perfusion MRI. *J Magn Reson Imaging* 2004; **19**: 758–770.

54. Wacker CM, Hartlep AW, Pfleger S *et al*. Susceptibility-sensitive magnetic resonance imaging detects human myocardium supplied by a stenotic coronary artery without a contrast agent. *J Am Coll Cardiol* 2003; **41**: 834–840.

55. Wacker CM, Bock M, Hartlep AW *et al*. Changes in myocardial oxygenation and perfusion under pharmacological stress with dipyridamole: Assessment using T_2^* and T_1 measurements. *Magn Reson Med* 1999; **41**: 686–695.

56. Friedrich MG, Niendorf T, Schulz-Menger J *et al*. Blood oxygen level-dependent magnetic resonance imaging

in patients with stress-induced angina. *Circulation.* 2003; **108**: 2219–2223.

57. Mostbeck GH, Caputo GR, Higgins CB. MR measurement of blood flow in the cardiovascular system. *AJR Am J Roentgenol* 1992; **159**: 453–461.

58. Rebergen SA, van der Wall EE, Doornbos J *et al.* Magnetic resonance measurement of velocity and flow: Technique, validation, and cardiovascular applications. *Am Heart J* 1993; **126**: 1439–1456.

59. Didier D, Ratib O, Friedli B *et al.* Cine gradient-echo MR imaging in the evaluation of cardiovascular diseases. *Radiographics* 1993; **13**: 561–573.

60. Suzuki J, Caputo GR, Kondo C *et al.* Cine MR imaging of valvular heart disease: Display and imaging parameters affect the size of the signal void caused by valvular regurgitation. *AJR Am J Roentgenol* 1990; **155**: 723–727.

61. Mohiaddin RH, Pennell DJ. MR blood flow measurement. Clinical application in the heart and circulation. *Cardiol Clin* 1998; **16**: 161–187.

62. Kondo C, Caputo GR, Semelka R *et al.* Right and left ventricular stroke volume measurements with velocity-encoded cine MR imaging: *In vitro* and *in vivo* validation. *AJR Am J Roentgenol* 1991; **157**: 9–16.

63. Hundley WG, Li HF, Lange RA *et al.* Assessment of left-to-right intracardiac shunting by velocity-encoded, phase-difference magnetic resonance imaging. A comparison with oximetric and indicator dilution techniques. *Circulation* 1995; **91**: 2955–2960.

64. Caputo GR, Kondo C, Masui T *et al.* Right and left lung perfusion: *In vitro* and *in vivo* validation with oblique-angle, velocity-encoded cine MR imaging. *Radiology* 1991; **180**: 693–698.

65. Li D, Paschal CB, Haacke EM *et al.* Coronary arteries: Three-dimensional MR imaging with fat saturation and magnetization transfer contrast. *Radiology* 1993; **187**: 401–406.

66. Manning WJ, Li W, Boyle NG *et al.* Fat-suppressed breath-hold magnetic resonance coronary angiography. *Circulation* 1993; **87**: 94–104.

67. Kim WY, Stuber M, Börnet P. Three-dimensional black-blood cardiac magnetic resonance coronary vessel wall imaging detects positive arterial remodelling in patients with non-significant coronary artery disease. *Circulation* 2002; **106**: 296.

68. Botnar R, Stuber M, Danias P *et al.* Coronary magnetic resonance angiography. In: Manning WJ & Pennell DJ, eds. *Cardiovascular Magnetic Resonance.* Churchill Livingstone, Philadelphia, 2001.

69. Botnar RM, Stuber M, Danias PG *et al.* Improved coronary artery definition with T$_2$-weighted, free-breathing, three-dimensional coronary MRA. *Circulation* 1999; **99**: 3139–3148.

70. Wielopolski PA, Manning WJ, Edelman RR. Single breath-hold volumetric imaging of the heart using magnetization-prepared 3-dimensional segmented echo planar imaging. *J Magn Reson Imaging* 1995; **5**: 403–409.

71. Slavin GS, Riederer SJ, Ehman RL. Two-dimensional multishot echo-planar coronary MR angiography. *Magn Reson Med* 1998; **40**: 883–889.

72. Fayad ZA, Fuster V. Clinical imaging of the high-risk or vulnerable atherosclerotic plaque. *Circ Res* 2001; **89**: 305–316.

73. Herfkens RJ, Higgins CB, Hricak H *et al.* Nuclear magnetic resonance imaging of atherosclerotic disease. *Radiology* 1983; **148**: 161–166.

74. Fayad ZA, Fuster V. Characterization of atherosclerotic plaques by magnetic resonance imaging. *Ann N Y Acad Sci* 2000; **902**: 173–186.

75. Fayad ZA, Nahar T, Fallon JT *et al. In vivo* magnetic resonance evaluation of atherosclerotic plaques in the human thoracic aorta: A comparison with transesophageal echocardiography. *Circulation* 2000; **101**: 2503–2509.

76. Yuan C, Beach KW, Smith LH Jr *et al.* Measurement of atherosclerotic carotid plaque size *in vivo* using high resolution magnetic resonance imaging. *Circulation* 1998; **98**: 2666–2671.

77. Wiesmann F, Robson MD, Francis JM *et al.* Visualization of the ruptured plaque by magnetic resonance imaging. *Circulation* 2003; **108**: 2542.

78. Coulden RA, Moss H, Graves MJ *et al.* High resolution magnetic resonance imaging of atherosclerosis and the response to balloon angioplasty. *Heart* 2000; **83**: 188–191.

79. Fayad Z, Fuster V, Nikolaou K *et al.* Computed tomography and magnetic resonance imaging for non-invasive coronary angiography and plaque imaging: Current and potential future concepts. *Circulation* 2002; **106**: 2026.

80. Fayad ZA, Fuster V, Fallon JT *et al.* Non-invasive *in vivo* human coronary artery lumen and wall imaging using black-blood magnetic resonance imaging. *Circulation* 2000; **102**: 506–510.

81. Botnar RM, Kim WY, Bornert P *et al.* 3D coronary vessel wall imaging utilizing a local inversion technique with spiral image acquisition. *Magn Reson Med* 2001; **46**: 848–854.

82. Toussaint JF, LaMuraglia GM, Southern JF *et al.* Magnetic resonance images of lipid, fibrous, calcified, hemorrhagic, and thrombotic components of human atherosclerosis *in vivo. Circulation* 1996; **94**: 932–938.

83. Hayes CE, Mathis CM, Yuan C. Surface coil phased arrays for high-resolution imaging of the carotid arteries. *J Magn Reson Imaging* 1996; **6**: 109–112.

84. Neubauer S, Ingwall JS. Verapamil attenuates ATP depletion during hypoxia: ^{31}P NMR studies of the isolated rat heart. *J Mol Cell Card* 1989; **21**: 1163–1178.

85. Ingwall JS. Phosphorus nuclear magnetic resonance spectroscopy of cardiac and skeletal muscles. *Am J Physiol* 1982; **242**: H729–744.

86. Neubauer S, Ertl G, Krahe T *et al.* Experimental and clinical possibilities of MR spectroscopy of the heart. *Z Kardiol* 1991; **80**: 25–36, in German.

87. Clarke K, Stewart LC, Neubauer S *et al.* Extracellular volume and trans-sarcolemmal proton movement during ischemia and reperfusion: a ^{31}P NMR spectroscopic study of the isovolumic rat heart. *NMR Biomed* 1993; **6**: 278–286.

88. Horn M, Weidensteiner C, Scheffer H *et al.* Detection of myocardial viability based on measurement of sodium content: A (23)Na-NMR study. *Magn Reson Med* 2001; **45**: 756–764.

89. Liao R, Nascimben L, Friedrich J *et al.* Decreased energy reserve in an animal model of dilated cardiomyopathy. Relationship to contractile performance. *Circ Res* 1996; **78**: 893–902.

90. Zhang J, Wilke N, Wang Y *et al.* Functional and bioenergetic consequences of postinfarction left ventricular remodeling in a new porcine model. MRI and ^{31}P-MRS study. *Circulation* 1996; **94**: 1089–1100.

91. Ugurbil K, Petein M, Madian R *et al.* High resolution proton NMR studies of perfused rat hearts. *FEBS Lett* 1984; **167**: 73–78.

92. Balschi JA, Hetherington HP, Bradley EL Jr *et al.* Water-suppressed one-dimensional ^{1}H NMR chemical shift imaging of the heart before and after regional ischemia. *NMR in Biomedicine* 1995; **8**: 79–86.

93. Balschi JA, Hai JO, Wolkowicz PE *et al.* ^{1}H NMR measurement of triacylglycerol accumulation in the postischemic canine heart after transient increase of plasma lipids. *J Mol Cell Cardiol* 1997; **29**: 471–480.

94. Bottomley PA, Weiss RG. Non-invasive localized MR quantification of creatine kinase metabolites in normal and infarcted canine myocardium. *Radiology* 2001; **219**: 411–418.

95. Schneider J, Fekete E, Weisser A *et al.* Reduced (1)H-NMR visibility of creatine in isolated rat hearts. *Magn Reson Med* 2000; **43**: 497–502.

96. Kreutzer U, Mekhamer Y, Chung Y *et al.* Oxygen supply and oxidative phosphorylation limitation in rat myocardium in situ. *Am J Physiol Heart Circ Physiol* 2001; **280**: H2030–2037.

97. Solomon MA, Jeffrey FM, Storey CJ *et al.* Substrate selection early after reperfusion of ischemic regions in the working rabbit heart. *Magn Reson Med* 1996; **35**: 820–826.

98. Malloy CR, Jones JG, Jeffrey FM *et al.* Contribution of various substrates to total citric acid cycle flux and anaplerosis as determined by ^{13}C isotopomer analysis and O$_2$ consumption in the heart. *Magma* 1996; **4**: 35–46.

99. Lewandowski ED. Cardiac carbon 13 magnetic resonance spectroscopy: On the horizon or over the rainbow? *J Nucl Cardiol* 2002; **9**: 419–428.

100. Burgess SC, Babcock EE, Jeffrey FM *et al.* NMR indirect detection of glutamate to measure citric acid cycle flux in the isolated perfused mouse heart. *FEBS Lett* 2001; **505**: 163–167.

101. Weiss RG. ^{13}C-NMR for the study of intermediary metabolism. *Magma* 1998; **6**: 132.

102. Kohler SJ, Perry SB, Stewart LC *et al.* Analysis of ^{23}Na NMR spectra from isolated perfused hearts. *Magn Reson Med* 1991; **18**: 15–27.

103. Clarke K, Cross HR, Keon CA *et al.* Cation MR spectroscopy (^{7}Li, ^{23}Na, ^{39}K and ^{87}Rb). *Magma* 1998; **6**: 105–106.

104. DeLayre JL, Ingwall JS, Malloy C *et al.* Gated sodium-23 nuclear magnetic resonance images of an isolated perfused working rat heart. *Science.* 1981; **212**: 935–936.

105. Kim RJ, Lima JAC, Chen EL *et al.* Fast ^{23}Na magnetic resonance imaging of acute reperfused myocardial infarction. Potential to assess myocardial viability. *Circulation* 1997; **95**: 1877–1885.

106. Neubauer S, Krahe T, Schindler R *et al.* ^{31}P magnetic resonance spectroscopy in dilated cardiomyopathy and coronary artery disease. Altered cardiac high-energy phosphate metabolism in heart failure. *Circulation* 1992; **86**: 1810–1818.

107. Bottomley PA. MR spectroscopy of the human heart: The status and the challenges. *Radiology* 1994; **191**: 593–612.

108. Shen W, Asai K, Uechi M *et al.* Progressive loss of myocardial ATP due to a loss of total purines during the development of heart failure in dogs: A compensatory role for the parallel loss of creatine. *Circulation* 1999; **100**: 2113–2118.

109. Yabe T, Mitsunami K, Inubushi T *et al.* Quantitative measurements of cardiac phosphorus metabolites in coronary artery disease by ^{31}P magnetic resonance spectroscopy. *Circulation* 1995; **92**: 15–23.

110. Bottomley PA, Hardy CJ, Roemer PB. Phosphate metabolite imaging and concentration measurements in human heart by nuclear magnetic resonance. *Magn Reson Med* 1990; **14**: 425–434.

111. Bottomley PA, Atalar E, Weiss RG. Human cardiac high-energy phosphate metabolite concentrations by 1D-resolved NMR spectroscopy. *Magn Reson Med* 1996; **35**: 664–670.

112. Meininger M, Landschutz W, Beer M. Concentrations of human cardiac phosphorus metabolites determined by SLOOP ^{31}P NMR spectroscopy. *Magn Reson Med* 1999; **41**: 657–663.

113. Pohmann R, von Kienlin M. Accurate phosphorus metabolite images of the human heart by 3D acquisition-weighted CSI. *Magn Reson Med* 2001; **45**: 817–826.

114. Boada FE, Gillen JS, Shen GX *et al.* Fast three dimensional sodium imaging. *Magn Reson Med* 1997; **37**: 706–715.

115. Pabst T, Sandstede J, Beer M *et al.* Optimization of ECG-triggered 3D (23)Na MRI of the human heart. *Magn Reson Med* 2001; **45**: 164–166.

116. Lee RF, Giaquinto R, Constantinides C *et al.* A broadband phased-array system for direct phosphorus and sodium metabolic MRI on a clinical scanner. *Magn Reson Med* 2000; **43**: 269–277.

117. Shellock FG. *Guide to MR Procedures and Metallic Objects: Update 2001* [7th edn]. Lippincott, Williams and Wilkins Healthcare, Philadelphia, 2001.

118. Vahlhaus C, Sommer T, Lewalter T *et al.* Interference with cardiac pacemakers by magnetic resonance imaging: Are there irreversible changes at 0.5 Tesla? *Pacing Clin Electrophysiol* 2001; **24**: 489–495.

119. Martin ET, Coman JA, Owen W *et al.* Cardiac pacemakers and MRI: Safe evaluation of 47 patients using a 1.5 Tesla MR system without altering pacemaker or imaging parameters. *JACC* 2004; **43**: 1315–1324.

120. Achenbach S, Moshage W, Diem B *et al.* Effects of magnetic resonance imaging on cardiac pacemakers and electrodes. *Am Heart J* 1997; **134**: 467–473.

121. Duru F, Luechinger R, Candinas R. MR imaging in patients with cardiac pacemakers. *Radiology* 2001; **219**: 856–858.

122. Shellock FG, Tkach JA, Ruggieri PM *et al.* Cardiac pacemakers, ICDs, and loop recorder: Evaluation of translational attraction using conventional ("longbore") and "short-bore" 1.5- and 3.0-Tesla MR systems. *J Cardiovasc Magn Reson* 2003; **5**: 387–397.

123. American Heart Association. *Heart and Stroke Statistical Update.* American Heart Association, Dallas, TX, 2002.

124. Roubin GS, Robinson KA, King SB, 3rd *et al.* Early and late results of intracoronary arterial stenting after coronary angioplasty in dogs. *Circulation.* 1987; **76**: 891–897.

125. Hug J, Nagel E, Bornstedt A *et al.* Coronary arterial stents: Safety and artifacts during MR imaging. *Radiology* 2000; **216**: 781–787.

126. Scott NA, Pettigrew RI. Absence of movement of coronary stents after placement in a magnetic resonance imaging field. *Am J Cardiol* 1994; **73**: 900–901.

127. Strohm O, Kivelitz D, Gross W *et al.* Safety of implantable coronary stents during ^{1}H-magnetic resonance imaging at 1.0 and 1.5 T. *J Cardiovasc Magn Reson* 1999; **1**: 239–245.

128. Schroeder AP, Houlind K, Pedersen EM *et al.* Magnetic resonance imaging seems safe in patients with intracoronary stents. *J Cardiovasc Magn Reson* 2000; **2**: 43–49.

129. Kramer CM, Rogers WJ Jr, Pakstis DL. Absence of adverse outcomes after magnetic resonance imaging early after stent placement for acute myocardial infarction: A preliminary study. *J Cardiovasc Magn Reson* 2000; **2**: 257–261.

130. Gerber TC, Fasseas P, Lennon RJ *et al.* Clinical safety of magnetic resonance imaging early after coronary artery stent placement. *J Am Coll Cardiol* 2003; **42**: 1295–1298.

131. Orford JL, Lennon R, Melby S *et al.* Frequency and correlates of coronary stent thrombosis in the modern era: Analysis of a single center registry. *J Am Coll Cardiol* 2002; **40**: 1567–1572.

132. Soulen RL, Budinger TF, Higgins CB. Magnetic resonance imaging of prosthetic heart valves. *Radiology* 1985; **154**: 705–707.

133. Francis JM, Pennell DJ. Treatment of claustrophobia for cardiovascular magnetic resonance: Use and effectiveness of mild sedation. *J Cardiovasc Magn Reson* 2000; **2**: 139–141.

CHAPTER 3

Multidetector and electron-beam computed tomography of the heart

Robert Detrano & Nathan D. Wong

Introduction

Both multidetector and electron beam computed tomography (CT) provide thin tomographic images of the heart. Though these technologies have some differences, they are similar in that they both combine the high spatial resolution of computed tomography with very rapid temporal resolution. This combination of features makes it possible to visualize small structures such as coronary arteries with or without contract enhancement. Since all CT scanning uses x-ray absorption to create images, natural contrast will depend on physical density and the abundance of atoms with differing atomic numbers. Iodine and calcium have high atomic numbers and will appear white in CT images. Hydrogen, which is abundant in fat, has a low atomic number and appears dark grey. Blood and soft tissue have similar density and consist of similar proportions of the same atoms (hydrogen, oxygen, carbon) and thus appear light grey. Lung contains air which is of very low physical density and appears pitch black. Computed tomography, therefore, can distinguish non-iodinated blood from air, fat and bone but not from muscle or other soft tissue. This distinction of blood and soft tissue would require mixing of high atomic number Iodine in contrast injection with blood in order to distinguish blood from soft tissue using CT. The accentuated absorption of x-rays by elements of high atomic number such as calcium and iodine allows excellent visualization of small amounts of arterial calcium as well as differentiation between the contrast enhanced lumina of medium size coronary arteries and their intima lined walls.

Technical aspects

Electron Beam CT (EBT) scanners use an x-ray source, which consists of a 210-degree arc ring of tungsten targets, which are activated by bombardment from a magnetically focused beam of electrons fired from an electron gun behind the scanner ring. It takes one twentieth of a second to complete a rotation of the electron beam using EBT scanners. Sub-second, non-electron beam, or multidetector computed tomographic (MDCT) scanners use a rapidly rotating x-ray tube and several rows of detectors, also rotating. The tube and detectors are fitted with slip rings that allow them to continuously move through multiple 360-degree rotations. Present versions complete a 360-degree rotation in about four tenths of a second. These exposure times can be decreased to as little as .2 s by utilizing only a portion of the 360-degree rotation. For coronary calcium non-contrast scanning, the EBT scanner can acquire only one tomogram at a time; the MDCT scanner can acquire from four to 64 tomograms at a time depending on the model and other settings.

Multidetector scanners have a helical or spiral mode which is made possible by using a slip-ring interconnect. This allows the x-ray tube and detectors to rotate continuously during image acquisition since no wires directly connect the rotating and stationary components of the system (i.e. no need to unwind the wires). While the entire gantry (x-ray source and detectors) continuously rotates, the table moves the patient through the imaging plane at a predetermined speed. The relative speed of the gantry rotation table motion is called the scan pitch. The smooth rapid table motion or pitch in

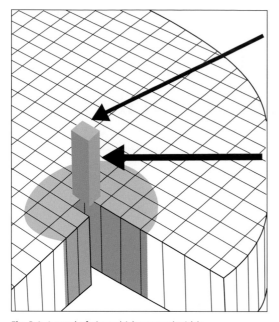

Fig. 3.1 A voxel of given thickness and width (narrow arrow).

helical scanning allows complete coverage of the cardiac anatomy in 15–25 s. A disadvantage of this method in cardiac scanning, however, is a small increase in radiation dose with respect to electron beam scanners.

Each individual tomogram can be thought of as a virtual slice of tissue consisting of blocks (voxels) containing numbers, each of which is proportional to the absorption of x-rays at that point and with a thickness and width determined by the reconstruction. Fig. 3.1 shows part of a tomogram.

Speed and time: The most challenging aspect of imaging of the heart is its inherent motion. General Electric's electron beam tomographic (EBT) scanner has a temporal resolution of 50–100 ms. A gantry rotation time of as little as 0.33 s with a temporal resolution of 83 ms is possible from the new 64-slice multidetector scanners.

The cephalad-caudad length of the heart that can be captured in one heartbeat at high spatial resolution by some scanners is now greater than 6 cm. Thus an average heart can be imaged in its entirety in about three to four heartbeats with some scanners.

Signal to noise: Signal-to-noise ratio is as important as temporal resolution. This refers to the sensitivity of the scanning instrument to detect real differences in radiographic density over random noise, which is present in all scan images. Noise is defined as the variability in pixel number in a physically homogeneous region of the object scanned. Noise levels are higher for the older EBT scanner, but have been greatly reduced using the new E-speed EBT model scanners though the cost of this reduction has been some modest increase in radiation dose.

Radiation exposure: There has never been any scientific evidence showing that diagnostic radiation exposure causes harmful health effects. However, conventional wisdom is that any radiation may be harmful and diagnostic exposure should be minimized. Table 3.1 shows the radiation exposure from various types of CT studies of the heart:

A few generalizations that can be made include:
1 There is little difference in radiation exposure between scanner types when axial sequential scanning is used.

Table 3.1 Radiation exposure to adult males during calcium scanning and CT angiography from various computed tomographic studies of the heart. Doses reported in milliSieverts.

Scanner Type	Exam	Mode	Approximate effective dose
EBT	coronary calcium	standard axial sequential	<1 mSv
MDCT (Siemens MDCT with kVp 120)	coronary calcium	standard xial Sequential	<1 mSv
MDCT	coronary calcium	helical (pitch = 1)	4–6 mSv
EBT	CT coronary angiography	axial with overlap	2–3 mSv
MDCT	CT coronary angiography	helical (pitch = 1)	~8.0 mSv

Sources: Unpublished data, MESA study; J.J. Carr, personal communication.

II Helical scanning will result in higher exposure than sequential scanning.

III Slice overlap increases dose.

It is important to be working with staff who are technically knowledgeable regarding cardiac scanning so that they can accurately explain risks and benefits to patients referred for scanning.

Clinical applications

Coronary calcium pathophysiology

Atherosclerotic calcification has many similarities to bone formation in cartilage plates [1] and occurs when other pathological manifestations of atherosclerosis are present. Gla-containing proteins that are involved in the transport of calcium out of vessel walls are involved in atherosclerotic calcification. Calcified plaque also contains mRNA for bone morphogenetic protein, a potent factor for osteoblastic differentiation as well as cells that are capable of osteoblastic transformation [2]. Osteoprotogerin, another bone protein has also been shown to be associated with calcification in arteries. Although calcification is found more frequently in advanced lesions, it may also occur in the lesions that are seen as early as the second decade of life. The relation of arterial calcification to the probability of plaque rupture is unknown. Though the extent of calcification is directly related to the volume of plaque, this relationship is far from perfect, and it is not known if the amount of calcium tracks the amount of plaque over time. Teleological speculations and some empirical evidence [3] suggest that calcification may represent an attempt to protect threatened myocardium by strengthening weakened atherosclerotic plaque that is prone to rupture.

Coronary calcium: Historical perspective
Fluoroscopy

Fluoroscopic image intensifiers have been standard equipment in hospitals for decades. The first reports on the use of non-invasive fluoroscopy for detecting coronary calcium appeared in the 1960s [4, 5]. There was a surge of interest, which culminated in the late 1980s with a meta-analysis [6] and the development of two modifications, which increased sensitivity and accuracy. [7, 8]. The meta-analysis concluded that though the sensitivity of fluoroscopy appeared to be low, its specificity was high and

its accuracy compared well to most forms of stress testing.

Computed tomography

In 1987 Reinmuller [9] reported CT for coronary calcium to be more sensitive but less specific than fluoroscopy for predicting angiographic stenoses. Masuda [10] and Timmins [11] also found CT to have increased sensitivity for stenoses. The increased contrast resolution of CT is the reason for its expected increase in sensitivity. Localization and quantification of calcifications is also more accurate with CT.

Electron beam computed tomography (EBT)

Reports on EBT's potential for imaging coronary calcifications began very early with the papers of Tannenbaum [12] and Agatston [13]. Several other investigators [14–16] reported accuracies for predicting angiographic stenoses that are comparable to those of exercise testing. We know of one meta-analysis which shows encouraging results in this regard [17].

Measures of coronary calcium

Fig. 3.2 shows a calcification in the left anterior descending coronary artery. All measures of coronary calcium depend on an inherent definition of a calcified lesion. Such definitions depend on two factors, a minimum brightness value (Hounsfield number) assigned to a pixel in the anatomic distribution of the coronary tree and a minimum number of adjacent or contiguous pixels that have that brightness value. The standard set by the Multiethnic

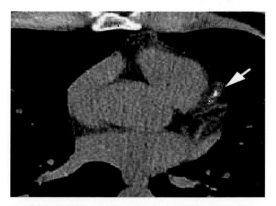

Fig. 3.2 Calcification in the left coronary artery (arrow, outlined in red).

(a)

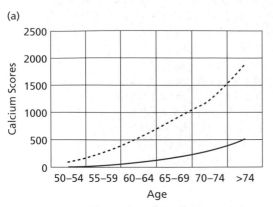

(b)

No. of Men	Age (yrs.)	5th	25th	50th	75th	90th
300	<35	0	0	0	0	5
807	35–39	0	0	0	0	35
1,551	40–44	0	0	0	3	142
2,040	45–49	0	0	0	25	312
2,473	50–54	0	0	5	88	630
2,062	55–59	0	0	36	223	1,163
1,333	60–64	0	2	95	441	1,807
841	65–69	0	19	201	684	2,480
490	70–74	0	28	302	942	3,390
272	>74	0	105	521	1,385	3,941
Total: 12,169						

Fig. 3.3 (a) Plot of 50th (solid line) and 75th (broken line) percentiles of coronary calcium scores in men. (b) Table of coronary artery percentile scores stratified by age. (Figure re-drawn with permission from: Reference 22, Mitchell TL, Pippin JJ, Devers SM *et al.* Age- and sex-based nomograms from coronary artery calcium scores as determined by electron beam computed tomography. *Am J Cardiol* 2001; **87**: 453–6.)

Study of Atherosclerosis (MESA) and Coronary Artery Risk Development in Young Adults (CARDIA) studies is a brightness value of greater than 130 Hounsfield units and four contiguous pixels using a 35 cm field of view [18].

The most popular measure of coronary calcium is the "Agatston" calcium score. This is an attenuation weighted volume of "plaques" whose pixel numbers exceed 130. A simpler and slightly more reproducible measure is the calcium area or volume. The calcium volume is the total volume of all voxels with Hounsfield numbers exceeding 130. Callister and Raya have developed an interpolated volume scoring method, which smooths adjacent voxel numbers between image slices [19]. They have found their method to be more reproducible, though other research has not found large differences in reproducibility between the different scoring measures [20]. Others have proposed the coronary calcium mass as a more reproducible and accurate measure.

Age and sex-based nomograms have been in use to assist in determining calcification amount [21]. A recent report on a total of 18,785 patients [22] showed coronary artery calcium percentile scores derived for men and women based on five year age intervals, and predictive scoring systems were derived based on the 50th and 75th percentiles of calcium scores (see Fig. 3.3 and Fig. 3.4).

Progression of coronary calcium

Serial coronary calcium studies to follow the progression of atherosclerosis would be useful if the following conditions were met:

I The progression of coronary calcium tracked the progression of unstable coronary plaque; as noted above, the extent to which this is true is still a matter of debate.

II The measurement error, defined as the rescan variability, was much lower than the real change over time.

Coronary calcium is known to progress [23, 24]. However, the extent to which this progression tracks the progression of atherosclerotic plaque is unknown. Unfortunately, many who investigate temporal changes in calcium score over time have not considered that our understanding of the significance of atherosclerotic calcification is poor. Furthermore, the ability to track progression of calcium will depend on the rescan variability compared to the expected rate of progression. If the former is much greater than the latter, then progression within a year or two will not be easy to detect in a single individual.

Examination of age dependent scores in cross-sectional data can most easily assess expected changes or progression over time. The approximate yearly increase in calcium score in cross-sectional research studies is between 20 and 35%. There are also pro-

(a)

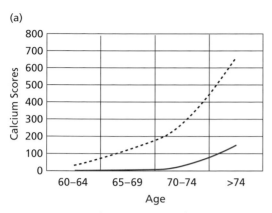

(b)

No. of Women	Age (yrs.)	5th	25th	50th	75th	90th
459	<40	0	0	0	0	1
726	40–44	0	0	0	0	7
1,102	45–49	0	0	0	0	37
1,421	50–54	0	0	0	0	81
1,143	55–59	0	0	0	6	203
771	60–64	0	0	0	35	445
532	65–69	0	0	8	114	791
276	70–74	0	0	28	244	1,268
186	>74	0	18	149	521	2,423
Total: 6,616						

Fig. 3.4 (a) Plot of 50th (solid line) and 75th (broken line) percentiles of coronary calcium scores in women. (b) Table of coronary artery percentile scores stratified by age. (Figure re-drawn with permission from: Reference 22,

Mitchell TL, Pippin JJ, Devers SM *et al.* Age- and sex-based nomograms from coronary artery calcium scores as determined by electron beam computed tomography. *Am J Cardiol* 2001; **87**: 453–6.)

spective studies showing similarly rapid progression of coronary calcium over time [25–27]. Statistical arguments suggest that even with this rapid rate of progression, at least three years would have to pass before perceived changes in calcification could be judged to be significant in a single individual. This limitation on the clinical use of CT calcium assessments is similar to that seen for other types of vascular imaging such as coronary angiography [28]. This drawback has far less effect on the utility of coronary calcium assessments for research studies when used in samples of at least 100 persons.

Screening and predicting events

The monograph by Morrison [29] contains an excellent definition of the purpose of screening for chronic diseases. "Screening for disease control can be defined as the examination of asymptomatic people in order to classify them as likely or not likely to have the disease that is the object of screening. The goal of screening is to reduce morbidity and mortality from disease among the people screened by early treatment of the cases discovered."

There is an aspect of this definition that receives little attention in much of the debate regarding calcium screening. This aspect is implied in the phrase "reduce morbidity and mortality". If this goal to reduce disease incidence cannot be achieved, then screening will not achieve its purpose and cannot be deemed effective. For example, cholesterol screening is effective only because lipoproteins are clinically

effective targets for preventive therapy; mammographic screening for breast cancer and occult blood screening for colon cancer have been proven to be effective in certain groups, not solely because they predict clinical disease and mortality but also because screening leads to a course of action proven to save lives.

Before we can endorse massive coronary calcium screening of the entire population, or even a subpopulation, of adults, we need to have a screening test that leads to effective preventive therapy when applied to asymptomatic persons. Thus the test must predict clinical disease in asymptomatic persons in a way that allows therapeutically effective decisions to be made based on the results.

It is sometimes argued that coronary calcium measurements can be helpful in certain subsets of persons, based on risk factor status and specifically on lipid levels. For example, some would very aggressively treat a 45-year-old man with reductase inhibitors, ACE inhibitors, and aspirin if his LDL-cholesterol were in the range between 100–130 mg/dl and he had a coronary calcium score of 400 (well above 90th percentile for age and gender). They would argue: "I know he has coronary disease. Therefore, he should be in a secondary prevention category and I should treat him as if he had suffered a myocardial infarction." Logical though it seems, this argument has an important flaw. The flaw lies in the expanded definition of coronary heart disease from "clinical to preclinical" disease. A calcium score of 400 has not been shown to be equivalent to a prior myocardial infarction. Those with prior infarctions have been proven to benefit from aggressive LDL-cholesterol lowering. However, even if a score of 400 in this person predicted a grave prognosis, we could not be sure that any benefit would be garnered from intervention.

Position of the professional societies

The American Heart Association and the American College of Cardiology have taken responsible positions on this issue in recommending that persons of intermediate coronary heart disease risk may be suitable candidates for screening if referred by their physician [30–32].

In this paradigm, a clinical examination including personal and family medical history, and blood pressure and lipid measurement should always be used to determine the indication for a coronary calcium exam. General screening of asymptomatic adults should be discouraged and coronary calcium studies should be restricted to those at intermediate risk who might benefit from aggressive risk factor modification and possibly to those with atypical chest pain.

Computed tomographic coronary angiography

For multislice CT systems, acquisition of up to 64 slices allows for scanning the entire heart within 10–20 s with a z axis resolution as low as 0.6 mm and a temporal resolution close to 200 ms. These new technological developments are driving a renewed interest in contrast enhanced cardiac CT. This section will review current and developing techniques and application of contrast enhanced CT angiography. CT angiography has the potential to address several important parameters related to atherosclerotic changes in the coronary arteries, including detection of non-calcified plaque.

Without the addition of an intravascular contrast agent, differentiation of the vessel wall from the vessel lumen is not possible in most instances with CT. This is due to the similar x-ray attenuation of blood and soft tissue. This multiplanar capability provides an ability to afford quantitative information on vessel lumen, relatively irrespective of stenosis orientation, with a single acquisition. In the next section we will consider current technical aspects of contrast enhanced CT imaging of the heart, review the published scientific literature, and conclude with areas of active research.

Technique

CT angiography allows imaging of the coronary arteries during arterial enhancement following the intravenous injection of contrast material. The test can be performed on an outpatient basis. Complications are rare (venous extravasation, anaphylactoid reactions to contrast and nephrotoxicity).

Scout images and planar tomograms are first acquired. The CT operator uses the scout images to prescribe subsequent scan volumes. The patient is positioned head first supine on the couch and moved slightly to the right in order to place the heart in the center of the scanning circle. Three ECG electrodes are placed and ECG gated 2.5–3 mm images are made for calcium screening and for navigation to find exact start and endpoints for the CTA coronary scan. This unenhanced scan is used to identify the location of coronary calcium, stents, catheters, foreign bodies, or other findings which partially obscure the contrast agent.

A non-ionic contrast medium is administered into an arm vein at a given concentration (e.g. 370 mg/ml). Approximately 120–150 ml is injected at a rate of 3.5–4.0 ml/s using an automatic injector. A semiautomated bolus-tracking technique is used to determine the transit time of contrast from the injection site to the ascending aorta. The transit time is then used as the delay time from the start of the contrast injection to imaging start for the CT coronary angiogram. Contrast enhanced EBT of the coronary arteries typically uses a sequential scan mode with prospective ECG triggering and overlapping 3 mm slices. 1–3 mm slice collimation is used for multislice scanners.

Debate remains as to the optimal trigger point within the RR interval. In one large study of 2,660 patients who underwent EBT scanning, motion artifact was least (<3% in all cases) when triggering ranged from 27–48% for heart rates of <50 to more than 100 beats/min [33]. In another study involving multidetector CT angiography, the left anterior descending artery was best visualized in mid-diastole at 60–70%, the right coronary artery in early diastole at 40%, and the left circumflex artery had optimal image quality most often at 50% [34].

MDCT systems can operate in either the sequential or helical mode. In the sequential mode, a 4, 8, 16, 32, or 64-slice scanner can acquire the same number of simultaneous data channels of image information. Thus a 64-channel system can acquire, within the same cardiac cycle up to 60 mm per heartbeat. In the helical or spiral mode of operation, a MDCT system can acquire several simultaneous data channels while there is continuous motion of the CT table. The relative motion of the rotating x-ray tube to the table speed is called the scan pitch and is particularly important for cardiac gating in the helical mode. By combining information from each of the detector rows, the effective temporal resolution of the images can currently be set at less than 100 ms, and the various cardiac phases can be reconstructed. An advantage of the helical acquisition mode is that there is a continuous model of the heart from base to apex, as opposed to the sequential/cine mode in which there are discrete slabs of slices which have been obtained in a "step and shoot" fashion.

Clinical studies

Dr. Stephan Achenbach and colleagues have evaluated the ability of contrast enhanced EBT to evaluate coronary artery bypass grafts [35], detect high-grade restenosis after percutaneous trans-luminal angioplasty (PTCA) [36], and determine patency of infarct related coronary vessels [37]. They have also compared EBT coronary angiography to catheter based coronary angiography in a study of 125 patients [38, 39]. The study was a direct comparison of the proximal and middle segments of the major coronary arteries, using the American Heart Association reporting system with both EBT and conventional coronary angiography. In this study, 25% of coronary vessels could not be evaluated (124/500 vessels), mostly because of respiratory artifacts and coronary calcifications. The number of patients with none of the four major coronary arteries of sufficient quality to evaluate was 15%. After excluding the 124 vessels which could not be evaluated, EBT angiography correctly categorized 69/75 (92%) coronary vessels as having high-grade stenoses or occlusions and 282/301 (94%) of vessels were normal or had stenoses of less than 75% reduction in vessel diameter as compared to the standard of conventional catheter based angiography (Fig. 3.5). Fig. 3.6 shows a normal CT angiogram for reference.

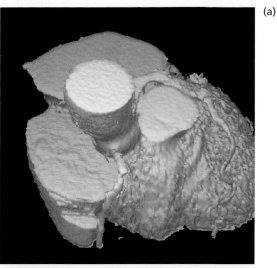
(a)

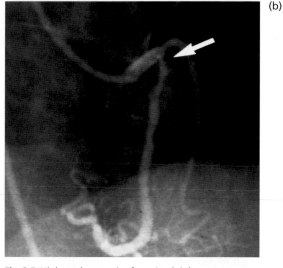
(b)

Fig. 3.5 High grade stenosis of proximal right coronary artery. Shaded surface display of a high grade stenosis of the right coronary artery is demonstrated with contrast-enhanced cardiac CT in (a) (Imatron C150) and compared with the conventional coronary angiogram in (b). (Figure reproduced with permission and by courtesy of S. Achenbach, Department of Internal Medicine II, Cardiology, University of Erlangen-Nuremberg from: Reference 39, Achenbach S, Moshage W, Ropers D, *et al.* Value of electron-beam computed tomography for the noninvasive detection of high-grade coronary-artery stenoses and occulsions. *N Engl J Med* 1998; **339**: 1964–1971.)

(a)

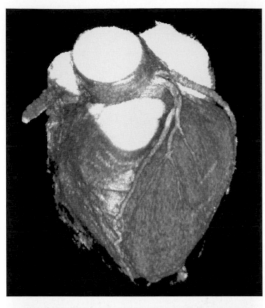

(b)

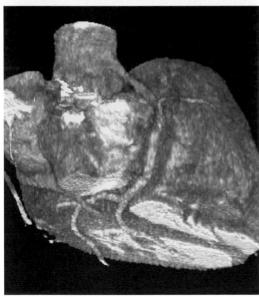

Fig. 3.6 Normal CT coronary angiography (Siemens Volume Zoom): (a) The left anterior descending coronary artery from origin to cardiac apex is demonstrated. The proximal extent of the left circumflex coronary, which originates directly from the ascending aorta, is also seen. (b) The same 3-dimensional data is viewed such that the origin and course of the right coronary artery is demonstrated in the atrioventricular groove. (Figure reproduced with permission and by courtesy of S. Achenbach, Department of Internal Medicine II, Cardiology, University of Erlangen-Nuremberg from: Reference 39, Achenbach S, Moshage W, Ropers D, *et al.* Value of electron-beam computed tomography for the noninvasive detection of high-grade coronary-artery stenoses and occulsions. *N Engl J Med* 1998; **339**: 1964–1971.)

Table 3.2 Sensitivity and specificity of CT angiography compared to coronary angiography.

Author	n	Sensitivity	Specificity
Kopp *et al.* [40]	102	86%	93%
Achenbach *et al.* [41]	64	91%	84%
Becker *et al.* [42]	48	82%	97%
Herzog *et al.* [44]	120	71%	92%

The authors noted that the majority of missed stenoses (false negatives) were located in the right and left circumflex coronary arteries, in the segments coursing perpendicular to the transverse imaging plane where the 3 mm slice thickness and volume averaging may be important factors.

Overall, published studies of MDCT coronary angiography in the detection and quantification of coronary lesions from various centers have shown a sensitivity of 75–90%, specificity of 90–95%, a positive predictive value of 0.7–0.9, and a negative predictive value of 0.8–0.9 for detection of hemodynamically significant stenoses (Table 3.2). However, in a number of studies, evaluation of the proximal arteries remains difficult.

The continued rapid technologic advancement of MDCT and EBT suggests that there will be further improvements in CT coronary angiography. A 16 channel MDCT system (Toshiba Aquilion 16) utilizes 16 detector rows to improve temporal resolution, reduce breath-hold time and reduce contrast dose (Fig. 3.7). Further improvements in image quality can be expected with 32 and 64-slice scanners now available. We will observe continued rapid advancement in CT for coronary angiography and a series of comparative studies evaluating these new CT techniques with existing measures of coronary heart disease.

Evaluation of plaque composition

Plaques occupying less than 40% of the area within the internal elastic membrane may escape detection by conventional coronary angiography, and it is often these non-stenotic plaques that cause the majority of myocardial infarctions. CT angiography may allow for the detection of early changes before narrowing of the luminal diameter. Direct compar-

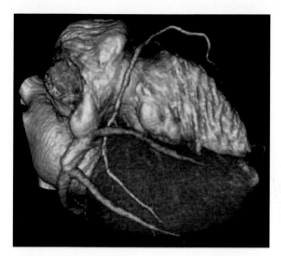

Fig. 3.7 Volume rendered image from 16-slice Toshiba Aquilion multidetector scanner showing distal RCA and veins. Severe coronary artherosclerosis, with significant obstructions affecting the distal left main, proximal LAD and first diagonal and the proximal RCA (with permission and courtesy of Toshiba, Inc.).

ison between multidetector CT angiography and intravascular ultrasound (IVUS) confirms that non-calcified plaques from CT angiography correspond to soft tissue material on IVUS which may either be fibrotic or lipid-rich plaques. Moreover, denser areas from IVUS correspond to heavily calcified areas on

CT angiography. Soft tissue plaques tend to obstruct the lumen of the coronary vessel whereas areas of extensive calcification are remodeled and may therefore be non-obstructive [42] (Fig. 3.8, Fig. 3.9 and Fig. 3.10). Others have also shown plaque composition detected by MDCT versus IVUS to yield identical results with regard to plaque composition and quantification of lesions [44].

Cardiac valves and chambers

Echocardiography remains the major modality for imaging cardiac valves. However, in cases where lung disease or body habitus make transthoracic echo difficult, CT can be used. Valve and mitral chordal thickening and valve stenosis can be identified using rapid CT. Vegetations and ring abscesses can also be detected. CT has been used to image paravalvular pathology [45].

CT can reliably detect left atrial thrombus. Tomada *et al.* [46] found that CT accurately detected left atrial thrombus. All patients with thrombus detected by CT had thrombus at surgery and 13 patients with no thrombus by CT were found to have no thrombus at surgery. Helgason *et al.* [47] compared EBT with transthoracic echocardiography in 40 patients presenting with stroke. CT detected evidence of left atrial or LV thrombus in 12 patients, while echo detected thrombus in only two patients.

Fig. 3.8 Correlation of CT angiography of the coronary arteries with intravascular ultrasound illustrates the ability of MDCT to demonstrate calcified and non-calcified coronary plaques. (Figure reproduced with permission from: Reference 42, Becker CR, Ohnesorge BM, Schoepf UJ *et al.* Current development of cardiac imaging with multidetector-row CT. *Eur J Radiol* 2000; **36**: 97–103.)

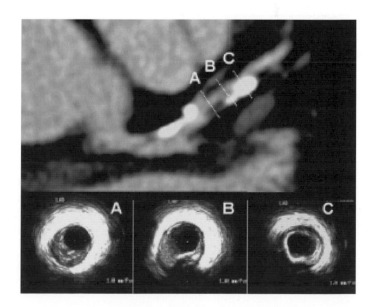

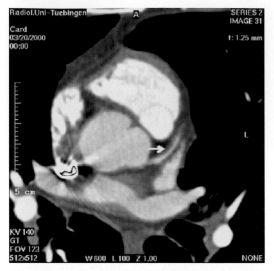

Fig. 3.9 Non-calcified, soft, lipid-rich plaque in left anterior descending artery (arrow) (Somatom Sensation 4, 120 ml Imeron 400). The plaque was confirmed by intravascular ultrasound. (Figurer reproduced with permission from: Reference 40, Kopp AF, Schroder S, Kuttner A *et al.* Multidetector row CT for non-invasive coronary angiograph patients. *Radiology* 2000; **217**(P): 375–380.

Assessing ventricular function and cardiomyopathies

CT plays a supportive role to echocardiography in assessing ventricular function. The entire left and right ventricles can be imaged throughout the cardiac cycle. Sufficient contrast enhancement is usually achieved with 30–40 ml of contrast medium injected in a peripheral arm vein. These images will accurately define the endocardial boundaries and allow precise measurements of ventricular volumes, ejection fraction and left ventricular mass [48, 49].

One interesting application is in the evaluation of patients with known cardiomyopathy, in whom the knowledge as to etiology might assist in management. Both EBT and MDCT have shown capability of distinguishing ischemic from non-ischemic cardiomyopathy by the detection of coronary calcium [50, 51].

Pericardial disease

Epicardial fat and the surrounding air filled lung provides natural contrast that permits easy identification of a normal pericardium. Thickening of the pericardium can easily be identified and this technology surpasses any other in identifying chronic pericarditis, particularly when it is calcific (Fig. 3.11). CT is thus ideal for differentiating constrictive pericarditis from restrictive cardiomyopathy. The presence of normal pericardial thickness, (i.e. 2–3 mm) excludes the diagnosis of constriction [52].

Congenital heart disease

Management of patients with congenital heart disease requires accurate information regarding structure and function of the cardiac chambers and

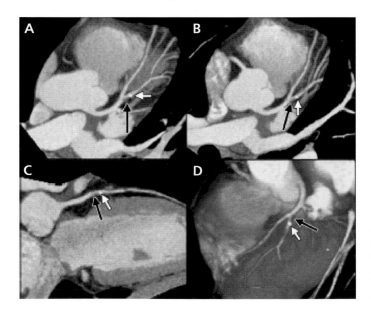

Fig. 3.10 CT angiogram of calcified coronary arteries. (Figure reproduced with permission from: Reference 43, Schoenhagen P, Halliburton S, Stillman A *et al.* Non-invasive imaging of coronary arteries: Current and future role of multidetector row CT. *Radiology* 2004; **232**: 7–17.)

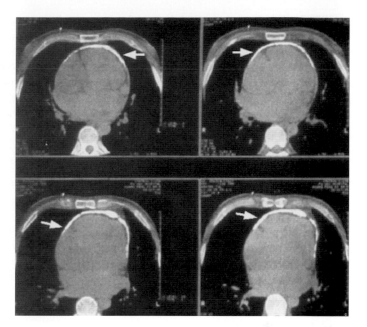

Fig. 3.11 Thick, calcified pericardium is clearly demonstrated (arrows).

great vessels. There have been many recent reports of the use of CT as a modality to define abnormalities in structure and function of the heart. However, the role of CT in this application remains largely supportive to angiography and echocardiography.

When imaging the hearts of infants and small children, it is essential to use a slice thickness that is small enough not to miss small structures such as the ductus arteriosus or anomalous coronary arteries. Most rapid scanners have the option of a 1.5 mm slice thickness or less. Another consideration is temporal resolution. The most prominent role of CT in the assessment of congenital heart lesions will involve structures that are inaccessible to the ultrasonic probe, such as the pulmonary artery and the aorta's ascending and descending branch and arch.

MDCT and EBT scanners should not require more than one injection of contrast to obtain high quality images of cardiac chambers and vessels. Most scanners operate in a mode that allows visualization of the wash-in and wash-out of contrast from the cardiac chambers. Shunt calculations can be done in a manner similar to that using indicator dilution methods in the cardiac catheterization laboratory. However, this is fraught with some difficulty due to beam hardening and other physical errors.

Specific problems for which CT is indicated, include determining the origin of the coronary arteries; visualization of the pulmonary arteries in cyanotic congenital heart disease; precise definition of aortic geometry in Marfan's disease, and partial or total anomalous pulmonary venous drainage. CT can also be used for visualization and assessment of patent ductus arteriosus and aortic coarctation [53–58].

Aortic disease

The thoracic aorta is an integral component of the cardiac CT exam and thoracic imaging in general. CT is the primary means of imaging the lung, thoracic trauma (blunt and penetrating), aneurysms and aortic dissections [59]. In the situation of an acute life-threatening event, CT can provided extensive information concerning the heart, aorta and great vessels. In addition, during the same exam, the brain and spinal canal can be evaluated. The entire global CT exam (head, cervical spine, chest, abdomen and pelvis) can be completed on modern MDCT systems in less than 15 min. These capabilities have made modern CT an indispensable tool in emergency departments and medical centers world wide and the development of the MDCT systems have further expanded these capabilities [60].

In the setting of chest trauma, CT can be extremely useful in diagnosis and as an aid to surgical management [61–64]. Contrast CT can rapidly identify aortic tears, intramural hematoma and dissection. In addition, the presence of mediastinal hematoma and other associated injuries can be assessed. These exams are performed in critically ill patients who may require mechanical ventilation, invasive monitoring, intravenous infusions pumps, and cardiac pacing. The well designed CT imaging suite is hospitable to life support equipment, which can remain in the room and operational throughout the imaging procedure.

CT is playing an increasingly important role in the diagnosis and management of thoracic aortic pathology [65, 66]. Although MRI and transesophageal echocardiography can provide exquisite and unique information, the robust nature of CT often make it the imaging modality of choice.

Contrast enhanced CT can identify and classify aortic dissections and aortic aneurysms.

Acknowledgement

The editorial assistance of Linda Neese is deeply appreciated.

References

1. Doherty TM, Detrano RC. Coronary calcification: A new perspective on an old problem. *Calcif Tissue Int.* 1994; **54**: 224–230.

2. Fraser JD, Price PA. Lung, heart and kidney express high levels of mRNA for the vitamin K dependent gal protein. *J Biol Chem* 1988; **263**: 11033–11036.

3. Cheng GC, Loree HM, Kamm RD *et al.* Distribution of circumferential stress in ruptured and stable atherosclerotic lesions. *Circulation* 1993; **87**: 1179–1187.

4. Jorgens J, Blank N, Wilcox WA. Cinefluorographic detection and recording of calcification within the heart. *Radiology* 1960; **74**: 550–554.

5. Lieber A, Jorgens J. Cinefluorography of coronary artery calcifications. *Amer J Roentgenolgy* 1961; **86**: 1063–1070.

6. Gianrossi R, Detrano R, Colombo A *et al.* Cardiac fluoroscopy for the diagnosis of coronary disease: A meta-analytic review. *Am Heart J.* **120**: 1179–1188, 1990.

7. Detrano R, Markovic D, Simpfendorfer C *et al.* Digital subtraction fluoroscopy: A new method of detecting coronary calcifications with improved sensitivity for the prediction of coronary disease. *Circulation* 1985; **71**: 725–732.

8. Molloi S, Detrano R, Ersahin A *et al.* Quantification of coronary artery calcium by dual energy digital subtraction fluoroscopy. *Med Phys* 1991; **18**: 295–298.

9. Reinmuller R, Lipton M. Detection of coronary artery calcification by computed tomography. *Dynam Cardiovasc Imaging* 1987; **1**: 139–145.

10. Masuda Y, Naito S, Aoyagi Y *et al.* Coronary artery calcification detected by CT. *Angiology* 1990; **41**: 1037–1047.

11. Timmins ME, Pinsk R, The functional significance of calcification of the coronary arteries as detected on CT. *J Thorac Imaging* 1991; **7**: 79–82.

12. Tannenbaum SR, Kondos GT. Detection of calcific deposits in coronary arteries by ultrafast computed tomography and correlation with angiography. *Am J Cardiol* 1989; **63**: 870–872.

13. Agatston AS, Janowitz WR, Hildner FJ *et al.* Quantification of coronary artery calcium using ultrafast computed tomography. *J Am Coll Cardiol* 1990; **15**: 827–832.

14. Detrano R, Hsiai T, Wang S *et al.* Prognostic value of coronary calcification and angiographic stenoses in patients undergoing angiography. *J Am Coll Cardiol* 1996; **27**: 285–290.

15. Breen JB, Sheedy PF, Schwartz RS *et al.* Coronary artery calcification detected with ultrafast CT as an indication of coronary artery disease. *Radiology* 1992; **185**: 435–439.

16. Fallavolita JA, Brody AS, Bunnell IL *et al.* Fast computed tomography detection of coronary artery calcification in the diagnosis of coronary artery disease: Comparison with angiography in patients <50 years old. *Circulation* 1994; **89**: 285–289.

17. Nallamothu BK, Saint S, Bielak LF. Electron-beam computed tomography in the diagnosis of coronary artery disease: A meta-analysis. *Arch Intern Med* 2001; **161**: 833–838.

18. Carr JJ, Nelson JC, Wong ND. Measuring calcified coronary plaque with cardiac CT in population based studies: The standardized protocol of the multi-ethnic study of atherosclerosis (MESA) and coronary artery risk development in young adults (CARDIA). *Radiology* 2005; **234**: 135–143.

19. Callister TQ, Cooil B, Raya SP. Coronary artery disease: Improved reproducibility of calcium scoring with an electron-beam CT volumetric method. *Radiology* 1998; **208**: 807–808.

20. Detrano RC, Anderson A, Nelson J. Effect of computed tomography scanner type and calcium measurement method on the re-scan reproducibility of coronary measurements—MESA study. *Radiology*, in press.

21. Janowitz WR, Agatston AS, Kaplan G. Differences in prevalence and extent of coronary artery calcium detected by ultrafast computed tomography in asymptomatic men and women. *Am J Cardiol* 1993; **72**: 247–254.

22. Mitchell TL, Pippin JJ, Devers SM *et al.* Age- and sex-based nomograms from coronary artery calcium scores as determined by electron beam computed tomography. *Am J Cardiol* 2001; **87**: 453–456.

23. Budoff MJ, Lane KL, Bakhsheshi H *et al.* Rates of progression of coronary calcium by electron beam tomography. *Am J Cardiol* 2000; **86**: 8–11.

24. Callister TQ, Raggi P, Cooil B *et al.* Effect of HMG-CoA reductase inhibitors on coronary artery disease as assessed by electron-beam computed tomography. *N Engl J Med* 1998; **339**: 1972–1978.

25. Wong ND, Kawakubo M, LaBree L *et al.* Control of lipids according to National Cholesterol Education Program (NCEP) criteria and coronary calcium progression. *Am J Cardiol* 2004; **94**: 431–436.

26. Maher JE, Bielak LF, Raz JA *et al.* Progression of coronary artery calcification: A pilot study. *Mayo Clin Pro* 1999; **74**: 347–355.

27. Kawakubo M, LaBree L, Xiang M *et al.* Ethnic differences in the extent, prevalence and progression of coronary calcium. *Ethn Dis* 2005; **15**: 198–204.

28. Zir LM. Observer variability in coronary angiography. *Int J Cardiol* 1983; **3**: 171–173.

29. Morrison A. *Screening in Chronic Disease.* Oxford University Press, New York, 1985: Ch1: 3.

30. O'Rourke RA, Brundage BH, Froelicher VF *et al.* American College of Cardiology/American Heart Association expert consensus document on electron-beam computed tomography for the diagnosis and prognosis of coronary artery disease. *Circulation* 2000; **101**: 126–140.

31. Smith S, Greenland P, Grundy S. Prevention conference 5: Beyond secondary prevention: Identifying the high risk patient for coronary prevention. *Circulation* 2000; **10**: 111–116.

32. Wilson PWF, Smith SC, Blumenthal RS *et al.* Task force #4: How do we select patients for atherosclerosis imaging? In: 34th Bethesda Conference: Can atherosclerosis imaging techniques improve the detection of patients at risk for ischemic heart disease? *J Am Coll Cardiol* 2003; **41**: 1898–1906.

33. Mao S, Budoff MJ, Bin L *et al.* Optimal ECG trigger point in electron beam CT studies: Three methods for minimizing motion artifact. *Acad Radiol* 2001; **8**: 1107–1115.

34. Kopp AF, Schroeder S, Kuettner A *et al.* Non-invasive coronary angiography with high resolution multidetector-row computed tomography. Results in 102 patients. *Eur Heart J* 2002; **23**: 1714–1725.

35. Achenbach S, Moshage W, Ropers D *et al.* Non-invasive, three-dimensional visualization of coronary artery bypass grafts by electron beam tomography. *Am J Cardiol* 1997; **79**: 856–861.

36. Achenbach S, Moshage W, Ropers D *et al.* Detection of high-grade restenosis after PTCA using contrast enhanced electron beam CT. *Circulation* 1997; **96**: 2785–2788.

37. Achenbach S, Moshage W, Ropers D *et al.* Contrast enhanced electron beam computed tomography to analyse the coronary arteries in patients after acute myocardial infarction. *Heart* 2000; **84**: 489–493.

38. Achenbach S, Moshage W, Ropers D *et al.* Non-invasive coronary angiography by retrospectively ECG-gated multislice spiral CT. *Circulation* 2000; **102**: 2823–2828.

39. Achenbach S, Moshage W, Ropers D *et al. N Engl J Med* 1998; **339**: 1964–1971.

40. Kopp AF, Schroder S, Kuttner A *et al.* Multidetector row CT for non-invasive coronary angiograph patients. *Radiology* 2000; **217**(P): 375–380.

41. Achenbach S, Giesler T, Ropers D *et al.* Detection of coronary artery stenoses by contrast enhanced retrospectively electrocardiographically gated, multislice spiral computed tomography. *Circulation* 2001; **103**: 2535–2358.

42. Becker CR, Ohnesorge BM, Schoepf UJ *et al.* Current development of cardiac imaging with multidetector-row CT *Eur J Radiol* 2000; **36**: 97–103.

43. Schoenhagen P, Halliburton S, Stillman A *et al.* Non-invasive imaging of coronary arteries: Current and future role of multidetector row CT. *Radiology* 2004; **232**: 7–17.

44. Schroder S, Flohr T, Kopp AF *et al.* Accuracy of density measurements within plaques located in artificial coronary arteries by multislice computed tomography: Results of a phantom study. *J Comput Assist Tomogr* 2001; **25**: 900–906.

45. Bleiweis MS, Milliken JC, Baumgartner FJ *et al.* Application of the ultrafast CT for diagnosis of perivalvular abscesses: Surgical implications. *Chest* 1994; **106**: 629–632.

46. Tomada H, Hoshiai M, Tagawa R *et al.* Evolution of left atrial thrombus with computed tomography. *Am Heart J* 1980; **100**: 306–310.

47. Helgason CM, Chomka E, Louie E *et al.* The potential role for ultrafast cardiac computed tomography in patients with stroke. *Stroke* 1989; **20**: 465–472.

48. Pietras RJ, Wolfkiel CJ, Veselik K. Validation of ultrafast computed tomographic left ventricular volume measurement. *Invest Radiol* 1991; **26**: 28–34.

49. Roig E, Chomka EV, Castaner A *et al.* Exercise ultrafast computed tomography for the detection of coronary artery disease. *J Am Coll Cardiol* 1989; **13**: 1073–1081.

50. Budoff MJ, Shavelle DM, Lamont DH *et al.* Usefulness of electron beam computed tomography scanning for distinguishing ischemic from non-ischemic cardiomyopathy. *J Am Coll Cardiol* 1998; **32**: 1173–1178.

51. Shemesh J, Tenenbaum A, Fisman EZ *et al.* Coronary calcium as a reliable tool for differentiating ischemic from non-ischemic cardiomyopathy. *Am J Cardiol* 1996; **77**: 191–194.

52. Oren RM, Grover-McKay M, Stanford W *et al.* Accurate preoperative diagnosis of pericardial constriction using

cine computed tomography. *J Am Coll Cardiol* 1993; **22**: 832–838.

53. Liptom M, Coulden R. Valvular heart disease. *Radiol Clin North Am* 1999; **37**: 319–39.

54. Taneja K, Sharma S, Kumar K *et al.* Comparison of computed tomography and cineangiography in the demonstration of central pulmonary arteries in cyanotic congenital heart disease. *Cardiovasc Intervent Radiol* 1996; **19**: 97–100.

55. Carrell T. Cardiovascular surgery in Marfan's syndrome. *Schweiz Med* 1997; **127**: 992–1006.

56. Shinozaki H, Shimizu K, Anno H *et al.* Total anomous pulmonary venous drainage in an adult diagnosed with helical computed tomography. *Intern Med* 1997; **36**: 912–916.

57. Sharma S, Mehta A, O'Donovan P. Computed tomography and magnetic resonance findings in long standing patent ductus. *Angiology* 1996; **47**: 393–398.

58. Becker C, Soppa C, Fink U *et al.* Spiral CT angiography and 3D reconstruction in patients with aortic coarctation. *Eur Radiol* 1997; **7**: 1473–1477.

59. Fishman JE. Imaging of blunt aortic and great vessel trauma. *J Thorac Imaging* 2000; **15**: 97–103.

60. Rubin GD, Shiau MC, Leung AN *et al.* Aorta and iliac arteries: Single versus multiple detector-row helical CT angiography. *Radiology* 2000; **215**: 670–676.

61. LeBlang SD, Dolich MO. Imaging of penetrating thoracic trauma. *J Thorac Imaging* 2000; **15**: 128–135.

62. Zinck SE, Primack SL. Radiographic and CT findings in blunt chest trauma. *J Thorac Imaging* 2000; **15**: 87–96.

63. Kouchoukos NT, Dougenis D. Surgery of the thoracic aorta. *N Engl J Med* 1997; **336**: 1876–1888.

64. Rubin GD. Helical CT angiography of the thoracic aorta. *J Thorac Imaging* 1997; **12**: 128–149.

65. Galla JD, Ergin MA, Lansman SL *et al.* Identification of risk factors in patients undergoing thoracoabdominal aneurysm repair. *J Card Surgery* 1997; **12** (2 suppl): 292–299.

66. Semba CP, Kato N, Kee ST *et al.* Acute rupture of the descending thoracic aorta: Repair with use of endovascular stent-grafts. *J Vasc Interv Radiol* 1997; **8**: 337–42.

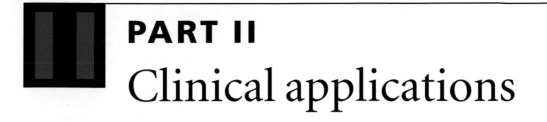

PART II
Clinical applications

CHAPTER 4

PET assessment of myocardial perfusion

Marcelo F. Di Carli

Introduction

Over the past two decades, the experimental and clinical use of positron emission tomography (PET) has significantly contributed to the knowledge of cardiac physiology and metabolism. Positron tomography has emerged from the experimental arena and currently plays an important role in clinical cardiology.

Coronary stenoses may be diagnosed and located through PET myocardial perfusion imaging in patients with suspected ischemic heart disease. In addition, the physiological severity of known coronary stenoses may be precisely characterized since PET enables absolute quantification of coronary flow reserve (CFR). The aim of this chapter is to provide a review of myocardial perfusion assessment with PET for identification and characterization of preclinical and clinical coronary artery disease (CAD), while recognizing that its clinical role continues to expand because of ongoing research.

Tracers for assessment of myocardial perfusion

While several tracers have been used for evaluating myocardial perfusion with PET, the most widely used are ^{13}N-ammonia, Rubidium-82 (^{82}Rb), and ^{15}O-labeled water.

^{13}N-ammonia

^{13}N-ammonia is a cyclotron product and has a physical half-life of 9.96 min. After injection, ^{13}N-ammonia rapidly disappears from the circulation, permitting the acquisition of images of excellent quality. Although the sequestration of ^{13}N-ammonia in the lungs is usually minimal, it may be increased in patients with depressed left ventricular systolic function or chronic pulmonary disease and, occasionally, in smokers. This may, in turn, adversely affect the quality of the images. In these cases, it may be necessary to increase the time between injection and image acquisition in order to optimize the contrast between myocardial and background activity.

Animal studies have shown that 95–100% of intravascular ^{13}N-ammonia traverses the capillary membrane into the interstitial space and ultimately into the myocyte [1]. Once inside the myocyte, ^{13}N-ammonia is incorporated into the glutamine pool and becomes metabolically trapped [1]. Only a small fraction diffuses back into the intravascular space [1]. Its retention by the myocardium has a non-linear and inverse relationship with blood flow. The fraction of ^{13}N-ammonia retained by the myocardium during its first pass is 0.83 when blood flow is 1 ml/min/g, and decreases to 0.60 as flow increases to 3 ml/min/g. As with other non-diffusible tracers, the net tissue extraction (the product of the retained fraction during first pass and the blood flow velocity) decreases as myocardial blood flow increases. For ^{13}N-ammonia, the relation between net tissue extraction and blood flow is linear for blood flow velocities up to 2.5 ml/min/g. At high flow rates, "metabolic trapping" of ^{13}N-ammonia becomes the rate-limiting step of tracer retention. This leads to underestimation of blood flow in high flow rates [2]. Therefore, in order to quantify myocardial blood flow using ^{13}N-ammonia, it becomes necessary to correct for flow-dependent changes in net tissue extraction.

82Rubidium

[82]Rb is a generator-produced radiotracer with a physical half-life of 76 seconds, and kinetics similar to [201]thallium [3]. Its parent radioinuclide is Strontium-82, which has a physical half-life of 23 days. Because of the distinct advantage of not requiring an on-site cylclotron, [82]Rb is the most widely used radionuclide for assessment of myocardial perfusion with PET. The short half-life of [82]Rb makes imaging challenging, but it allows for rapid sequential perfusion imaging. Optimal myocardial to blood pool contrast is achieved within 90 seconds after injection. However, this time is usually longer ($\geq$120 s) in patients with low ejection fraction.

After intravenous injection, [82]Rb rapidly crosses the capillary membrane [3]. Myocardial uptake of [82]Rb requires active transport via the Na/K ATP transporter, which is dependent on coronary blood flow [4]. Similar to other non-diffusible tracers, the net extraction fraction of [82]Rb decreases in a non-linear fashion with increasing myocardial blood flow [4–6]. The single-capillary transit extraction fraction of [82]Rb exceeds 50%.

15O-water

[15]O-water is cyclotron produced and has a physical half-life of 2.07 min. ^{15}O-water is a freely diffusible agent with very high myocardial extraction across a wide range of myocardial blood flows [3]. The degree of extraction is independent of flow and is not affected by the metabolic state of the myocardium [3]. Because it is a freely diffusible tracer, however, imaging is challenging because of its high concentration in the blood pool. This requires subtraction of the blood pool counts from the original image in order to visualize the myocardium. This can be accomplished by acquiring a second set of images after a single inhalation 40–50 mCi of ^{15}O-carbon monoxide (CO). [15]CO binds irreversibly to hemoglobin forming ^{15}O-carboxyhemoglobin, thereby allowing delineation and digital subtraction of blood pool activity. The cumbersome nature of the procedure required to subtract blood pool activity of ^{15}O-water in order to visualize the myocardium has limited the use of this tracer in the clinical setting.

Selecting a perfusion tracer for clinical cardiac PET

Although in many ways ^{15}O-water is an ideal flow tracer, its use in the clinical setting remains limited. Besides requiring an on-site cyclotron, obtaining diagnostic images requires an impractical image subtraction procedure. The advantages of ^{13}N-ammonia are its higher first-pass tissue extraction (65–70%) compared to Rubidium-82 (60–65%) [1, 5–7]; and a longer half-life, which allows longer imaging times and better count statistics, as well as injection during treadmill exercise and subsequent imaging of the trapped radionuclide in the myocardium. However, the main disadvantage of ^{13}N-ammonia vis-à-vis [82]Rb is the need for an on-site cyclotron that makes it costly and impractical. Also, its longer physical half-life makes rest-stress protocols more inefficient than with [82]Rb (~90 min vs 25 min respectively). Finally, increased uptake in the liver and, occasionally, in the lungs (e.g. heart failure, smokers) can significantly affect image quality. Fig. 4.1 and Fig. 4.2 demonstrate that, with modern PET scanners, comparable image quality can be obtained with both ^{13}N-ammonia and [82]Rb.

Imaging protocols

Fig. 4.3 and Fig. 4.4 illustrate several protocols that are commonly used in clinical practice [8]. Image acquisition starts with careful positioning of the patient in the PET or PET/CT gantry. Patients should be made as comfortable as possible in order to minimize movement during the study. After the patient is positioned appropriately, the precise location of the heart in the thorax should be determined. This can be done using a short transmission image acquired either with a Germanium-68 external radioactive ring or, in centers with a combined PET/CT unit, with a CT scout image. Once the heart is localized, a transmission image (~15–40 s with CT, or 5–15 min with an external radioactive source depending on the scanner and the age of the radioactive source) is obtained in order to have a direct measurement of photon attenuation.

After the scout and transmission scans, [82]Rb (40–60 mCi) or ^{13}N-ammonia (~20 mCi) is

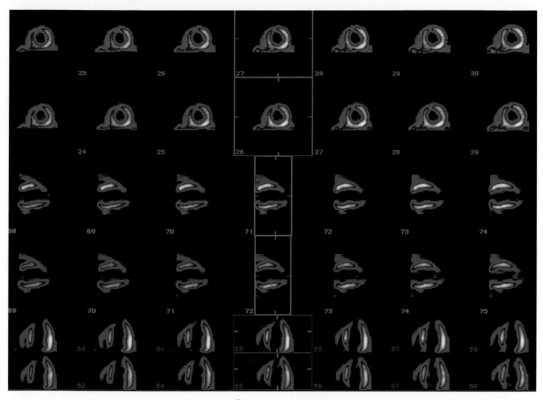

Fig. 4.1 Myocardial perfusion images obtained with ¹³N-ammonia during vasodilator-stress and at rest. Images demonstrate a severe perfusion deficit in the mid left anterior descending territory, which is fixed reflecting scarred myocardium.

injected at rest. Imaging begins 90–120 s after ⁸²Rb injection or three to five minutes after ¹³N-ammonia injection (single frame acquisition), to allow for clearance of radioactivity from the lungs and blood pool, and it extends for five or 20 min, respectively. Alternatively, imaging can begin with the infusion of ⁸²Rb or ¹³N-ammonia and continued for seven to eight minutes or 20 min (multiframe or dynamic image sequence), respectively. The latter approach is generally used for quantification of myocardial blood flow (ml/min/g). After resting imaging, a pharmacologic stress is performed (e.g. vasodilator stress with adenosine or dipyridamole, or dobutamine), and at peak stress a second injection of ⁸²Rb (40–60 mCi) or ¹³N-ammonia (~20 mCi) is again administered. Since all PET radiotracers decay by emitting photons with similar energy (511 keV), counts in the field of view should decrease to background levels before new images with a second radiotracer injec-

tion may be obtained. For ⁸²Rb (physical half-life: 76 s), stress testing can be performed without delay after completion of the resting study. For ¹³N-ammonia (physical half-life: 9.96 min), however, stress testing is delayed for approximately 30 min after completion of the resting study to allow for radioactive decay of the first dose of ¹³N-ammonia to background levels. Stress images are then obtained in the same manner as with the resting study. Attenuation correction of the stress images is generally performed with a separate transmission image that is obtained after stress imaging is complete (especially for PET/CT scanners). This second transmission scan is important because the heart will tend to change position within the chest due to the different breathing pattern during pharmacologic stress. When studies are acquired with a single frame format, image acquisition can be ECG gated to allow assessment of regional and global left ventricular function. Due to its ultra-short half-life,

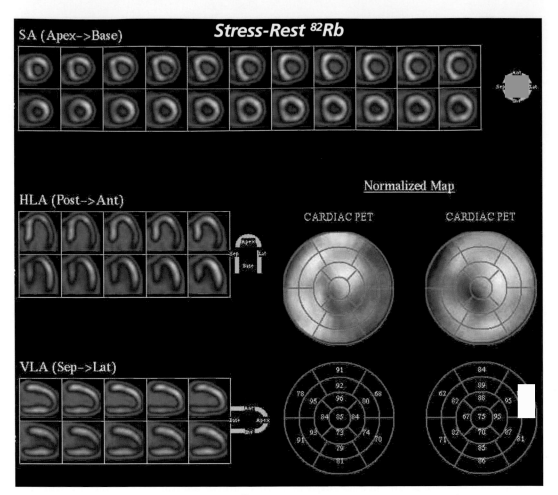

Fig. 4.2 Myocardial perfusion images obtained with ^{82}Rb during vasodilator-stress and at rest. Images demonstrate a mild-moderate perfusion deficit in the left circumflex territory, which is reversible reflecting myocardial ischemia.

^{82}Rb allows peak stress gated imaging, which may be helpful in identifying patients with extensive coronary artery disease (CAD) as left ventricular ejection fraction changes during pharmacologic stress have similar implications to those during exercise (Fig. 4.5 and Fig. 4.6). However, when images are obtained using a multiframe sequence, a separate ^{82}Rb or ^{13}N-ammonia injection is necessary to obtain ECG gated images. The time required for completing a rest and stress myocardial perfusion study varies between 25 and 120 min depending on the radionuclide, imaging protocol, and PET or PET/CT scanner used (Fig. 4.3 and Fig. 4.4).

Pharmacologic interventions to evaluate coronary microvascular function

Vascular smooth muscle cell function

Changes in arteriolar resistance in response to agents such as adenosine or dipyridamole are largely mediated by direct vascular smooth muscle relaxation and, thus, measurements of myocardial blood flow (MBF) during peak hyperemia are thought to reflect primarily endothelium-independent vasodilation. However, there is evidence that 20–40% of the maximal vasodilator response caused by adenosine or dipyridamole is related to the release

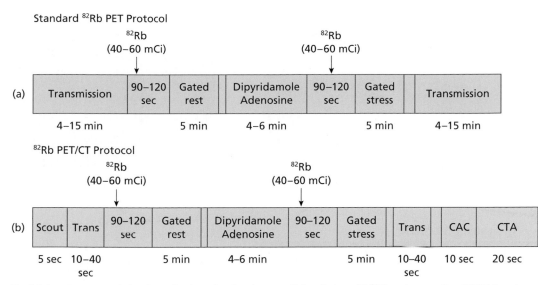

Fig. 4.3 Imaging protocols for the evaluation of regional myocardial perfusion with ^{82}Rb and conventional PET (a), and PET/CT (b) scanners.

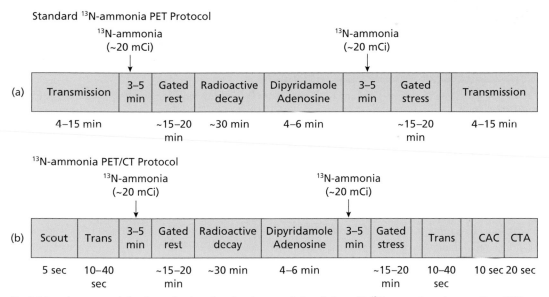

Fig. 4.4 Imaging protocols for the evaluation of regional myocardial perfusion with ^{13}N-ammonia and conventional PET (a), and PET/CT (b) scanners.

of nitric oxide (NO) from intact endothelium due to increased shear stress on endothelial cells caused by the hyperemic response. In humans, blockade of NO production by L-N^{G}-monomethyl arginine (an inhibitor of NO synthase) during continuous infusion of adenosine reduces forearm and cor-

onary blood flow by approximately 20–40% [9, 10]. This implicates a flow-dependent, predominantly endothelium-mediated mechanism at the level of the resistance and the epicardial vessels as contributor to the hyperemic flow response. Thus, the vasodilator response to agents such as adenosine

End Diastolic Volume

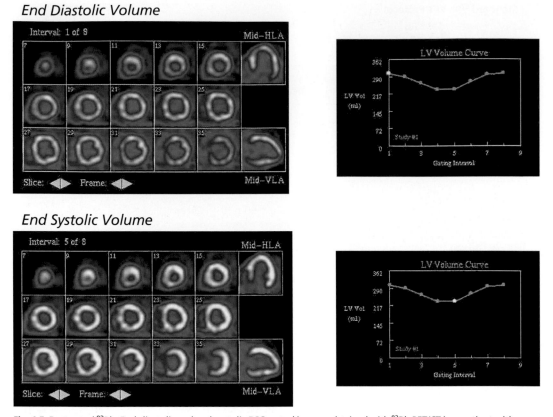

End Systolic Volume

Fig. 4.5 Rest gated ^{82}Rb. End-diastolic and end-systolic ECG-gated images obtained with ^{82}Rb PET/CT in a patient with cardiomyopathy.

and dipyridamole assesses the integrated effects of both vascular smooth muscle and endothelial cell function. It also implicates endothelial dysfunction as a major determinant of the reduced hyperemic response in patients with risk factors for CAD. Furthermore, it suggests that significant improvements in pharmacologically stimulated hyperemic responses as observed after interventions aimed at risk factor modification may also be attributed to improvements in endothelial function and in NO bioavailabity [11–13].

Vascular endothelial cell function

Acetylcholine is considered the classic stimulus to evaluate endothelial-dependent vasoreactivity. It requires intracoronary injections and, thus, it is always employed with invasive techniques such as coronary angiography to measure endothelium-

mediated vasodilation in both epicardial and resistance vessels [14–15]. Endothelium-mediated coronary vasoreactivity may also be determined by the cold pressor test (CPT) [14–15]. A significant correlation between the coronary vasomotor response to intracoronary acetylcholine and that to CPT has been demonstrated in patients with mild atherosclerosis [16]. Therefore, CPT has been proposed as a non-invasive tool to probe endothelium-dependent coronary vasomotion. Sympathetic stimulation by the CPT induces norepinephrine release from cardiac and peripheral sympathetic-nerve endings. The direct effect of norepinephrine (α1, α2, and β1 receptor agonist) on smooth muscle cells is vasoconstriction, which is mediated by activation of α1 and α2-adrenoceptors. When endothelial function is normal, this vasoconstrictor effect is opposed by endothelial α2 adrenoceptor-

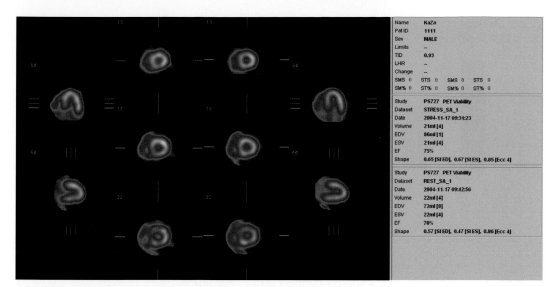

Fig. 4.6 ECG-gated images obtained with [82]Rb PET/CT at rest and during peak vasodilator-stress in a patient without evidence of obstructive CAD.

mediated stimulation of NO release [17]. In contrast, when endothelial cell function is abnormal, the vasoconstrictive response to norepinephrine predominates [14].

Evaluation of patients with known or suspected coronary artery disease

Preclinical CAD

The significant advances in our understanding of the mechanisms that initiate and facilitate the progression of coronary atherosclerosis have greatly improved our ability to target therapies aimed at prevention, halting progression, or promoting regression of atherosclerosis before it becomes clinically overt. Thus, cardiovascular medicine is witnessing a dramatic shift from the "traditional" paradigm of diagnosing obstructive CAD, to a "new" paradigm in which the central goal is to detect patients who are at risk for developing CAD or who already have preclinical (albeit not obstructive) disease.

In this paradigm shift, the traditional relative assessments of regional myocardial perfusion will likely be insufficiently sensitive to identify preclinical CAD and, thus, be of limited clinical value. It is now clear that endothelial dysfunction is an early event in atherosclerosis that precedes the development of structural changes in the coronary arteries, and that it is magnified in the presence of coronary risk factors and obstructive CAD. Consequently, endothelial dysfunction and its resulting consequences on coronary vasoreactivity is an attractive diagnostic target, especially for methods that can quantify coronary vasodilator dysfunction noninvasively such as PET. Detection of patients at risk may offer an opportunity for early medical intervention aimed at halting the progression of atherogenesis, and ultimately lead to a reduction in cardiovascular events.

Relation between risk factors and coronary vasoreactivity as measured by PET

There is mounting and consistent evidence that patients with coronary risk factors including dyslipidemia, diabetes, hypertension, and smoking demonstrate abnormal coronary vasodilator function as measured by PET (Fig. 4.7) [18]. Importantly, these

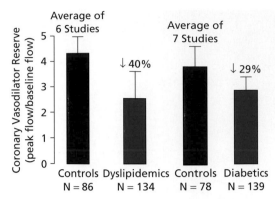

Fig. 4.7 Bar graph illustrating average coronary flow reserve as determined by PET in patients with dyslipidemia (left) and diabetes (right) without clinically overt CAD. (Figure reproduced with permission from: Reference 18, Campisi R, Di Carli MF. Assessment of coronary flow reserve and microcirculation: A clinical perspective. *J Nucl Cardiol* 2004; **11**: 3–11.)

abnormalities are present in patients without clinically overt (obstructive) CAD. These abnormalities in vascular function have been linked with endothelial dysfunction, an early event in atherogenesis. Thus, PET measures of coronary vasodilator function may be useful surrogate markers of atherosclerotic disease activity. Such measurements of impaired coronary vasoreactivity, in patients with and without obstructive CAD, may also have important prognostic implications [19–23].

Furthermore, the available evidence also suggests that these measures of coronary vasoreactivity are useful markers for monitoring therapeutic responses [12, 24–27]. For example, lipid-lowering

therapy with HMG-CoA reductase inhibitors (statins) consistently improves coronary vasodilator function in patients with and without obstructive CAD (Table 4.1). This improvement in coronary vasodilator function has important clinical implications because it may reduce ischemic burden and improve symptoms in patients with obstructive CAD [28]. The beneficial effects of statins on vascular function have been linked to improved endothelial function, decreased platelet aggregability and thrombus deposition, and reduced vascular inflammation.

Clinical CAD

PET has proven to be a powerful and efficient noninvasive imaging modality for evaluating regional myocardial perfusion in patients with known or suspected obstructive CAD. Several technical advantages account for the improved diagnostic power of PET including: (1) routine measured (depth independent) attenuation correction, which decreases false positives and, thus, increases specificity; (2) high spatial and contrast resolution (heart-to-background ratio) that allows improved detection of small perfusion defects, thereby decreasing false negatives and increasing sensitivity (Fig. 4.8), and (3) high temporal resolution that allows fast dynamic imaging of tracer kinetics, which makes absolute quantification of myocardial perfusion (in ml/min/g of tissue) possible. In addition, the use of short-lived radiopharmaceuticals allows fast, sequential assessment of regional myocardial perfusion (e.g. rest and stress), thereby improving laboratory efficiency and patient throughput (Fig. 4.1 and Fig. 4.2).

Table 4.1 Effects of HMG-CoA reductase inhibitor treatment on myocardial perfusion in patients with and without obstructive CAD.

Author	Methodology	Endpoint	Magnitude of benefit
Baller [24]	PET	↑ in hyperemic MBF	↑ 31%
Janatuinen [25]	PET	↑ in hyperemic MBF	↑ 27%
Guethlin [12]	PET	↑ in hyperemic MBF	↑ 35%
Huggins [26]	PET	↑ in hyperemic MBF	↑ 46%
Yokoyama [13]	PET	↑ in hyperemic MBF	↑ 20%
Schwartz [28]	SPECT	↓ PD size and severity	↓ 22%

MBF: myocardial blood flow; PD size: perfusion defect. (Table reprinted with permission from: Reference 18, Campisi R, Di Carli MF. Assessment of coronary flow reserve and microcirculation: A clinical perspective. *J Nucl Cardiol* 2004; **11**: 3–11.)

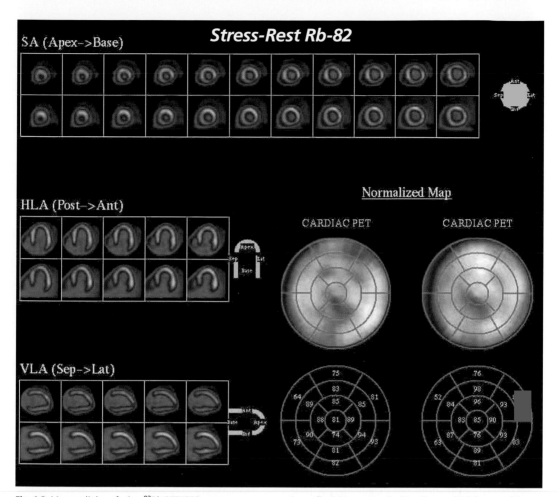

Fig. 4.8 Myocardial perfusion ^{82}Rb PET/CT images obtained during vasodilator-stress and at rest. Images demonstrate a small and mild perfusion deficit in the left circumflex/obtuse marginal territory, which is reversible, reflecting myocardial ischemia.

Although these technical advantages have been recognized for a long time, the use of PET for routine detection of CAD has only gained momentum in recent years. Recent FDA approval of PET radiotracers (i.e. ^{82}Rb, ^{13}N-ammonia, and ^{18}F-FDG) and the subsequent changes in reimbursement are responsible for much of the recent growth in clinical cardiac PET.

Diagnostic accuracy of PET for detection of obstructive CAD

The performance of PET in the detection of obstructive CAD has been documented in seven studies, including one with 663 patients (Table 4.2)

[8]. In these studies, regional myocardial perfusion was assessed with ^{13}N-ammonia or ^{82}Rb: the average sensitivity for detecting >50% angiographic stenosis was 89% (range, 83–100%), whereas the average specificity was 86% (range, 73–100%).

Comparative studies of PET versus SPECT

Only two studies have performed a head to head comparison of the diagnostic accuracy of ^{82}Rb PET and ^{201}thallium SPECT in the same patient population [8]. Go and colleagues compared PET and SPECT in 202 patients [34]. Their

Table 4.2 Sensitivity and specificity of PET for detecting obstructive CAD.

Year	Author	Radiotracer	Prior MI (%)	Sensitivity (%)	Specificity (%)
1992	Marwick [29]	^{82}Rb	49	90 (63/70)	100 (4/4)
1992	Grover-McKay [30]	^{82}Rb	13	100 (16/16)	73 (11/15)
1991	Stewart [35]	^{82}Rb	42	83 (50/60)	86 (18/21)
1990	Go [34]	^{82}Rb	47	93 (142/152)	78 (39/50)
1989	Demer [31]	^{82}Rb/^{13}N-ammonia	34	83 (126/152)	95 (39/41)
1988	Tamaki [32]	^{13}N-ammonia	75	98 (47/48)	100 (3/3)
1986	Gould [33]	^{82}Rb/^{13}N-ammonia	NR	95 (21/22)	100 (9/9)
	Total			**89**	**86**

Table reproduced with permission from: Reference 8, Di Carli MF. Advances in positron emission tomography. *J Nucl Cardiol* 2004; **11**: 719–732.

results showed a higher sensitivity with PET (76% vs 93%), and no significant changes for specificity (80% vs 78% for SPECT and PET, respectively). In another study, Stewart *et al.* compared PET and SPECT in 81 patients [35]. They observed a higher specificity for PET (53% vs 83% for SPECT and PET, respectively), and no significant differences in sensitivity (84% vs 86% for SPECT and PET, respectively). Diagnostic accuracy was higher with PET (89% vs 78%).

Using measurements of coronary flow reserve to evaluate the extent of CAD

Most reports evaluating the diagnostic performance of myocardial perfusion PET to detect angiographic stenoses, however, examined imaging results in terms of sensitivity and specificity rather than as a continuous spectrum of severity [36]. In patients with CAD, non-invasive measurements of coronary blood flow and flow reserve by PET are inversely and non-linearly related to stenosis severity as defined by quantitative angiography. Importantly, coronary lesions of intermediate severity have a differential coronary flow reserve that decreases as stenosis severity increases; this can be detected by PET, thus allowing better definition of the functional importance of known coronary epicardial stenosis (Fig. 4.9) [37–39]. Fig. 4.10 illustrates the potential use of measurements of myocardial blood flow and coronary vasodilator reserve to better delineate the extent of underlying CAD. In patients with so called "balanced" ischemia or diffuse CAD, measurements of coronary vasodi-

lator reserve would uncover areas of myocardium at risk that would be generally missed by performing only relative assessments of myocardial perfusion. It is generally accepted that while the relative assessment of myocardial perfusion with SPECT remains a sensitive means for detecting CAD, the approach often uncovers only the territory supplied by the most severe stenosis. This is based on the fact that in patients with CAD coronary vasodilator reserve is often abnormal even in territories supplied by non-critical angiographic stenoses [40, 41], thereby reducing the heterogeneity of flow between "normal" and "abnormal" zones.

Two recent reports illustrate the potential clinical value of measures of coronary vasodilator reserve as assessed by PET to delineate the extent of underlying CAD. Yoshinaga *et al.* compared the clinical value of measures of coronary vasodilator reserve as assessed by PET to relative assessments of myocardial perfusion by SPECT in 27 patients with CAD [41]. They showed good agreement between SPECT defects and PET measures of vasodilator reserve in only 16 of 58 (28%) myocardial regions supplied by coronary stenosis >50% as assessed by quantitative angiography. The remaining 42 of 58 (72%) regions with angiographic stenoses showed no regional perfusion defects by SPECT but a definitely abnormal vasodilator reserve by PET. Similarly, Parkash *et al.* recently reported on the value of quantification of coronary flow reserve versus the traditional relative assessment of myocardial perfusion to delineate the extent of CAD in a relatively small group of 23 patients [42]. In patients with

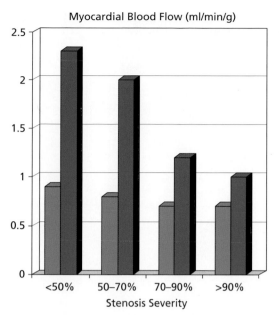

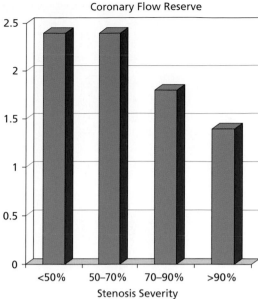

Fig. 4.9 Relation between myocardial blood flow and coronary vasodilator reserve, and coronary stenoses severity on quantitative coronary angiography. (Figure reproduced with permission from: Reference 18, Campisi R, Di Carli MF. Assessment of coronary flow reserve and microcirculation: A clinical perspective. *J Nucl Cardiol* 2004; **11**: 3–11.)

3-vessel CAD, they found that defect sizes were significantly larger using quantification methods as compared with the traditional method (44 ± 18% vs 69 ± 24%). In patients with single vessel CAD, defect sizes were smaller using quantification methods than with the traditional method (10 ± 12% vs 18 ± 17%). Thus, this is clearly an area of great clinical interest and future studies are warranted to evaluate the added value of quantitative flow measurements for the non-invasive diagnosis of CAD.

PET measurements of myocardial perfusion to monitor progression and regression of coronary artery disease

Lipid-lowering trials in patients with coronary atherosclerosis have demonstrated no progression or only modest regression of anatomic coronary artery stenoses compared to control patients [43–46]. Despite the lack of, or modest, regression in coronary artery stenoses, these studies have reported a proportionately greater decrease in coronary events in treated than in control patients [43–47]. This has led to the hypothesis that stabilization of atherosclerotic plaques, reduction of inducible

myocardial ischemia (caused by an improvement in coronary vasodilator function), or both effects combined, may be more closely related to improved clinical outcomes than the anatomic change in plaque burden. There is mounting evidence that the functional abnormalities in coronary vascular function described above can be improved by therapeutic interventions designed to improve the risk factor profile, and that these changes can be measured non-invasively with PET.

Conclusions

Positron emission tomography provides accurate diagnosis of the extent, severity and anatomic location of coronary artery disease. A review of the current literature indicates that the sensitivity and specificity of myocardial perfusion with pharmacological stress vary from 90–95% in both men and women. An additional advantage of PET is its ability to quantify regional perfusion and coronary flow reserve. Experimental and clinical evidence indicates that these measurements of coronary flow reserve have a non-linear inverse correlation with

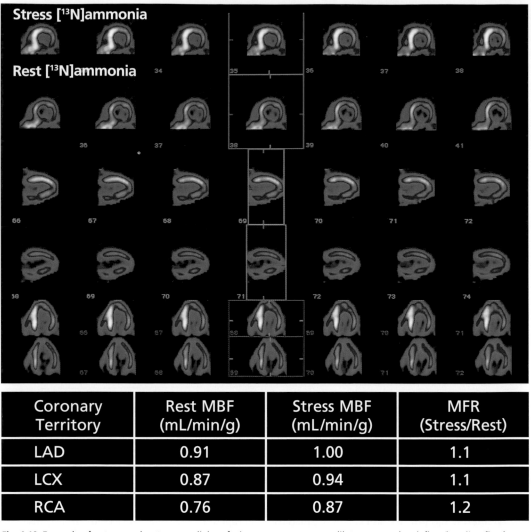

Coronary Territory	Rest MBF (mL/min/g)	Stress MBF (mL/min/g)	MFR (Stress/Rest)
LAD	0.91	1.00	1.1
LCX	0.87	0.94	1.1
RCA	0.76	0.87	1.2

Fig. 4.10 Example of a stress and rest myocardial perfusion PET study with ^{13}N-ammonia as the flow tracer. The images (top panel) demonstrate a moderate sized, severe, and fixed perfusion deficit in the inferior and inferolateral walls, consistent with myocardial infarction. The quantitative data (lower panel) demonstrate impaired coronary vasodilator reserve (peak flow/baseline flow) in all three coronary territories. Subsequent coronary angiography demonstrated significant 3-vessel CAD. This case illustrates the potential use of blood flow quantitation to better delineate the extent of CAD.

the anatomic severity of stenosis. These measurements are useful for assessing the functional implications of coronary stenoses of intermediate severity (50–80%), especially in patients with extensive CAD.

The high relative cost of positron emission tomography requires a careful selection of patients. The great sensitivity and, above all, the high specificity of PET for diagnosing coronary heart dis-

ease, make it a particularly useful tool for the assessment of obese patients and women with a low-intermediate probability of having coronary disease. This important clinical role is expected to grow with the availability of PET/CT scanners that allow a true integration (fusion) of structure and function. This will allow a comprehensive examination of the heart's anatomy and function in ways never before possible.

References

1. Schelbert HR, Phelps ME, Huang SC et al. ^{13}N-ammonia as an indicator of myocardial blood flow. *Circulation* 1981; **63**: 1259–1272.

2. Hutchins GD, Schwaiger M, Rosenspire KC et al. Non-invasive quantification of regional blood flow in the human heart using ^{13}N-ammonia and dynamic positron emission tomographic imaging. *J Am Coll Cardiol* 1990; **15**: 1032–1042.

3. Schelbert HR. Evaluation of myocardial blood flow in cardiac disease. In: Skorton DJ, Schelbert HR, Wolf GL, Brundage BH, eds. *Cardiac Imaging. A Companion to Braunwald's Heart Disease.* W B Saunders, Philadelphia, 1991: 1093–1112.

4. Selwyn AP, Allan RM, L'Abbate A et al. Relation between regional myocardial uptake of Rubidium-82 and perfusion: Absolute reduction of cation uptake in ischemia. *Am J Cardiol* 1982; **50**: 112–121.

5. Mullani NA, Goldstein RA, Gould KL et al. Myocardial perfusion with Rubidium-82. I. Measurement of extraction fraction and flow with external detectors. *J Nucl Med* 1983; **24**: 898–906.

6. Goldstein RA, Mullani NA, Marani SK et al. Myocardial perfusion with Rubidium-82. II. Effects of metabolic and pharmacologic interventions. *J Nucl Med* 1983; **24**: 907–915.

7. Yoshida K, Mullani N, Gould KL. Coronary flow and flow reserve by PET simplified for clinical applications using Rubidium-82 or ^{13}N-ammonia. *J Nucl Med* 1996; **37**: 1701–1712.

8. Di Carli MF. Advances in positron emission tomography. *J Nucl Cardiol* 2004; **11**: 719–732.

9. Smits P, Williams SB, Lipson DE et al. Endothelial release of nitric oxide contributes to the vasodilator effect of adenosine in humans [published erratum appears in *Circulation* 1996; **93**: 1942]. *Circulation* 1995; **92**: 2135–2141.

10. Buus NH, Bottcher M, Hermansen F et al. Influence of nitric oxide synthase and adrenergic inhibition on adenosine-induced myocardial hyperemia. *Circulation* 2001; **104**: 2305–2310.

11. Czernin J, Barnard RJ, Sun KT et al. Effect of short term cardiovascular conditioning and low fat diet on myocardial blood flow and flow reserve. *Circulation* 1995; **92**: 197–204.

12. Guethlin M, Kasel AM, Coppenrath K et al. Delayed response of myocardial flow reserve to lipid-lowering therapy with fluvastatin. *Circulation* 1999; **99**: 475–481.

13. Yokoyama I, Momomura S, Ohtake T et al. Improvement of impaired myocardial vasodilatation due to diffuse coronary atherosclerosis in hypercholesterolemics after lipid-lowering therapy. *Circulation* 1999; **100**: 117–122.

14. Nabel EG, Ganz P, Gordon JB et al. Dilation of normal and constriction of atherosclerotic coronary arteries caused by the cold pressor test. *Circulation* 1988; **77**: 43–52.

15. Zeiher AM, Drexler H, Wollschlaeger H et al. Coronary vasomotion in response to sympathetic stimulation in humans: Importance of the functional integrity of the endothelium. *J Am Coll Cardiol* 1989; **14**: 1181–1190.

16. Zeiher AM, Drexler H, Wollschlager H et al. Endothelial dysfunction of the coronary microvasculature is associated with coronary blood flow regulation in patients with early atherosclerosis. *Circulation* 1991; **84**: 1984–1992.

17. Kichuk MR, Seyedi N, Zhang X et al. Regulation of nitric oxide production in human coronary microvessels and the contribution of local kinin formation. *Circulation* 1996; **94**: 44–51.

18. Campisi R, Di Carli MF. Assessment of coronary flow reserve and microcirculation: A clinical perspective. *J Nucl Cardiol* 2004; **11**: 3–11.

19. Schindler TH, Hornig B, Buser PT et al. Prognostic value of abnormal vasoreactivity of epicardial coronary arteries to sympathetic stimulation in patients with normal coronary angiograms. *Arterioscler Thromb Vasc Biol* 2003; **23**: 495–501.

20. Schindler TH, Nitzsche EU, Munzel T et al. Coronary vasoregulation in patients with various risk factors in response to cold pressor testing: Contrasting myocardial blood flow responses to short and long term vitamin C administration. *J Am Coll Cardiol* 2003; **42**: 814–822.

21. Halcox JP, Schenke WH, Zalos G et al. Prognostic value of coronary vascular endothelial dysfunction. *Circulation* 2002; **106**: 653–658.

22. Schachinger V, Zeiher AM. Prognostic implications of endothelial dysfunction: Does it mean anything? *Coron Artery Dis* 2001; **12**: 435–443.

23. Al Suwaidi J, Reddan DN, Williams K et al. Prognostic implications of abnormalities in renal function in patients with acute coronary syndromes. *Circulation* 2002; **106**: 974–980.

24. Baller D, Notohamiprodjo G, Gleichmann U et al. Improvement in coronary flow reserve determined by positron emission tomography after six months of cholesterol-lowering therapy in patients with early stages of coronary atherosclerosis. *Circulation* 1999; **99**: 2871–2875.

25. Janatuinen T, Laaksonen R, Vesalainen R et al. Effect of lipid-lowering therapy with pravastatin on myocardial blood flow in young mildly hypercholesterolemic adults. *J Cardiovasc Pharmacol* 2001; **38**: 561–568.

26. Huggins GS, Pasternak RC, Alpert NM et al. Effects of short term treatment of hyperlipidemia on coronary vasodilator function and myocardial perfusion in regions

having substantial impairment of baseline dilator reverse. *Circulation* 1998; **98**: 1291–1296.

27. Yokoyama I, Yonekura K, Inoue Y *et al.* Long term effect of simvastatin on the improvement of impaired myocardial flow reserve in patients with familial hypercholesterolemia without gender variance. *J Nucl Cardiol* 2001; **8**: 445–451.

28. Schwartz RG, Pearson TA, Kalaria VG *et al.* Prospective serial evaluation of myocardial perfusion and lipids during the first six months of pravastatin therapy: Coronary artery disease regression single photon emission computed tomography monitoring trial. *J Am Coll Cardiol* 2003; **42**: 600–610.

29. Marwick TH, Nemec JJ, Stewart WJ *et al.* Diagnosis of coronary artery disease using exercise echocardiography and positron emission tomography: Comparison and analysis of discrepant results. *J Am Soc Echocardiogr* 1992; **5**: 231–238.

30. Grover-McKay M, Ratib O, Schwaiger M *et al.* Detection of coronary artery disease with positron emission tomography and Rubidium-82. *Am Heart J* 1992; **123**: 646–652.

31. Demer LL, Gould KL, Goldstein RA *et al.* Assessment of coronary artery disease severity by positron emission tomography. Comparison with quantitative arteriography in 193 patients. *Circulation* 1989; **79**: 825–835.

32. Tamaki N, Yonekura Y, Senda M *et al.* Value and limitation of stress thallium-201 single photon emission computed tomography: Comparison with ^{13}N-ammonia positron tomography. *J Nucl Med* 1988; **29**: 1181–1188.

33. Gould KL, Goldstein RA, Mullani NA *et al.* Non-invasive assessment of coronary stenoses by myocardial perfusion imaging during pharmacologic coronary vasodilation. VIII. Clinical feasibility of positron cardiac imaging without a cyclotron using generator-produced Rubidium-82. *J Am Coll Cardiol* 1986; **7**: 775–789

34. Go RT, Marwick TH, MacIntyre WJ *et al.* A prospective comparison of Rubidium-82 PET and thallium-201 SPECT myocardial perfusion imaging utilizing a single dipyridamole stress in the diagnosis of coronary artery disease. *J Nucl Med* 1990; **31**: 1899–1905.

35. Stewart RE, Schwaiger M, Molina E *et al.* Comparison of Rubidium-82 positron emission tomography and thallium-201 SPECT imaging for detection of coronary artery disease. *Am J Cardiol* 1991; **67**: 1303–1310.

36. Van Train KF, Garcia EV, Maddahi J *et al.* Multicenter trial validation for quantitative analysis of same-day rest-stress technetium-99m-sestamibi myocardial tomograms. *J Nucl Med* 1994; **35**: 609–618.

37. Di Carli MF, Czernin J, Hoh CK *et al.* Relation among stenosis severity, myocardial blood flow, and flow reserve in patients with coronary artery disease. *Circulation* 1995; **91**: 1944–1951.

38. Uren NG, Melin JA, De Bruyne B *et al.* Relation between myocardial blood flow and the severity of coronary-artery stenosis. *N Engl J Med* 1994; **330**: 1782–1788.

39. Beanlands RS, Muzik O, Melon P *et al.* Non-invasive quantification of regional myocardial flow reserve in patients with coronary atherosclerosis using ^{13}N-ammonia positron emission tomography. Determination of extent of altered vascular reactivity. *J Am Coll Cardiol* 1995; **26**: 1465–1475.

40. Uren NG, Crake T, Lefroy DC *et al.* Reduced coronary vasodilator function in infarcted and normal myocardium after myocardial infarction. *N Engl J Med* 1994; **331**: 222–227.

41. Yoshinaga K, Katoh C, Noriyasu K *et al.* Reduction of coronary flow reserve in areas with and without ischemia on stress perfusion imaging in patients with coronary artery disease: A study using oxygen 15-labeled water PET. *J Nucl Cardiol* 2003; **10**: 275–283.

42. Parkash R, deKemp RA, Ruddy TDT *et al.* Potential utility of Rubidium-82 PET quantification in patients with 3-vessel coronary artery disease. *J Nucl Cardiol* 2004; **11**: 440–449.

43. Ornish D, Brown SE, Scherwitz LW *et al.* Lifestyle changes and heart disease. *Lancet* 1990; **336**: 741–742.

44. Brown G, Albers JJ, Fisher LD *et al.* Regression of coronary artery disease as a result of intensive lipid-lowering therapy in men with high levels of apolipoprotein B. *N Engl J Med* 1990; **323**: 1289–1298.

45. Kane JP, Malloy MJ, Ports TA *et al.* Regression of coronary atherosclerosis during treatment of familial hypercholesterolemia with combined drug regimens. *JAMA* 1990; **264**: 3007–3012.

46. Gould KL, Ornish D, Scherwitz L *et al.* Changes in myocardial perfusion abnormalities by positron emission tomography after long term, intense risk factor modification. *JAMA* 1995; **274**: 894–901.

47. Watts GF, Lewis B, Brunt JN *et al.* Effects on coronary artery disease of lipid-lowering diet, or diet plus cholestyramine, in the St Thomas' Atherosclerosis Regression Study (STARS). *Lancet* 1992; **339**: 563–569.

CHAPTER 5

PET: Metabolism, innervation and receptors

Frank M. Bengel & Markus Schwaiger

Introduction

Thanks to the almost unlimited availability of biomolecules for labeling with positron-emitting isotopes, quantitative imaging of biologic processes has been a major strength and a key element of cardiac PET. Combination of multiple tracers allows for a detailed investigation of molecular tissue properties. Substrate metabolism and autonomic innervation of the myocardium are biologic targets which have been studied extensively in the clinical setting using PET. Not only did these studies refine the basic understanding of physiologic interrelations, pathogenetic mechanisms and therapeutic interventions, metabolic imaging has also been the driving force in development of the field of clinical assessment of myocardial viability. The broad spectrum of probes for biologic tissue targets is likely to contribute to further clinical developments in several areas in the future.

This chapter gives an overview of the current state of PET for imaging of myocardial metabolism, innervation and receptors. Available tracers and their biologic targets are summarized along with their clinical application and their future potential.

Assessment of myocardial metabolism

Myocardial energy metabolism depends on the oxidation of various substrates (Fig. 5.1), and several PET radiopharmaceuticals have been developed for its investigation (Table 5.1). Combination of these metabolic tracers allows for detailed insights into substrate utilization and metabolic regulation of the myocardium. Additionally, assessment of myocardial viability as the most important clinical application of PET has emerged from studies of myocardial metabolism.

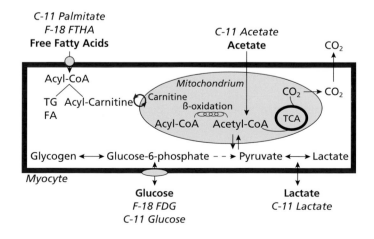

Fig. 5.1 Pathways of myocardial metabolism which can be investigated by PET, including tracers for the specific pathways.

Table 5.1 PET radiopharmaceuticals for clinical metabolic imaging.

Tracer	Biologic target
F-18 fluorodeoxyglucose (FDG)	glucose transport, hexokinase
C-11 glucose	glucose metabolism
C-11 acetate	oxidative metabolism (TCA cycle turnover)
C-11 palmitate	fatty acid metabolism
F-18 thioheptadecanoic acid (FTHA)	fatty acid uptake
C-11 lactate	lactate utilization

Imaging the regulation of substrate metabolism

Under fasting conditions, free fatty acids represent the major source for cardiac ATP production [1, 2]. Free fatty acids are avidly extracted by myocardium and long chain acyl-CoA is rapidly formed. The activated form of fatty acids may then be used for synthesis of triglycerides or phospholipids, but the majority of acyl-CoA is transported via the carnitine shuttle into mitochondria for β-oxidation. Short chained acetyl-CoA is the end product of β-oxidation and enters the tricarboxylic acid cycle as final common pathway for oxidative metabolism of all substrates.

In presence of high free fatty acid levels and low plasma insulin, only small amounts of glucose are taken up by myocardium. In the postprandial state, glucose transport is enhanced and glycolytic flux is increased. But even after carbohydrate loading, only about 30–50% of overall substrate metabolism in the heart depends on glucose [3]. Lactate as a substrate can become a significant contributor to myocardial energy metabolism during physical exercise, when plasma levels increase [4].

Aside from the physiologic increase of glycolysis in the postprandial state, glycolysis plays an important role during myocardial ischemia and following reperfusion. Experimental studies have shown that glucose transport and metabolism are upregulated during myocardial ischemia with production and release of lactate [5, 6]. However, following ischemic episodes, glycolysis remains enhanced with evidence of oxidative and non-oxidative utilization of exogenous glucose. There is evidence that enhanced myocardial oxidative glucose metabolism persists after ischemic episodes, most likely because of an upregulation and increased expres-

sion of glucose transporter proteins, especially GLUT 1 [7].

Fatty acid metabolism

The first radiopharmaceutical used for PET assessment of regional cardiac metabolism was C-11 palmitate. Experimental studies with changing cardiac workload or cardiac substrate availability demonstrated changes in C-11 palmitate kinetics [8]. Similarly, ischemia induced by atrial pacing resulted in a decreased myocardial turnover of C-11 palmitate [9]. Because of the complex metabolic fate and the multiple pathways involved, precise interpretation of the kinetics of C-11 palmitate has been difficult. An approach for quantitative analysis has been introduced, which allows for calculation of rates of fatty acid uptake and oxidation [10], but applications have been limited to mechanistic studies in small, well-selected patient groups.

Overall oxidative metabolism

C-11 acetate is a probe of overall oxidative metabolism which avoids the complexity of substrate interaction, defining the relative contribution of long chain fatty acids and carbohydrates. Acetate is extracted proportionally to myocardial blood flow, then converted intracellularly to C-11 acetyl-CoA and enters the tricarboxylic acid (TCA)-cycle in the mitochondria. Radioactivity equilibrates within TCA-cycle intermediates and clears from the myocardium in the form of C-11 CO_2 (Fig. 5.2). Several studies have indicated that C-11 acetate kinetics, as assessed by dynamic PET imaging are only sparsely affected by substrate interactions, and thus allow for quantification of myocardial oxygen consumption [11–14]. When combined with measures of cardiac contractile performance, C-11

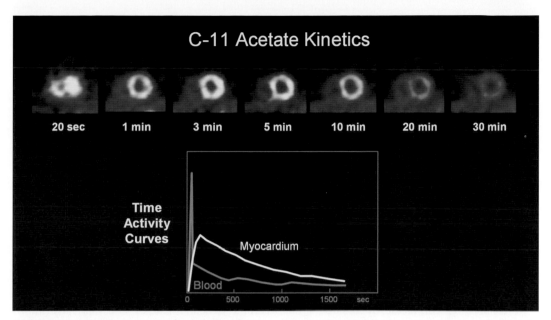

Fig. 5.2 Dynamic imaging sequence after injection of C-11 acetate. A representative short axis slice is depicted at various times after injection, showing wash-out of tracer from the myocardium, which reflects turnover in the tricarboxylic acid cycle. Time activity curves are depicted at the bottom, which are used for obtaining quantitative indexes of oxidative metabolism.

acetate PET can be used for a non-invasive estimation of cardiac efficiency (defined as the relation between work and oxygen consumption) [15]. This approach is of special interest in heart failure [16], where it can be used to measure effects of drugs such as beta-blockers or dobutamine [15, 17], and thereby to optimize medical therapy.

Glucose metabolism

F-18 deoxyglucose traces transmembranous transport, as well as phosphorylation of exogenous glucose [18, 19]. F-18 deoxyglucose-6-phosphate does not enter any further metabolic pathways but accumulates in myocardium proportional to glucose transport and phosphorylation [20, 21]. However, FDG molecules display different affinities for glucose transport and phosphorylation than the glucose molecule. To account for this discrepancy, a correction term is necessary for quantification of exogenous glucose utilization of the myocardium by FDG. This correction term, the lumped constant, is assumed to be constant under physiologic and most pathophysiologic conditions, although some data indicate that under rapidly changing conditions the lumped constant may actually change as a function of altered affinities for glucose transport, as well as for the hexokinase reaction [22]. Exogenous glucose utilization can be quantified using a simple fitting procedure of FDG myocardial kinetics and parametric display of regional metabolic data [23].

More recently, synthesis of C-11 glucose has been described. This tracer follows the entire metabolic pathways of glucose, suggesting that modeling of kinetics is complex and difficult. An algorithm for quantification has been described [24], but application remains limited to very few centers.

With a combination of available metabolic imaging techniques, detailed insights into the role of substrate utilization and metabolic regulation can be obtained. Peterson *et al.*, for example combined C-11 glucose, C-11 palmitate and C-11 acetate. They found increased myocardial oxygen consumption and decreased efficiency in obese young women. Insulin resistance was also observed, which was associated with increased myocardial fatty acid utilization. It was concluded that these findings may contribute to the development of impaired cardiac performance in obesity [25]. Another option is to combine assessment of myocardial metabolism with PET measurements in other organs such as liver, peripheral muscle or adipose tissue [26]. Although limited primarily to research, these approaches show that PET provides great flexibility for a detailed assessment of metabolism in heart and other organs in health and disease.

Myocardial viability

Patients with severe ventricular dysfunction undergo bypass surgery or angioplasty with considerable risk of procedure-related morbidity and mortality [27]. But it is these patients who seem to benefit most from interventional therapy [27–31]. The decision to proceed with revascularization in those patients is thus critical, and accurate methods to identify individuals who benefit most are required to justify the potential risks.

Reversibility of contractile dysfunction is an important factor contributing to the beneficial effect of revascularization. It is well known that contractile dysfunction in patients with coronary disease does not necessarily reflect scar tissue [32, 33]. Several non-invasive imaging techniques have been developed to identify tissue viability in dysfunctioning myocardium and to thereby determine which patients with ventricular dysfunction are the most appropriate candidates for revascularization [34]. At the same time, experimental investigations were initiated to reproduce clinical observations in the animal laboratory and to define the pathophysiology of reversible left ventricular dysfunction [35].

Pathophysiologic concepts

"Stunned myocardium" is characterized by persisting myocardial dysfunction in absence of irreversible damage despite restoration of near normal blood flow [36]. Contractile dysfunction in this setting is completely reversible, as can be observed clinically, e.g. following thrombolysis for acute myocardial infarction or after exercise induced ischemia [35, 37]. In addition to "acute" stunning as a consequence of a single ischemic episode, the term has also been extended to chronic left ventricular dysfunction associated with repetitive episodes of ischemia, then referred to as "repetitive stunning" [35, 38].

Clinical observations of reversible left ventricular dysfunction in patients with chronic coronary artery disease have led to the introduction of the term "hibernating myocardium" [33]. The initial concept of hibernation included the hypothesis of reduced resting perfusion due to severe coronary stenosis leading to an adaptive downregulation of contractile function which is reversible after re-establishment of normal perfusion [33, 39]. Uncoupling of contractile work and myocardial blood flow is thought to be part of this adaptation. Energy can be saved and the tolerance to ischemia can be increased at the expense of regional dysfunction. It is also hypothesized that these adaptive processes are associated with dedifferentiation of myocytes, decreased expression of contractile proteins and accumulation of glycogen [40–42].

Although Rahimtoola [33] initially described hibernating myocardium by a chronic reduction of blood flow as a culprit for dysfunction, implying chronic ischemia, studies with PET have shown that blood flow either can be normal or only slightly decreased in dysfunctioning viable myocardium [43]. Measurements of the perfusible tissue fraction also indicated that dysfunctioning myocardium may not be limited by oxygen supply under resting conditions [44, 45]. Based on these results, there is ongoing discussion as to whether reversible left ventricular dysfunction in severe ischemic heart disease reflects "repetitive stunning" or "hibernation" [32]. The clinical situation in most patients is characterized by heterogeneous ischemic injury, consisting of necrosis/scar in the subendocardium surrounded by viable but compromised tissue. The dynamic nature of ischemic heart disease renders these segments ischemic during daily life activities, which may lead to repetitive stunning. On the other hand, severe flow restriction may result in chronic hypoperfusion fulfilling the original criteria of hibernation. One can speculate that both conditions coexist in patients with advanced CAD and impairment of left ventricular function [46]. From a clinical point of view, the pathophysiological discussion is less important because many studies have shown that revascularization results in functional improvement of both stunned and hibernating myocardium [46].

Methodologic considerations

The level of myocardial blood flow alone identifies reversible contractile dysfunction only incompletely.

The situation is conclusive at both ends of the spectrum of flow, because normal levels are consistent with stunning and severely reduced levels indicate irreversible injury. An intermediate degree of flow reduction, however, can be associated with either reversibility or irreversibility of contractile dysfunction because myocardial hibernation may be present in addition to necrosis or tissue fibrosis [47].

If functional recovery is to occur following revascularization, cellular homeostasis, energy metabolism and membrane integrity must be preserved. Metabolic activity as the source for energy is a particular aspect of myocardial viability which can be targeted by PET imaging. Preserved metabolism in a dysfunctional area indicates viability and thus reversibility, while reduction of metabolism in parallel to flow reduction reflects scar and/or fibrosis and thus irreversible injury.

F-18 FDG myocardial imaging is the most frequent clinical application of cardiac PET [48, 49]. For assessment of myocardial viability, F-18 FDG is combined with resting perfusion measurements using either a second PET tracer in the same session, or (if performed at a place remote from a cyclotron and not equipped with a perfusion tracer generator) in combination with perfusion SPECT. Residual metabolic activity is an indicator of myocardial viability, and thus of reversibility of contractile dysfunction.

Standardization of the metabolic environment is necessary for clinical myocardial FDG imaging [50], because myocardial FDG uptake depends on glucose and insulin plasma concentrations as well as the rate of glucose utilization. There are several accepted methods for improvement of myocardial FDG PET image quality. Oral glucose loading is commonly used to stimulate insulin secretion and myocardial glucose utilization. It enhances the image quality, with more homogeneously distributed FDG uptake than observed during the fasting state [51]. Euglycemic hyperinsulinemic clamping is a more sophisticated approach that mimics the postabsorptive steady state [52, 53]. It has become an alternative to oral glucose loading for enhancing glucose utilization [53], because it yields images of consistently high diagnostic quality, even in patients with diabetes. Finally, several studies [54–57] have demonstrated that oral administration of

a nicotinic acid or its derivatives is another effective way to improve FDG image quality (55).

Clinical impact

In early studies, qualitative evaluation of PET flow studies demonstrated decreased ^{13}N-ammonia and increased FDG uptake (mismatch) in viable myocardium, which have been considered the scintigraphic hallmark of hibernation [58] (Fig. 5.3). Using information on both blood flow and glucose metabolism, sensitive and specific identification of viable myocardium can be performed. This was first shown by Tillisch et al. [58] who demonstrated that maintained FDG uptake in dysfunctioning segments with reduced flow is associated with functional recovery after revascularization, while segments with concordantly decreased flow and metabolism did not recover after restoration of blood flow. Subsequently, a large number of similar studies confirmed the predictive value of FDG imaging for recovery of contractile function after revascularization [58–65].

The importance of PET studies of tissue viability goes beyond the predictive value for functional recovery. Di Carli et al., for example have demonstrated that the per cent of mismatch identified preoperatively not only predicts recovery of function, but also relates to an improvement in heart failure symptoms and daily life activity [66]. If patients with a mismatch pattern are revascularized, a significant improvement in NYHA class has been observed [67]. Whereas, if they are treated medically, changes in NYHA class are not significant. More importantly, the pattern of blood flow and glucose metabolism contains predictive information about long term survival after surgery. Retrospective data analysis revealed a high incidence of cardiovascular complications in chronic CAD patients with regionally decreased blood flow, but maintained FDG uptake which did not undergo revascularization [67, 68]. The "mismatch" pattern identifies a subgroup of patients at increased risk for cardiovascular complications. The prognostic information appears to be independent of traditional markers such as left ventricular ejection fraction or NYHA classification, which were not different among the investigated subgroups. A study by Beanlands et al. consistently showed higher preoperative mortality, if revascularization was delayed for more than 35

(a)

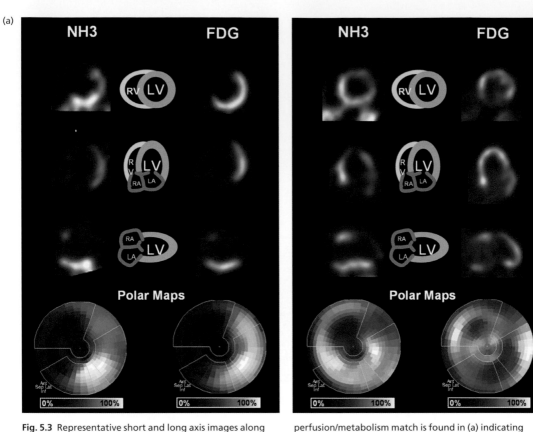

(b)

Fig. 5.3 Representative short and long axis images along with polar maps of perfusion (using N-13 NH₃) and metabolism (using F-18 FDG) in two patients with advanced coronary artery disease and left ventricular dysfunction. A perfusion/metabolism match is found in (a) indicating extensive scar, while a mismatch is found in (b) indicating hibernating myocardium.

days after identification of a PET mismatch pattern [69], supporting the notion that mismatch is an unstable state which requires immediate attention. Haas *et al.* confirmed the impact of PET on peri- and postoperative outcome by comparing two groups of patients with 3-vessel disease and impaired LV-function [70]. Patients selected for revascularization based on PET exhibited significantly lower perioperative complications and better long term outcome compared to a group of patients who underwent revascularization without prior viability assessment.

The potential of PET for sensitive prediction of functional recovery together with the significant prognostic information are likely to influence patient management and therapy planning. As reported by Beanlands *et al.*, PET altered clinical decision making in 57% of 87 patients with chronic

left ventricular dysfunction. Forty-two per cent of patients initially scheduled for bypass surgery were assigned to medical treatment after PET, and approximately half of the patients who were initially assigned for conservative therapy then underwent revascularization. Moreover, 63% of patients assigned for cardiac transplantation were submitted to bypass surgery after PET [71].

Hence, if PET metabolic imaging is used to guide clinical decision making and to select the appropriate therapy based on individual patient risk and likelihood for recovery, costly procedures such as bypass surgery and cardiac transplantation may be avoided if the patient is likely to have no benefit. Thereby, the use of viability imaging may contribute to an overall reduction of costs in the workup of patients with chronic coronary disease and impaired left ventricular function. Because of the significance of the clinical problem and the amount of health costs involved, large prospective randomized trials are necessary and are currently under way, the hope being that they will provide further evidence of the clinical usefulness of viability imaging.

Comparison with other imaging modalities

Numerous investigations exist which compare FDG PET with results of alternative tests, including electrocardiography, thallium-201 and Tc-99m flow agent imaging, stress echocardiography and MRI [34, 72]. Observations of discrepant results between FDG distribution and thallium-201 redistribution pattern have been observed and showed limitations of thallium-201 redistribution imaging for assessment of tissue viability, which are partly overcome by reinjection techniques [73]. The use of Tc-99m sestamibi also provides clinically useful information on tissue viability [74], especially when combined with nitrate application [75]. When comparing scintigraphic data with those obtained after positive inotropic interventions (imaged by echocardiography or magnetic resonance), it appears that tracer retention provides more sensitive markers of viable myocardium, while assessment of contractile reserve is associated with higher specificity for reversible myocardial dysfunction [34].

A more recent, very attractive test for detection of myocardial scar is magnetic resonance imaging of the late enhancement of gadolinium DTPA. This technique allows for accurate visualization of extent, location and transmurality of scar [76]. It compares well to PET for scar detection [77], but seems to detect non-transmural tissue damage with a higher sensitivity. The value of scar detection by late enhancement MRI for predicting functional recovery is good [78] but the clinical importance of non-transmural scar remains a problem. Because of the balance and transition between cell survival and cell death, hibernating myocardium as indicated by PET perfusion/metabolism mismatch may be present or absent in areas of non-transmural scar [79]. Imaging of scar alone does not allow for separation between these two different biologic states. This emphasizes the uniqueness of the PET imaging, which is very closely related to tissue biology.

Imaging of myocardial innervation

The autonomic nervous system consists of sympathetic and parasympathetic innervation. Their major neurotransmitters—norepinephrine and acetylcholine—which define stimulatory and inhibitory effects of each system, are different. Sympathetic and parasympathetic innervation of the heart facilitate its electrophysiologic and hemodynamic adaptation to changing cardiovascular demands by controlling electrophysiologic stimulation and conduction, along with contractile performance. The importance of alterations of the autonomic nervous system for cardiac pathophysiology has been increasingly emphasized. PET techniques provide non-invasive information about global and regional myocardial autonomic innervation (Fig. 5.4). They have substantially facilitated and refined the understanding of cardiac disease mechanisms.

Tracers of sympathetic innervation

Available tracers of sympathetic innervation are either true catecholamines or catecholamine analogues (Table 5.2), and differ in their specificity for the presynaptic uptake-1 transporter and vesicular storage inside the nerve terminal. Their usefulness is defined by low complexity of radiochemical synthesis, but also by the resulting specific radioactivity and chemical purity. Low specific activity and/or chemical impurity result in exposure to non-labeled catecholamines during tracer injection, which competes with the radiotracer for specific uptake and storage, and which increases the likelihood of pharmacologic adrenergic effects.

C-11 meta-hydroxyephedrine (HED) is the most frequently used PET tracer for mapping of sympathetic neurons. It is synthesized by N-methylation of metaraminol, which reliably yields HED at high specific activity [80]. HED is resistant to metabolism by mitochondrial monoamine oxidase (MAO) or catechol-O-methyl transferase (COMT) enzymes, and has a high affinity to uptake-1. Non-specific myocardial uptake is low, as demonstrated in isolated perfused rat hearts following desipramine blockade [81]. Although vesicular storage seems to occur, binding inside vesicles is low because of a higher lipophilicity of HED compared to norepinephrine. Addition of desipramine

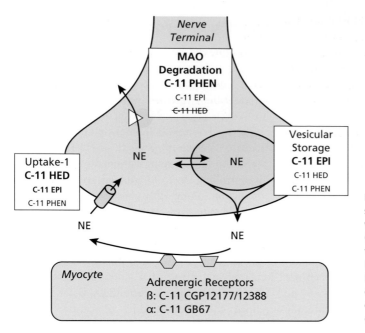

Fig. 5.4 Schematic display of a sympathetic nerve terminal along with the pathway of norepinephrine (NE), and specific tracers of neuronal function (HED = hydroxyephedrine, EPI = epinephrine, PHEN = phenylephrine, MAO = mitochondrial monoamine oxidase; size of writing reflects contribution of pathway to kinetics of respective tracer).

Table 5.2 PET radiopharmaceuticals for clinical neuronal imaging.

Tracer	Biologic target
C-11 hydroxyephedrine	presynaptic catecholamine uptake
C-11 epinephrine	presynaptic catecholamine uptake and storage
C-11 phenylephrine	presynaptic catecholamine uptake and metabolism
F-18 fluorodopamine	presynaptic sympathetic function

or norepinephrine to perfusate following application of HED in isolated rat hearts resulted in accelerated HED wash-out, suggesting that cardiac HED retention is dependent on reuptake by the norepinephrine transporter. HED is thus believed to undergo continuous release and reuptake by sympathetic neurons.

Epinephrine is radiolabeled with C-11 by N-methylation of norepinephrine at high yield and high specific activity [82]. C-11 epinephrine has been used in some clinical studies. It is handled in the myocardium in a manner similar to norepinephrine. It has high affinity for uptake-1, and although it is vulnerable to cytosolic MAO degradation, efficient vesicular intraneuronal storage causes very slow clearance of radioactivity from the heart. In isolated perfused rat hearts, addition of desipramine to the perfusate following C-11

epinephrine administration results in much less acceleration of tracer wash-out compared to C-11 HED [83], suggesting that C-11 epinephrine is a tracer of neuronal uptake and vesicular storage while C-11 HED largely reflects uptake-1 only.

Phenylephrine is a sympathomimetic amine which can be labeled with C-11 at high specific activity [84]. Human experience with C-11 phenylephrine has been reported [85], but remains limited. In contrast to HED, phenylephrine is sensitive to MAO degradation. Studies in isolated perfused rat hearts have shown that C-11 phenylephrine is transported by uptake-1 at a slower rate than HED. Intraneuronally it is rapidly transported into storage vesicles, diffuses out of vesicles at a rate slower than HED, but is then metabolized by MAO in neuronal cytosol [86]. Following injection of C-11 phenylephrine, there is thus considerable myocardial radioactivity wash-out, which is detectable during imaging and reflects MAO activity.

These available C-11-labeled tracers may be combined to identify differential effects of disease on processes of norepinephrine uptake, vesicular storage and metabolism in presynaptic adrenergic nerve terminals.

Because it permits measurement of tracer uptake and clearance, F-18 fluorodopamine has been proposed as a tracer of cardiac sympathetic innervation and function [87]. It has been used in a number of human studies to characterize cardiac innervation in disease conditions. Myocardial uptake of F-18 fluorodopamine occurs mainly via presynaptic uptake-1 and can be blocked by desipramine, as demonstrated in experimental [87] and human studies [88]. Following uptake into the neuron, fluorodopamine is sequestered into storage vesicles and ß-hydroxylated to fluoronorepinephrine. Due to the half-life of 110 min for F-18, tracer clearance from the heart can be surveyed over a longer period of time than with C-11 labelled tracers (half-life 20 min). Comparative studies of the kinetics of fluorodopamine and fluoronorepinephrine revealed a faster myocardial wash-out for fluorodopamine. These data suggested that myocardial activity clearance after fluorodopamine injection is largely attributed to inefficient beta-hydroxylation and subsequent degradation by neuronal MAO [89]. Additionally, rapid extraneuronal degradation has been observed. Soon after injection, radioactivity in blood corresponds mainly to radiolabeled metabolites [90]. For synthesis at sufficient specific activity, which is albeit lower compared to, e.g. C-11 HED, a complex no-carrier-added nucleophilic approach has been developed [91].

Other tracers of sympathetic neurons have been tested, but experience currently remains limited to a few experimental studies, and clinical application has not been reported.

Tracers of parasympathetic innervation

PET imaging of cardiac parasympathetic neurons is complicated because density of cholinergic neurons within the ventricular myocardium is low compared to sympathetic neurons. Additionally, design of a cholinergic tracer is difficult. Parasympathetic neurotransmitter uptake and storage mechanisms are highly specific for acetylcholine, and

cholinergic substances are rapidly degraded in blood and tissue.

Vesamicol is a compound which specifically binds to receptors on parasympathetic neuronal vesicles and inhibits storage of acetylcholine. F-18 fluoroethoxybenzovesamicol has been evaluated for cardiac imaging [92], but specific binding in isolated perfused rat hearts was low, and non-specific binding and wash-out were high. Additionally, there was considerable flow dependency of uptake, so that the usefulness of the tracer for clinical cardiac PET imaging was considered to be low [92]. No other tracers for presynaptic parasympathetic innervation have been established to date, confirming that this component of autonomic innervation is not easily accessible.

Neuroimaging in heart disease

The transplanted heart

Due to transsection of nerve fibers at surgery, the transplanted heart is initially completely denervated. First evidence of allograft reinnervation was derived from HED PET measurements, which showed reappearance of significant regional tracer retention in basal anterior myocardium [93]. Further studies have demonstrated a continuous increase of extent and intensity of reinnervation with time after transplantation (Fig. 5.5), but complete restoration of sympathetic innervation has never been observed [94, 95].

Because of heterogeneous reinnervation, the transplanted heart is a good model for determining physiologic effects of sympathetic innervation *in vivo* by an intraindivdual comparison of innervated and denervated myocardium. Di Carli *et al.* observed a significant improvement of flow response to cold in innervated compared to denervated vascular territories, while there was no difference for the response to adenosine. These results demonstrated the importance of sympathetic innervation for regulation of endothelial-dependent vascular reactivity [96]. Other studies have focussed on the effect of innervation on myocardial substrate utilization, and found higher utilization of glucose at equal rates of overall oxidative metabolism in denervated compared to reinnervated myocardium of allografts, suggesting a metabolic switch from free fatty acids to glucose under conditions of denervation

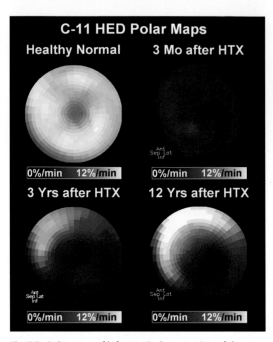

C-11 HED Polar Maps

Healthy Normal   3 Mo after HTX

0%/min   12%/min   0%/min   12%/min

3 Yrs after HTX   12 Yrs after HTX

0%/min   12%/min   0%/min   12%/min

Fig. 5.5 Polar maps of left ventricular retention of the catecholamine analogue C-11 hydroxyephedrine (HED) in a healthy individual and three patients at different times after cardiac transplantation (HTX).

[97]. Finally, the effect of reinnervation on exercise performance was determined in a group of 29 transplant recipients by HED PET and standardized exercise radionuclide angiography. Restoration of sympathetic innervation was associated with improved responses of heart rate and global as well as regional contractile function to exercise. These results support the functional importance of reinnervation in transplanted hearts, and suggest a clinical benefit for the transplant recipient through enhanced exercise capacity [98].

Ischemic syndromes

The sensitivity of cardiac sympathetic nerve terminals to ischemia has been supported by early experimental observations of a sustained reduction of cardiac uptake of F-18 metaraminol following short time periods of coronary occlusion [99]. A first study in patients early after myocardial infarction by Allman *et al.* showed that the area of reduced HED retention exceeded the perfusion defect—a finding that was especially pronounced in non-Q-wave infarcts [100]. The hypothesis of a higher

sensitivity of sympathetic neurons to ischemia compared to cardiomyocytes is further supported by observations of regionally reduced HED retention in the absence of resting perfusion defects in patients with advanced coronary artery disease but no evidence of myocardial infarction [101]. Whether the amount of sympathetic denervation in ischemic heart disease is linked with a higher incidence of ventricular arrhythmia and/or remodeling, and thus with an adverse outcome, needs to be evaluated.

Heart failure

The hyperadrenergic state in congestive heart failure causes desensitization and downregulation of cardiac beta-adrenergic receptors and alterations of postsynaptic signal transduction, which impair myocardial performance [102]. Presynaptic cardiac sympathetic innervation is also involved in this pathophysiologic process. Reduced global myocardial HED retention, which correlated with clinical markers of heart failure such as impaired ejection fraction and NYHA class, as well as with elevation of plasma catecholamine levels, has been described [103] (Fig. 5.6). Results of *in vivo* HED PET have been validated against *ex vivo* measurements in tissue of explanted hearts after transplantation in patients with terminal heart failure due to idiopathic dilated cardiomyopathy. Regional HED retention was significantly correlated with *ex vivo* tissue, norepinephrine content, and uptake-1 density, but not uptake-1 affinity [104]. Although the pathogenetic cause for altered presynaptic innervation in the failing heart are not yet fully elucidated, further consequences and correlates of impaired cardiac uptake-1 integrity have been identified with the help of quantitative neurotransmitter PET. Alterations of myocardial HED retention were globally and regionally associated with impaired contractile function as measured by gated blood pool SPECT, suggesting a common pathogenetic pathway [105]. Overall oxidative metabolism, determined by C-11 acetate PET, was not directly correlated with these findings [105], but a significant correlation between impaired presynaptic innervation and myocardial efficiency was identified in the failing heart [106].

Reduction of functioning local presynaptic catecholamine uptake sites as demonstrated by

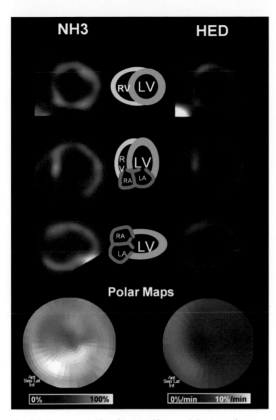

Fig. 5.6 Representative short and long axis images along with polar maps of perfusion (using N-13 NH₃) and sympathetic innervation (using C-11 HED) in a patient with dilated cardiomyopathy and terminal heart failure. Global reduction of HED retention reflects extensive alterations of presynaptic sympathetic innervation.

neurotransmitter imaging is likely to increase the myocardial overexposure to catecholamines and may facilitate progress and further deterioration of congestive heart failure. It has thus been speculated that alterations of sympathetic innervation are of prognostic value. Consistent with other studies using SPECT with I-123 MIBG, a prognostic value has also been suggested for quantitative HED PET imaging in heart failure. Pietila *et al.* found that reduced global HED retention was an independent predictor of adverse outcome in 46 patients with NYHA class II–III heart failure and an average ejection fraction of 35% [107].

Arrhythmia

Based on observations that stress and catecholamine infusion can induce ventricular arrhythmia in certain heart diseases, and based on experimental observations of a supersensitivity in myocardial areas with impaired sympathetic neuronal function, a role for the cardiac sympathetic nervous system in the pathogenesis of arrhythmia has been proposed. The relationship between myocardial denervation and ventricular refractoriness has been investigated by Calkins *et al.* using C-11 HED PET and intra-operative electrophysiologic measurements during placement of an implantable defibrillator in sustained ventricular tachycardia. The refractory period in areas with reduced HED retention was significantly longer than in areas with normal HED retention, documenting effects of innervation on myocardial electrophysiology [108].

Specific arrhythmogenic diseases have also been evaluated with regard to involvement of the sympathetic nervous system. In right ventricular outflow tract tachycardia, Schafers *et al.* used the beta-receptor ligand C-11 CGP12177 and C-11 HED for combined pre- and postsynaptic sympathetic assessment of the left ventricle, observing a reduction of both. They concluded that myocardial beta-adrenoceptor downregulation occurs subsequently to increased local synaptic catecholamine levels caused by impaired catecholamine reuptake in this form of arrhythmogenic disease [109]. Arrhythmogenic right ventricular cardiomyopathy was studied by the same group using the same technique. This time, only postsynaptic beta-receptor density was significantly reduced, while presynaptic HED uptake tended towards reduction only. The authors speculated that a secondary beta-receptor downregulation may occur after increased local synaptic norepinephrine levels caused by increased firing rates of the efferent neurons or as result of impaired presynaptic catecholamine reuptake [110]. A potential prognostic value for alterations of the sympathetic nervous system remains to be evaluated in future studies along with potential alleviating effects of therapeutic approaches.

Other neuropathies

Diabetes mellitus may be complicated by neuropathy, which often involves the autonomic nervous system. Using HED PET, Allman *et al.* first described a pattern of regional myocardial denervation characterizing cardiac diabetic neuropathy, which correlated with conventional markers of autonomic dysfunction [111]. Other studies have contributed to the establishment of a link between diabetic autonomic neuropathy and impairments of myocardial blood flow. Stevens *et al.* found significant reductions of global myocardial blood flow and flow reserve during adenosine-mediated vasodilation in neuropathic diabetic subjects compared to non-neuropathic diabetic and non-diabetic subjects [112]. Di Carli *et al.*, on the other hand, reported impaired flow response to adenosine in diabetic patients with and without PET-defined cardiac neuropathy compared to normals, while the flow response to sympathetic stimulation by the endothelial-dependent cold pressor test was further reduced in diabetic patients with neuropathy than in those without and in normal controls [113].

Idiopathic Parkinson's disease as well as atypical Parkinsonian syndromes such as multiple system atrophy can be associated with peripheral autonomic dysfunction. In idiopathic Parkinson's disease, this is thought to be caused primarily by postganglionic sympathetic dysfunction and in multiple system atrophy by predominantly central and preganglionic degeneration. Using HED in a small group of seven patients, Berding *et al.* confirmed the latter hypothesis and found reduced myocardial catecholamine uptake in idiopathic Parkinson's disease, which was especially pronounced when the neurologic disease was accompanied by orthostatic hypotension [114]. In another study, using F-18 fluorodopamine, serial imaging over a period of two years confirmed progressive loss of myocardial innervation as part of the neurodegeneration of Parkinson's disease [115].

F-18 fluorodopamine was also used to classify dysautonomias according to their involvement of the cardiac sympathetic nervous system. Patients with sympathetic neurocirculatory failure—based either on pure autonomic failure with no signs of central neurodegeneration or on classical Parkinsonism—showed no myocardial F-18 fluorodopamine uptake, while patients with sympathetic neurocirculatory failure based on the Shy-Drager syndrome (central neurodegeneration unresponsive to treatment with levodopa) showed increased levels of fluorodopamine uptake, indicating intact sympathetic terminals and absent nerve traffic [116].

Table 5.3 PET radiopharmaceuticals for clinical receptor imaging.

Tracer	Biologic target
C-11 CGP12177	beta-adrenergic receptor (non-selective)
C-11 CGP12388	beta-adrenergic receptor (non-selective)
C-11 GB67	alpha-adrenergic receptor
C-11 MQNB	muscarinic receptor

Targeting of cardiovascular receptors

Various myocardial receptors have been identified as playing a role in cardiovascular pathophysiology, and thus represent attractive targets for imaging. Several receptor ligands have been labeled successfully with positron-emitting radioisotopes and tested for clinical imaging (Table 5.3). Attractive targets for myocardial receptor imaging comprise not only the autonomic adrenergic and cholinergic systems, but also opiate, endothelin, angiotensin and adenosine receptor systems.

But the use of receptor-targeted tracers has been limited to few studies in the past and is yet waiting for its clinical breakthrough. Low selectivity and affinity of the probes, along with high non-specific binding, lack of hydrophilicity (to avoid binding to internalized inactive receptors), and pharmacologic/toxicologic effects have been frequently encountered limitations. Additionally, the often complicated and less reliable tracer synthesis has precluded a more widespread application of receptor ligands for cardiac PET. These difficulties will need to be overcome in the future in order to realize a potential clinical application.

Tracers of muscarinic receptors

The first myocardial receptors to be targeted with PET were muscarinic receptors [117]. For this purpose, a hydrophilic, non-metabolized antagonist, methylquinuclidinyl benzilate (MQNB) has been labeled with C-11. Left ventricular myocardial uptake of MQNB was higher in case of a lower heart rate as an indicator of parasympathetic activity, suggesting that binding reflects the physiologically active form of the muscarinic receptor [118]. A mathematical model has been established which allows for quantification of receptor concentration, association and dissociation constants [119]. Application of the tracer in humans, however, has been limited to a few studies [120–122]. Development of further muscarinic receptor ligands, which are more potent than MQNB, is still limited to the experimental setting [123].

Tracers of adrenergic receptors

At present, the only adrenoreceptor ligand which has been applied in several, albeit small clinical studies, is C-11 CGP12177, a non-selective, hydrophilic ß-receptor antagonist. Non-specific uptake in rats was low and plasma clearance was fast, suggesting feasibility for clinical imaging [124]. A graphical method, which circumvents issues related to metabolites, has been established for quantification in humans [125]. This approach requires a dual-injection protocol with doses of high and low specific activity. Synthesis of this tracer, however, is laborious and requires C-11 phosgen as a precursor, which has prevented a broader clinical application until now. *In vivo* studies in the failing heart confirmed downregulation of beta-receptors, which was associated with decreased contractile responsiveness to dobutamine, indicating a direct link between changes in the receptor number and its biological function [119]. Muscarinic receptor density, measured by PET and C-11 MQNB, was found to be upregulated as a potential adaptive mechanism [122].

CGP12388 is a recently introduced non-selective ß-adrenoceptor antagonist, which is more easily labelled with C-11 than CGP12177 [126]. Studies in isolated perfused rat heart have shown independency of flow and little non-specific binding [127], and *in vivo* quantification of receptor density has been successfully performed in humans [128]. This ligand is thus promising (Fig. 5.7), but the robustness of its application will need to be demonstrated in further clinical studies.

The prazosin derivative C-11 GB67 has been suggested as a ligand for imaging of α_1-receptors. Subtype selectivity and specific uptake in rat hearts were high, and visualization of myocardium in humans was possible, suggesting that the tracer is promising for further evaluation [129]. A variety of other subtype-specific or non-specific tracers for adrenergic receptors have been tested experimentally, but were found too unsuitable for clinical imaging mainly because of high non-specific binding or lipophilicity [130–134].

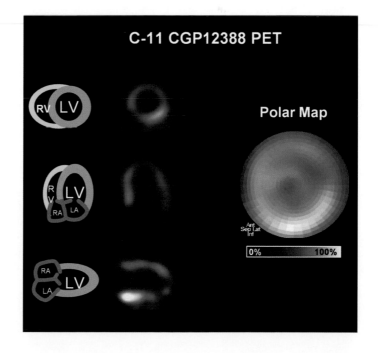

Fig. 5.7 Representative short and long axis images along with a polar map of the distribution of the non-selective beta-adrenergic receptor ligand C-11 CGP12388 in a healthy human.

Summary and future perspectives

The application of PET as a tool to study biologic mechanisms such as metabolism, neuronal function and receptors has substantially improved understanding of pathophysiologic processes in the heart. Clinical applications for assessment of myocardial viability have emerged in the past and knowledge derived from cardiac PET imaging has been successfully transferred to other imaging techniques, leading to their refinement.

In the future, the spectrum of target molecules for imaging will broaden and allow for an increasingly specific molecular tissue characterization. Combination of PET with morphologic imaging strategies will then allow for *in vivo* characterization and localization of molecular mechanisms not only in myocardium but also in the coronary tree. The vision is an integrated approach to the study of disease processes from molecular-biologic and physiologic to morphologic features in the cardiovascular system.

References

1. Liedtke AJ. Alterations of carbohydrate and lipid metabolism in the acutely ischemic heart. *Prog Cardiovasc Dis* 1981; **23**: 321–336.
2. Taegtmeyer H. Myocardial metabolism. In: Phelps M, Mazziotta J, Schelbert H, eds. *Positron Emission Tomography and Autoradiography: Principles and Applications for the Brain and Heart.* Raven Press, New York, 1986: 149–195.
3. Depre C, Vanoverschelde JL, Taegtmeyer H. Glucose for the heart. *Circulation* 1999; **99**: 578–588.
4. Gertz EW, Wisneski JA, Stanley WC *et al.* Myocardial substrate utilization during exercise in humans. Dual carbon-labeled carbohydrate isotope experiments. *J Clin Invest* 1988; **82**: 2017–2025.
5. Opie LH. Effects of regional ischemia on metabolism of glucose and fatty acids. Relative rates of aerobic and anaerobic energy production during myocardial infarction and comparison with effects of anoxia. *Circ Res* 1976; **38**: 152–174.
6. Kalff V, Schwaiger M, Nguyen N *et al.* The relationship between myocardial blood flow and glucose uptake in ischemic canine myocardium determined with fluorine-18-deoxyglucose. *J Nucl Med* 1992; **33**: 1346–1353.
7. Brosius F, Lui Y, Nguyen N *et al.* Persistent myocardial ischemia increases GLUT 1 transporter expression in both ischemic and non-ischemic heart regions. *J Mol Cell Cardiol* 1997; **29**: 1675–1685.
8. Schelbert HR, Henze E, Sochor H *et al.* Effects of substrate availability on myocardial C-11 palmitate kinetics by positron emission tomography in normal subjects and patients with ventricular dysfunction. *Am Heart J* 1986; **111**: 1055–1064.
9. Grover-McKay M, Schelbert HR, Schwaiger M *et al.* Identification of impaired metabolic reserve by atrial pacing in patients with significant coronary artery stenosis. *Circulation* 1986; **74**: 281–292.
10. Bergmann SR, Weinheimer CJ, Markham J *et al.* Quantitation of myocardial fatty acid metabolism using PET. *J Nucl Med* 1996; **37**: 1723–1730.
11. Gropler RJ, Siegel BA, Geltman EM. Myocardial uptake of carbon-11-acetate as an indirect estimate of regional myocardial blood flow. *J Nucl Med* 1991; **32**: 245–251.
12. Buck A, Wolpers HG, Hutchins GD *et al.* Effect of carbon-11-acetate recirculation on estimates of myocardial oxygen consumption by PET. *J Nucl Med* 1991; **32**: 1950–1957.
13. Buxton DB, Schwaiger M, Nguyen A *et al.* Radiolabeled acetate as a tracer of myocardial tricarboxylic acid cycle flux. *Circ Res* 1988; **63**: 628–634.
14. Brown MA, Myers DW, Bergmann SR. Validity of estimates of myocardial oxidative metabolism with carbon-11 acetate and positron emission tomography despite altered patterns of substrate utilization. *J Nucl Med* 1989; **30**: 187–193.
15. Beanlands RS, Bach DS, Raylman R *et al.* Acute effects of dobutamine on myocardial oxygen consumption and cardiac efficiency measured using carbon-11 acetate kinetics in patients with dilated cardiomyopathy. *J Am Coll Cardiol* 1993; **22**: 1389–1398.
16. Bengel FM, Permanetter B, Ungerer M *et al.* Non-invasive estimation of myocardial efficiency using positron emission tomography and C-11 acetate—comparison between the normal and failing human heart. *Eur J Nucl Med* 2000; **27**: 319–326.
17. Beanlands RS, Nahmias C, Gordon E *et al.* The effects of beta(1)-blockade on oxidative metabolism and the metabolic cost of ventricular work in patients with left ventricular dysfunction: A double-blind, placebo-controlled, positron-emission tomography study. *Circulation* 2000; **102**: 2070–2075.
18. Phelps ME, Huang SC, Hoffman EJ *et al.* Tomographic measurement of local cerebral glucose metabolic rate in humans with (F-18)2-fluoro-2-deoxy-D-glucose: validation of method. *Ann Neurol* 1979; **6**: 371–388.
19. Sokoloff L, Reivich M, Kennedy C *et al.* The (14C) deoxyglucose method for the measurement of local cerebral glucose utilization: Theory, procedure and

normal values in the conscious and anesthetized albino rat. *J Neurochem* 1977; **28**: 897–916.

20. Krivokapich J, Huang SC, Selin CE *et al.* Fluorodeoxyglucose rate constants, lumped constant, and glucose metabolic rate in rabbit heart. *Am J Physiol* 1987; **252**: H777–H787.

21. Krivokapich J, Huang SC, Phelps ME *et al.* Estimation of rabbit myocardial metabolic rate for glucose using fluorodeoxyglucose. *Am J Physiol* 1982; **243**: H884–H894.

22. Hariharan R, Bray M, Ganim R *et al.* Fundamental limitations of [^{18}F]2-deoxy-2-fluoro-D-glucose for assessing myocardial glucose uptake. *Circulation* 1995; **91**: 2435–2444.

23. Patlak CS, Blasberg RG. Graphical evaluation of blood-to-brain transfer constants from multiple-time uptake data. Generalizations. *J Cereb Blood Flow Metab* 1985; **5**: 584–590.

24. Herrero P, Weinheimer CJ, Dence C *et al.* Quantification of myocardial glucose utilization by PET and 1-carbon-11-glucose. *J Nucl Cardiol* 2002; **9**: 5–14.

25. Peterson LR, Herrero P, Schechtman KB *et al.* Effect of obesity and insulin resistance on myocardial substrate metabolism and efficiency in young women. *Circulation* 2004; **109**: 2191–2196.

26. Nuutila P, Knuuti MJ, Raitakari M *et al.* Effect of antilipolysis on heart and skeletal muscle glucose uptake in overnight fasted humans. *Am J Physiol* 1994; **267**: E941–946.

27. Passamani E, Davis KB, Gillespie MJ *et al.* A randomized trial of coronary artery bypass surgery: Survival of patients with a low ejection fraction. *N Engl J Med* 1985; **312**: 1665–1671.

28. Kaul T, Agnohotri A, Fields B *et al.* Coronary artery bypass grafting in patients with an ejection fraction of twenty per cent or less. *J Thorac Cardiovasc Surg* 1996; **111**: 1001–1012.

29. Miller D, Stinson E, Alderman E. Surgical treatment of ischemic cardiomyopathy: Is it ever too late? *Am J Surg* 1981; **141**: 688–693.

30. Mickleborough L, Maruyama H, Takagi Y *et al.* Results of revascularization in patients with severe left ventricular dysfunction. *Circulation* 1995; **92**: 73–79.

31. Luciani G, Faggian T, Razzolini R *et al.* Severe ischemic left ventricular failure: coronary operation or heart transplantation. *Ann Thorac Surg* 1993; **55**: 719–723.

32. Wijns W, Vatner S, Camici P. Hibernating myocardium. *N Engl J Med* 1998; **339**: 173–181.

33. Rahimtoola SH. The hibernating myocardium. *Am Heart J* 1989; **117**: 211–221.

34. Bax JJ, Wijns W, Cornel JH *et al.* Accuracy of currently available techniques for prediction of functional recovery after revascularization in patients with left ventricular dysfunction due to chronic coronary artery disease: Comparison of pooled data. *J Am Coll Cardiol* 1997; **30**: 1451–1460.

35. Kloner R, Bolli R, Marban E *et al.* Medical and cellular implications of stunning, hibernation, and preconditioning: An NHLBI workshop. *Circulation* 1998; **97**: 1848–1867.

36. Heyndricks GR, Millard RW, McRitchie RJ *et al.* Regional myocardial function and electrophysiological alterations after brief coronary artery occlusion in conscious dogs. *J Clin Invest* 1975; **56**: 978–985.

37. Bolli R. Myocardial "stunning" in man. *Circulation* 1992; **86**: 1671–191.

38. Kloner RA, Allen J, Cox TA *et al.* Stunned left ventricular myocardium after exercise treadmill testing in coronary artery disease. *Am J Cardiol* 1991; **68**: 329–334.

39. Heusch G. Hibernating myocardium. *Physiol Rev* 1998; **78**: 1055–1085.

40. Elsässer A, Schlepper M, Klovekorn WP *et al.* Hibernating myocardium: an incomplete adaptation to ischemia. *Circulation* 1997; **96**: 2920–2931.

41. Schwarz ER, Schoendube FA, Kostin S *et al.* Prolonged myocardial hibernation exacerbates cardiomyocyte degeneration and impairs recovery of function after revascularization. *J Am Coll Cardiol* 1998; **31**: 1018–1026.

42. Depre C, Vanoverschelde JL, Gerber B *et al.* Correlation of functional recovery with myocardial blood flow, glucose uptake, and morphologic features in patients with chronic left ventricular ischemic dysfunction undergoing coronary artery bypass grafting. *J Thorac Cardiovasc Surg* 1997; **113**: 371–378.

43. Vanoverschelde JL, Wijns W, Depre C *et al.* Mechanisms of chronic regional postischemic dysfunction in humans. New insights from the study of non-infarcted collateral-dependent myocardium. *Circulation* 1993; **87**: 1513–1523.

44. Iida H, Tamura Y, Kitamura K *et al.* Histochemical correlates of ^{15}O-water-perfusable tissue fraction in experimental canine studies of old myocardial infarction. *J Nucl Med* 2000; **41**: 1737–1745.

45. Yamamoto Y, de Silva R, Rhodes C *et al.* A new strategy for the assessment of viable myocardium and regional myocardial blood flow using ^{15}O-water and dynamic positron emission tomography. *Circulation* 1992; **86**: 167–178.

46. Haas F, Augustin N, Holper K *et al.* Time course and extent of improvement of dysfunctioning myocardium in patients with coronary artery disease and severely depressed left ventricular function after revascularization: correlation with positron emission tomographic findings. *J Am Coll Cardiol* 2000; **36**: 1927–1934.

47. Gewirtz H, Fischman AJ, Abraham S *et al.* Positron emission tomographic measurements of absolute regional myocardial blood flow permits identification of non-viable myocardium in patients with chronic myocardial infarction. *J Am Coll Cardiol* 1994; **23**: 851–859.

48. Bacharach SL, Bax JJ, Case J *et al.* PET myocardial glucose metabolism and perfusion imaging: part 1—guidelines for data acquisition and patient preparation. *J Nucl Cardiol* 2003; **10**: 543–556.

49. Schelbert HR, Beanlands R, Bengel F *et al.* PET myocardial perfusion and glucose metabolism imaging: part 2—guidelines for interpretation and reporting. *J Nucl Cardiol* 2003; **10**: 557–571.

50. Knuuti J, Schelbert HR, Bax JJ. The need for standardisation of cardiac FDG PET imaging in the evaluation of myocardial viability in patients with chronic ischaemic left ventricular dysfunction. *Eur J Nucl Med Mol Imaging* 2002; **29**: 1257–1266.

51. Berry JJ, Baker JA, Pieper KS *et al.* The effect of metabolic milieu on cardiac PET imaging using fluorine-18-deoxyglucose and nitrogen-13-ammonia in normal volunteers. *J Nucl Med* 1991; **32**: 1518–1525.

52. DeFronzo RA, Tobin JD, Andres R. Glucose clamp technique: a method for quantifying insulin secretion and resistance. *Am J Physiol* 1979; **237**: E214–223.

53. Knuuti MJ, Nuutila P, Ruotsalainen U *et al.* Euglycemic hyperinsulinemic clamp and oral glucose load in stimulating myocardial glucose utilization during positron emission tomography. *J Nucl Med* 1992; **33**: 1255–1262.

54. Knuuti MJ, Yki-Jarvinen H, Voipio-Pulkki LM *et al.* Enhancement of myocardial [fluorine-18]fluorodeoxyglucose uptake by a nicotinic acid derivative. *J Nucl Med* 1994; **35**: 989–998.

55. Schinkel AF, Bax JJ, Valkema R *et al.* Effect of diabetes mellitus on myocardial ^{18}F-FDG SPECT using acipimox for the assessment of myocardial viability. *J Nucl Med* 2003; **44**: 877–883.

56. Schroder O, Hor G, Hertel A *et al.* Combined hyperinsulinaemic glucose clamp and oral acipimox for optimizing metabolic conditions during ^{18}F-fluorodeoxyglucose gated PET cardiac imaging: comparative results. *Nucl Med Commun* 1998; **19**: 867–874.

57. Stone CK, Holden JE, Stanley W *et al.* Effect of nicotinic acid on exogenous myocardial glucose utilization. *J Nucl Med* 1995; 36: 996–1002.

58. Tillisch J, Brunken R, Marshall R *et al.* Reversibility of cardiac wall motion abnormalities predicted by positron tomography. *N Engl J Med* 1986; **314**: 884–888.

59. Tamaki N, Yonekura Y, Yamashita K *et al.* Value of rest-stress myocardial positron tomography using nitrogen-13-ammonia for the preoperative prediction of reversible asynergie. *J Nucl Med* 1989; **30**: 1302–1310.

60. Tamaki N, Ohtani H, Yamashita K *et al.* Metabolic activity in the areas of new fill-in after thallium-201 reinjection: comparison with positron emission tomography using fluorine-18-deoxyglucose. *J Nucl Med* 1991; **32**: 673–678.

61. Vom Dahl J, Eitzman DT, al-Aouar ZR *et al.* Relation of regional function, perfusion, and metabolism in patients with advanced coronary artery disease undergoing surgical revascularization. *Circulation* 1994; **90**: 2356–2366.

62. Marwick TH, MacIntyre WJ, Lafont A *et al.* Metabolic responses of hibernating and infarcted myocardium to revascularization. A follow-up study of regional perfusion, function, and metabolism. *Circulation* 1992; **85**: 1347–1353.

63. Lucignani G, Paolini G, Landoni C *et al.* Presurgical identification of hibernating myocardium by combined use of technetium-99 m hexakis 2-methoxy-isobutylisonitrile single photon emission tomography and fluorine-18 fluoro-2-deoxy-D-glucose positron emission tomography in patients with coronary artery disease. *Eur J Nucl Med* 1992; **19**: 874–881.

64. Gropler RJ, Geltman EM, Sampathkumaran K *et al.* Comparison of carbon-11-acetate with fluorine-18-fluorodeoxyglucose for delineating viable myocardium by positron emission tomography. *J Am Coll Cardiol* 1993; **22**: 1587–1597.

65. Carrel T, Jenni R, Haubold-Reuter S *et al.* Improvement of severely reduced left ventricular function after surgical revascularization in patients with preoperative myocardial infarction. *Eur J Cardiothorac Surg* 1992; **6**: 479–484.

66. Di Carli MF, Asgarzadie F, Schelbert HR *et al.* Quantitative relation between myocardial viability and improvement in heart failure symptoms after revascularization in patients with ischemic cardiomyopathy. *Circulation* 1995; **92**: 3436–3444.

67. Di Carli MF, Davidson M, Little R *et al.* Value of metabolic imaging with positron emission tomography for evaluating prognosis in patients with coronary artery disease and left ventricular dysfunction. *Am J Cardiol* 1994; **73**: 527–533.

68. Eitzman D, Al-Aouar Z, Kanter H *et al.* Clinical outcome of patients with advanced coronary artery disease after viability studies with positron emission tomography. *J Am Coll Cardiol* 1992; **20**: 559–565.

69. Beanlands R, Hendry P, Masters R *et al.* Delay in revascularization is associated with increased mortality rate in patients with severe left ventricular dysfunction and viable myocardium on fluorine 18-fluorodeoxyglucose

positron emission tomography imaging. *Circulation* 1998; **98** (19 suppl): II51–56.

70. Haas F, Haehnel CJ, Picker W *et al.* Preoperative positron emission tomographic viability assessment and perioperative and postoperative risk in patients with advanced ischemic heart disease. *J Am Coll Cardiol* 1997; **30**: 1693–1700.

71. Beanlands RS, deKemp RA, Smith S *et al.* ^{18}F-fluorodeoxyglucose PET imaging alters clinical decision making in patients with impaired ventricular function. *Am J Cardiol* 1997; **79**: 1092–1095.

72. Baer FM, Voth E, Schneider CA *et al.* Comparison of low-dose dobutamine-gradient-echo magnetic resonance imaging and positron emission tomography with [18F]fluorodeoxyglucose in patients with chronic coronary artery disease. A functional and morphological approach to the detection of residual myocardial viability. *Circulation* 1995; **91**: 1006–1015.

73. Dilsizian V, Rocco TP, Freedman NM *et al.* Enhanced detection of ischemic but viable myocardium by the reinjection of thallium after stress-redistribution imaging. *N Engl J Med* 1990; **323**: 141–146.

74. Udelson JE, Coleman PS, Metherall J *et al.* Predicting recovery of severe regional ventricular dysfunction: comparison of resting scintigraphy with thallium-201 and technetium-99 m-sestamibi. *Circulation* 1994; **89**: 2552–2561.

75. Cornel JH, Arnese M, Forster T *et al.* Potential and limitations of Tc-99 m sestamibi scintigraphy for the diagnosis of myocardial viability. *Herz* 1994; **19**: 19–27.

76. Kim RJ, Wu E, Rafael A *et al.* The use of contrast-enhanced magnetic resonance imaging to identify reversible myocardial dysfunction. *N Engl J Med* 2000; **343**: 1445–1453.

77. Klein C, Nekolla SG, Bengel FM *et al.* Assessment of myocardial viability with contrast-enhanced magnetic resonance imaging: comparison with positron emission tomography. *Circulation* 2002; **105**: 162–167.

78. Selvanayagam JB, Kardos A, Francis JM *et al.* Value of delayed-enhancement cardiovascular magnetic resonance imaging in predicting myocardial viability after surgical revascularization. *Circulation* 2004; **110**: 1535–1541.

79. Knuesel PR, Nanz D, Wyss C *et al.* Characterization of dysfunctional myocardium by positron emission tomography and magnetic resonance: relation to functional outcome after revascularization. *Circulation* 2003; **108**: 1095–1100.

80. Rosenspire KC, Haka MS, van Dort ME *et al.* Synthesis and preliminary evaluation of carbon-11-meta-hydroxyephedrine: A false transmitter agent for heart neuronal imaging. *J Nucl Med* 1990; **31**: 1328–1334.

81. DeGrado TR, Hutchins GD, Toorongian SA *et al.* Myocardial kinetics of carbon-11-meta-hydroxyephedrine: Retention mechanisms and effects of norepinephrine. *J Nucl Med* 1993; **34**: 1287–1293.

82. Chakraborty PK, Gildersleeve DL, Jewett DM *et al.* High yield synthesis of high specific activity R-(-)-[11C]epinephrine for routine PET studies in humans. *Nucl Med Biol* 1993; **20**: 939–944.

83. Nguyen NT, DeGrado TR, Chakraborty P *et al.* Myocardial kinetics of carbon-11-epinephrine in the isolated working rat heart. *J Nucl Med* 1997; **38**: 780–785.

84. Del Rosario RB, Jung YW, Caraher J *et al.* Synthesis and preliminary evaluation of [11C]-(-)-phenylephrine as a functional heart neuronal PET agent. *Nucl Med Biol* 1996; **23**: 611–616.

85. Raffel DM, Corbett JR, del Rosario RB *et al.* Clinical evaluation of carbon-11-phenylephrine: MAO-sensitive marker of cardiac sympathetic neurons. *J Nucl Med* 1996; **37**: 1923–1931.

86. Raffel DM, Wieland DM. Influence of vesicular storage and monoamine oxidase activity on [11C]phenylephrine kinetics: studies in isolated rat heart. *J Nucl Med* 1999; **40**: 323–330.

87. Goldstein DS, Chang PC, Eisenhofer G *et al.* Positron emission tomographic imaging of cardiac sympathetic innervation and function. *Circulation* 1990; **81**: 1606–1621.

88. Goldstein DS, Eisenhofer G, Dunn BB *et al.* Positron emission tomographic imaging of cardiac sympathetic innervation using 6 [18F] fluorodopamine: initial findings in humans. *J Am Coll Cardiol* 1993; **22**: 1961–1971.

89. Ding YS, Fowler JS, Gatley SJ *et al.* Mechanistic positron emission tomography studies of 6 [18F] fluorodopamine in living baboon heart: Selective imaging and control of radiotracer metabolism using the deuterium isotope effect. *J Neurochem* 1995; **65**: 682–690.

90. Goldstein DS, Holmes C. Metabolic fate of the sympathoneural imaging agent 6 [18F] fluorodopamine in humans. *Clin Exp Hypertens* 1997; **19**: 155–161.

91. Ding YS, Fowler JS, Gatley SJ *et al.* Synthesis of high specific activity 6 [18F] fluorodopamine for positron emission tomography studies of sympathetic nervous tissue. *J Med Chem* 1991; **34**: 861–863.

92. DeGrado TR, Mulholland GK, Wieland DM *et al.* Evaluation of (-)[18F]fluoroethoxybenzovesamicol as a new PET tracer of cholinergic neurons of the heart. *Nucl Med Biol* 1994; **21**: 189–195.

93. Schwaiger M, Hutchins GD, Kalff V *et al.* Evidence for regional catecholamine uptake and storage sites in the transplanted human heart by positron emission tomography. *J Clin Invest* 1991; **87**: 1681–1690.

94. Bengel FM, Ueberfuhr P, Ziegler SI *et al.* Serial assessment of sympathetic reinnervation after orthotopic heart transplantation. A longitudinal study using PET and C-11 hydroxyephedrine. *Circulation* 1999; **99**: 1866–1871.

95. Bengel FM, Ueberfuhr P, Hesse T *et al.* Clinical determinants of ventricular sympathetic reinnervation after orthotopic heart transplantation. *Circulation* 2002; **106**: 831–835.

96. Di Carli MF, Tobes MC, Mangner T *et al.* Effects of cardiac sympathetic innervation on coronary blood flow. *N Engl J Med* 1997; **336**: 1208–1215.

97. Bengel FM, Ueberfuhr P, Ziegler SI *et al.* Non-invasive assessment of the effect of cardiac sympathetic innervation on metabolism of the human heart. *Eur J Nucl Med* 2000; **27**: 1650–1657.

98. Bengel FM, Ueberfuhr P, Schiepel N *et al.* Effect of sympathetic reinnervation on cardiac performance after heart transplantation. *N Engl J Med* 2001; **345**: 731–738.

99. Schwaiger M, Guibourg H, Rosenspire K *et al.* Effect of regional myocardial ischemia on sympathetic nervous system as assessed by fluorine-18-metaraminol. *J Nucl Med* 1990; **31**: 1352–1357.

100. Allman KC, Wieland DM, Muzik O *et al.* Carbon-11 hydroxyephedrine with positron emission tomography for serial assessment of cardiac adrenergic neuronal function after acute myocardial infarction in humans. *J Am Coll Cardiol* 1993; **22**: 368–375.

101. Bulow HP, Stahl F, Lauer B *et al.* Alterations of myocardial presynaptic sympathetic innervation in patients with multivessel coronary artery disease but without history of myocardial infarction. *Nucl Med Commun* 2003; **24**: 233–239.

102. Bristow MR. The autonomic nervous system in heart failure. *N Engl J Med* 1984; **311**: 850–851.

103. Hartmann F, Ziegler S, Nekolla S *et al.* Regional patterns of myocardial sympathetic denervation in dilated cardiomyopathy: An analysis using carbon-11 hydroxyephedrine and positron emission tomography. *Heart* 1999; **81**: 262–270.

104. Ungerer M, Hartmann F, Karoglan M *et al.* Regional *in vivo* and *in vitro* characterization of autonomic innervation in cardiomyopathic human heart. *Circulation* 1998; **97**: 174–180.

105. Bengel FM, Permanetter B, Ungerer M *et al.* Relationship between altered sympathetic innervation, oxidative metabolism and contractile function in the cardiomyopathic human heart; a non-invasive study using positron emission tomography. *Eur Heart J* 2001; **22**: 1594–1600.

106. Bengel FM, Permanetter B, Ungerer M *et al.* Alterations of the sympathetic nervous system and metabolic performance of the cardiomyopathic heart. *Eur J Nucl Med Mol Imaging* 2002; **29**: 198–202.

107. Pietila M, Malminiemi K, Ukkonen H *et al.* Reduced myocardial carbon-11 hydroxyephedrine retention is associated with poor prognosis in chronic heart failure. *Eur J Nucl Med* 2001; **28**: 373–376.

108. Calkins H, Allman K, Bolling S *et al.* Correlation between scintigraphic evidence of regional sympathetic neuronal dysfunction and ventricular refractoriness in the human heart. *Circulation* 1993; **88**: 172–179.

109. Schafers M, Lerch H, Wichter T *et al.* Cardiac sympathetic innervation in patients with idiopathic right ventricular outflow tract tachycardia. *J Am Coll Cardiol* 1998; **32**: 181–186.

110. Wichter T, Schafers M, Rhodes CG *et al.* Abnormalities of cardiac sympathetic innervation in arrhythmogenic right ventricular cardiomyopathy: Quantitative assessment of presynaptic norepinephrine reuptake and postsynaptic beta-adrenergic receptor density with positron emission tomography. *Circulation* 2000; **101**: 1552–1558.

111. Allman KC, Stevens MJ, Wieland DM *et al.* Non-invasive assessment of cardiac diabetic neuropathy by carbon-11 hydroxyephedrine and positron emission tomography. *J Am Coll Cardiol* 1993; **22**: 1425–1432.

112. Stevens MJ, Dayanikli F, Raffel DM *et al.* Scintigraphic assessment of regionalized defects in myocardial sympathetic innervation and blood flow regulation in diabetic patients with autonomic neuropathy. *J Am Coll Cardiol* 1998; **31**: 1575–1584.

113. Di Carli MF, Bianco-Batlles D, Landa ME *et al.* Effects of autonomic neuropathy on coronary blood flow in patients with diabetes mellitus. *Circulation* 1999; **100**: 813–819.

114. Berding G, Schrader CH, Peschel T *et al.* [N-methyl (11)C]meta-hydroxyephedrine positron emission tomography in Parkinson's disease and multiple system atrophy. *Eur J Nucl Med Mol Imaging* 2003; **30**: 127–131.

115. Li ST, Dendi R, Holmes C *et al.* Progressive loss of cardiac sympathetic innervation in Parkinson's disease. *Ann Neurol* 2002; **52**: 220–223.

116. Goldstein DS, Holmes C, Cannon RO 3rd *et al.* Sympathetic cardioneuropathy in dysautonomias. *N Engl J Med* 1997; **336**: 696–702.

117. Syrota A, Paillotin G, Davy JM *et al.* Kinetics of *in vivo* binding of antagonist to muscarinic cholinergic receptor in the human heart studied by positron emission tomography. *Life Sci* 1984; **35**: 937–945.

118. Syrota A, Comar D, Paillotin G *et al.* Muscarinic cholinergic receptor in the human heart evidenced under physiological conditions by positron emission tomography. *Proc Natl Acad Sci USA* 1985; **82**: 584–588.

119. Merlet P, Delforge J, Syrota A *et al.* Positron emission tomography with 11C CGP-12177 to assess beta-

adrenergic receptor concentration in idiopathic dilated cardiomyopathy. *Circulation* 1993; **87**: 1169–1178.

120. Delahaye N, Le Guludec D, Dinanian S *et al.* Myocardial muscarinic receptor upregulation and normal response to isoproterenol in denervated hearts by familial amyloid polyneuropathy. *Circulation* 2001; **104**: 2911–2916.

121. Le Guludec D, Delforge J, Syrota A *et al. In vivo* quantification of myocardial muscarinic receptors in heart transplant patients. *Circulation* 1994; **90**: 172–178.

122. Le Guludec D, Cohen-Solal A, Delforge J *et al.* Increased myocardial muscarinic receptor density in idiopathic dilated cardiomyopathy: An *in vivo* PET study. *Circulation* 1997; **96**: 3416–3422.

123. Visser TJ, van Waarde A, Jansen TJ *et al.* Stereoselective synthesis and biodistribution of potent [11C]-labeled antagonists for positron emission tomography imaging of muscarinic receptors in the airways. *J Med Chem* 1997; **40**: 117–124.

124. Law MP. Demonstration of the suitability of CGP 12177 for *in vivo* studies of beta-adrenoceptors. *Br J Pharmacol* 1993; **109**: 1101–1109.

125. Delforge J, Syrota A, Lancon JP *et al.* Cardiac beta-adrenergic receptor density measured *in vivo* using PET, CGP 12177, and a new graphical method. *J Nucl Med* 1991; **32**: 739–748.

126. Elsinga PH, van Waarde A, Jaeggi KA *et al.* Synthesis and evaluation of (S)-4-(3-(2′-[11C]isopropylamino)-2-hydroxypropoxy)-2H-benzimidazol-2-one ((S)-[11C]CGP 12388) and (S)-4-(3-((1′-[^{18}F]-fluoroisopropyl)amino)-2-hydroxypropoxy)-2H-benzimidazol-2-one ((S)-[18F]fluoro-CGP 12388) for visualization of beta-adrenoceptors with positron emission tomography. *J Med Chem* 1997; **40**: 3829–3835.

127. Momose M, Reder S, Raffel DM *et al.* Evaluation of cardiac beta-adrenoreceptors in the isolated perfused rat heart using (S)-11C-CGP12388. *J Nucl Med* 2004; **45**: 471–477.

128. Doze P, Elsinga PH, van Waarde A *et al.* Quantification of beta-adrenoceptor density in the human heart with (S)-[11C]CGP 12388 and a tracer kinetic model. *Eur J Nucl Med Mol Imaging* 2002; **29**: 295–304.

129. Law MP, Osman S, Pike VW *et al.* Evaluation of [11C]GB67, a novel radioligand for imaging myocardial alpha 1-adrenoceptors with positron emission tomography. *Eur J Nucl Med* 2000; **27**: 7–17.

130. Van Waarde A, Elsinga PH, Brodde OE *et al.* Myocardial and pulmonary uptake of S-1′-[^{18}F]fluorocarazolol in intact rats reflects radioligand binding to beta-adrenoceptors. *Eur J Pharmacol* 1995; **272**: 159–168.

131. Van Waarde A, Meeder JG, Blanksma PK *et al.* Suitability of CGP-12177 and CGP-26505 for quantitative imaging of beta-adrenoceptors. *Int J Rad Appl Instrum B* 1992; **19**: 711–718.

132. Visser TJ, van der Wouden EA, van Waarde A *et al.* Synthesis and biodistribution of [11C]procaterol, a beta2-adrenoceptor agonist for positron emission tomography. *Appl Radiat Isot* 2000; **52**: 857–863.

133. Riemann B, Schafers M, Law MP *et al.* Radioligands for imaging myocardial alpha- and beta-adrenoceptors. *Nuklearmedizin* 2003; **42**: 4–9.

134. Riemann B, Law MP, Kopka K *et al.* High non-specific binding of the beta(1)-selective radioligand 2-(125)I-ICI-H. *Nuklearmedizin* 2003; **42**: 173–180.

CHAPTER 6

MR angiography: Coronaries and great vessels

Patricia Nguyen & Phillip Yang

Introduction

Non-invasive diagnostic imaging of the coronary arteries and great vessels has been one of the most important clinical goals in cardiovascular medicine. The current gold standard for imaging the coronary arteries and great vessels is invasive angiography. Over one million invasive diagnostic coronary angiograms are performed each year to evaluate coronary artery atherosclerosis, with up to 20% of studies showing no evidence of significant disease [1]. The major limitation of this invasive technique is the associated morbidity and mortality ranging from 0.02 to 0.1% [2]. Similarly, in great vessel MR angiography (GV-MRA), the associated morbidity has relegated invasive angiography to a secondary, confirmatory role [3]. Invasive angiography also requires ionizing radiation and provides only projection images of the lumen. Thus, only limited information is available to determine atherosclerotic plaque burden, vascular function, and three-dimensional anatomical relationships between structures.

Magnetic resonance imaging (MRI) is a promising method for non-invasive imaging of the coronary arteries and great vessels. Submillimeter resolution, exquisite soft tissue contrast, and arbitrary imaging planes are now possible without ionizing radiation [4]. MRI provides flexible imaging capability by combining the chemical sensitivity of nuclear magnetic resonance with high spatial and temporal resolution. The potential of MRI lies in its comprehensive ability to detect physical and chemical processes including flow, motion, morphology, and tissue composition. While the potential of MRI has been at least partially realized in GV-MRA, routine clinical implementation of coronary MR angiography (C-MRA) has not been widespread [5]. Challenges still remain, including scan time, reliability, and robustness of C-MRA. This chapter addresses the challenges facing both C-MRA and GV-MRA by examining the recent technical advances, resultant clinical implementation, and future development.

Challenges

Optimal spatial and temporal resolution, accurate motion compensation, wide anatomical coverage, and high signal and contrast to noise ratios are the inherent challenges in C-MRA [6]. Improvement in one imaging parameter usually occurs at the expense of another. Imaging the coronaries is challenging because of their small size (<4 mm), tortuosity, competing MR signals from adjacent tissues, and the constant dysynchrony between cardiac and respiratory motions [6]. Other factors that have limited clinical application of both C-MRA and GV-MRA, especially in the acute setting, include restricted patient access, need for transportation to the scanner, longer examination time, and the question of adequate cardiac and respiratory monitoring during the scan [7]. New technical developments may facilitate routine application of MRA in the clinical setting.

Technical advances in C-MRA (coronary MRA)

Hardware development
Improvements in the gradient, receiver coil design, and the magnetic field (strength, homogeneity and capability) have been critical in C-MRA.

A major advance has been the development of high performance gradient systems. Higher peak gradient strength and slew rate have enabled imaging with higher temporal and spatial resolution [8]. In spiral C-MRA, for example earlier gradient systems (amplitude 10 mT/m with a slew rate of 16 mT/m /ms) have yielded a spatial resolution of 1.1–1.3 mm [9]; whereas, the newer high performance gradient system (amplitude 40 mT/m with a slew rate of 150 mT/m/ms) have yielded a resolution in the range of 0.5–0.6 mm [10]. The latest high performance gradient system can reach an amplitude of 45 mT/m with a slew rate of 200 mT/m/ms.

Another area of recent innovation is receiver coil design. Fayad *et al.* [11] developed a load-optimized phased array coil with the ability to selectively image the area of interest, minimizing noise volume and eliminating the need for coil repositioning. Using various configurations of coil shape, size, and quantity may enhance signal-to-noise ratio (SNR) and ease of use [12]. A study using a planar array of two smaller four inch coils dedicated to C-MRA enabled real time (RT) coil selection for the target coronary and resulted in higher SNR in the distal and posterior vessels, as shown in Fig. 6.1 [13]. The use of cylindrical arrays as opposed to planar arrays may provide additional gains in SNR [14]. More recently, several groups have utilized multi-channel coil arrays to achieve higher SNR in parallel imaging [15].

Imaging at higher fields has also improved SNR although the gains are not directly proportional to increases in field strength [16]. Imaging at higher fields also presents new technical challenges. The readout duration is limited by larger susceptibility effects, leading to off-resonance blurring [17, 18]. RF pulses and TE need to be shortened to improve both flow characteristics and T_2 signal loss [19, 20]. Slice profile may worsen, leading to partial volume effect. Magnetic field inhomogeneity could also lead to significant difficulties depending on the imaging sequence. Imaging parameters, including timing and flip angles, need to be adjusted [21].

Despite these technical challenges, high field imaging holds promise. Multiple imaging techniques for C-MRA have been successfully implemented at 3 Tesla [22]. Feasibility was first demonstrated using a 3D-segmented gradient echo (GRE) with respiratory navigator, yielding an in-plane resolution

of 0.7–1.0 mm and an average time per scan of seven minutes [23]. Despite the sensitivity of spiral imaging to off-resonance and field inhomogeneity, a recent comparison of spiral GRE C-MRA at 1.5 and 3 T showed a significant improvement in overall SNR, contrast-to-noise ratio (CNR), and image quality of the coronary anatomy at 3 T [22]. Comparative 1.5 T vs 3 T images are shown in Fig. 6.2 [22].

Software development

Significant improvement in MRA has also resulted from the development of motion compensation techniques, pulse sequences, k-space acquisition strategies, and methods to enhance CNR. Sequence implementation has been performed in 2D as well as 3D. More recent innovations, including parallel and real time imaging, have led to further enhancement of MRA.

Motion compensation techniques

New techniques for motion compensation have been developed which may improve image quality and scan efficiency. Accurate cardiac and respiratory gating is critical for coronary MRA. Cardiac gating, as well as patient monitoring, requires precise ECG triggering which can be challenging in the MR environment. Gating via vector ECG that uses multiple ECG channels simultaneously to reconstruct a vector cardiogram may minimize MR-related artifacts [24].

Respiratory motion compensation has also evolved from simple breath-hold, which is adequate for 2D implementation, to more complex free-breathing and navigator-echo techniques, necessary for the prolonged data acquisition time in 3D implementation. As early as 1993, a free-breathing method using averages of multiple acquisitions was developed, enabling acquisition of a thick volume [25]. The development of navigator sequences followed, whereby consistency of heart position can be monitored during scan acquisition [26, 27]. The positional data can correct the raw data during image reconstruction. Another approach uses the diminished variance algorithm (DVA) [28], which analyzes the histogram of the respiratory positions from a complete set of data and then reacquires the data from the most consistent locations. The data obtained during the breath-hold can be used

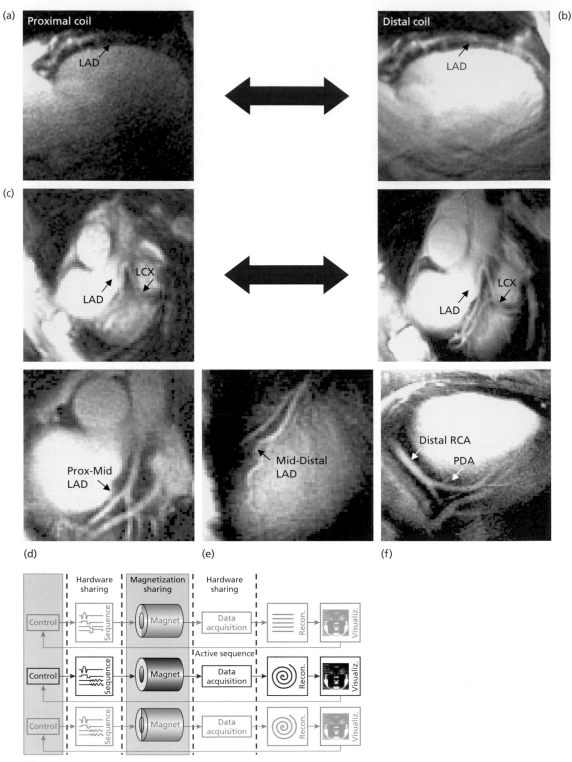

Fig. 6.1 (a) Real time images of the left anterior descending artery (LAD) and left circumflex artery (LCX) demonstrating dynamic selection of proximal (a) and distal coils (b), as well as, dynamic optimization of scan plane localization during breath-hold (c). High resolution images of the proximal– mid LAD (d), mid-distal LAD (e) and distal right coronary artery (RCA) and posterior descending artery (PDA) (f). (g) Structure of the adaptive real time architecture that enables dynamic selection of different pulse sequences and coils.

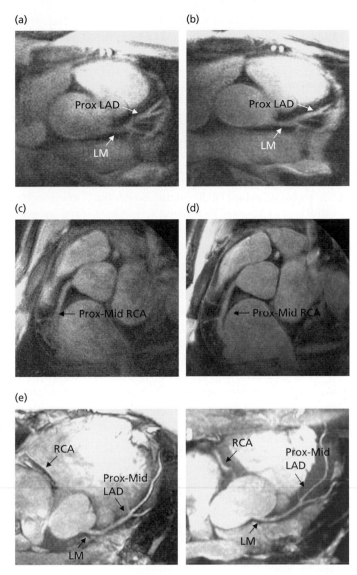

Fig. 6.2 Comparative images of the left main (LM) and left anterior descending artery (LAD) at 1.5 T (a) and 3 T (b) and the right coronary artery (RCA) at 1.5 T (c) and 3 T (d) using 2D breath-hold spiral gradient echo (GRE). (e) Comparative images of the LAD using 3D breath-hold steady state free precession (SSFP). Higher signal-to-noise ratio (SNR) and anatomic coverage was achieved at 3 T. (Figure reproduced courtesy of: Reference 22, Yang PC, Nguyen P, Shimakawa A *et al.* Spiral MR coronary angiography at 1.5 T and 3 T—clinical comparisons. *J Cardiovasc Magn Reson* 2004; **6**: 877–884, and V. S. Deshpande, Northwestern University, Chicago.)

to update free-breathing data accordingly. Other methods to compensate for respiratory motion include retrospective or prospective sorting of the images to accept images acquired within a certain gating window (±3–5 mm) [29–31]. These advanced methods, designed to improve patient comfort and compliance have not, however, consistently preserved the image quality [32, 33].

More recently, a novel approach for both cardiac and respiratory gating has been developed. Larson *et al.* [34] introduced a promising new approach called self gating that may make ECG gating, breath-holding and navigator techniques obsolete. In self gating, motion synchronization signal is extracted directly from the same MR signals used for image reconstruction, making ECG gating unnecessary. A study in seven volunteers showed no significant difference in image quality of cine MR obtained by self gating and conventional ECG gating techniques. In addition, self gating can eliminate the need for breath-holding and navigator techniques [34]. Using self gating, low resolution images are acquired during the free-breathing acquisition and are then compared to target expiration images. Only raw data-producing images with high correlation to the target images are included in the final high resolution reconstruction. The self gating technique produced no significant differences in image quality compared to breath-held techniques [35]; however, demonstration in C-MRA has not yet been published.

Pulse sequence design

Pulse sequence design has evolved from black blood, spine echo (SE) sequences to bright blood sequences such as GRE and steady state free precession (SSFP). The SE sequence generates images in which blood pool appears dark relative to surrounding soft tissue such as the myocardium [36]. In SE, an initial pulse (TE 20–30 ms) excites the sensitive proton, followed by a second T_2-weighted refocusing pulse (TE 50–90 ms) to produce a coherent signal [37]. Implementation of SE for C-MRA began in the 1980s but was met with limited success. Although SE was occasionally successful imaging the coronary ostia, reliable assessment of anomalous vessels or atherosclerosis was not feasible. In an early study by Lieberman *et al.* [38], ECG gated SE could visualize portions of the native coronary arteries in only 30% of 23 subjects. In a similar study, Paulin *et al.* [39] visualized the origin of the left main coronary artery in all six subjects while only 67% of the right coronary ostia were seen.

Improved visualization with a shorter acquisition can be achieved with fast SE. In fast SE, a long train of echoes is acquired by using a series of 180° RF pulses [40]. A superior black blood effect can be achieved by applying pre-inversion pulses (additional RF pulses outside the plane used to suppress signal of inflowing blood and to nullify the blood signal) [41]. In 1991, Wang *et al.* [42] adopted a fast, breath-hold inversion recovery technique for C-MRA that overcame the respiratory artifacts associated with previous attempts at coronary imaging. Multiple phase encodes per cardiac cycle and incremental flip angle compensated for spin saturation. Successful imaging of the left anterior descending and diagonal branches were achieved. Adding a second prepulse to null the fat signal (dual inversion) has resulted in higher SNR, CNR and spatial resolution [43]. Ten years later, Stuber *et al.* [44] developed a fast, dual inversion, navigator-gated SE sequence with 400 mm in-plane resolution for C-MRA as shown in Fig. 6.3.

In contrast to the SE and dual inversion FSE sequences, the GRE sequence produces an increased signal intensity of blood pool (bright blood). The bright blood signal on GRE images results from

(a)

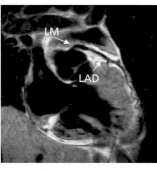

(b)

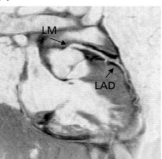

(c)

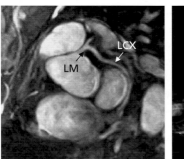

(d)

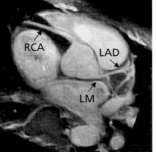

Fig. 6.3 Sample images using different pulse sequences: (a) 3D double oblique free-breathing dual inversion fast spin echo, black-blood coronary MRA of a left coronary system in a healthy subject reformatted in the original data set. The same image data are displayed video inverted (b). The figure shows the left main coronary artery (LM) and the left anterior descending artery (LAD). (c) Breath-hold 3D steady state free precession (SSFP) of the left circumflex (LCX). Breath-hold 3D gradient echo (GRE) with segmented k-space localization and echo-plantar imaging (EPI) acquisition using volume coronary angiography with targeted scans (VCATS) of the left main (LM), left anterior descending artery (LAD) and right coronary artery (RCA) (d). (Figure reproduced courtesy of: Reference 44, Stuber M, Botnar R, Spuentrup E *et al.* Three-dimensional high resolution fast spin echo coronary magnetic resonance angiography. *Magn Reson Med* 2001; **45**: 206–211, and T. Martin and T. Foo, Oklahoma Heart Institute, Tulsa, OK, and P Wielopolski, University Hospital, Rotterdam, The Netherlands.)

flow related enhancement obtained by applying RF pulses to saturate a volume of tissue. With a short TR (20–40 ms) and a low flip angle, maximal signal is emitted by inflowing blood [45, 46]. The first robust approach to C-MRA utilized GRE, initially described in an isolated heart and an *in vivo* animal model by Burstein *et al.* [47] and subsequently in humans by Edelman *et al.* [48]. Currently, GRE is the chosen acquisition scheme in the vast majority of reported C-MRA studies [25, 49–55].

A second bright blood technique, SSFP [56], achieves high tissue contrast yet maintains high temporal resolution. Unlike GRE, SSFP does not depend on the inflow of unsaturated spins or blood to produce contrast; thus, the signal loss associated with slow flow, resulting from saturation effects common in GRE, does not occur with SSFP [37]. SSFP enhances the contrast between blood and myocardium through preservation of both longitudinal and transverse magnetizations by refocusing the gradients in all three axes [57]. The steady state achieved by the magnetization provides high quality images using both T_1 and T_2 relaxation times [58, 59].

The concept of SSFP was proposed years ago [56], but the technique was extremely sensitive to field inhomogeneities and, thus, not applicable to cardiac imaging [60]. With recent improvement in gradient capabilities, short TRs on the order of 3–4 ms have been achieved. Combined with improved field capabilities, SSFP has become practical for cardiac imaging. Deshpande *et al.* [60] first demonstrated increase in SNR (55%), CNR (178%) and anatomical coverage using 3D-SSFP compared to 3D-GRE in volunteers. Several modifications to the original sequence have been made to improve image quality, including addition of intrinsic/extrinsic contrast [61, 62], asymmetric sampling (gradient echo occurs before the center of the readout period) [63], and parallel imaging [64].

K-space acquisition

In an effort to improve scan efficiency, k-space acquisition strategies have evolved from rectilinear segmented k-space to more complex echo planar and spiral imaging [9, 65].

Over the last decade, rectilinear segmented k-space imaging has dominated C-MRA [42, 48]. In rectilinear segmented k-space, multiple phase encoding steps are acquired during the cardiac cycle. Suc-

cessful visualization of native coronary arteries has been demonstrated in numerous studies using 2D-segmented k-space [25, 49–55]. However, limited anatomical coverage was shown using this technique.

Echo-planar imaging (EPI) was developed over two decades ago to improve scan efficiency [66]. Instead of acquiring multiple segmented k-space lines per cardiac cycle, EPI acquires the complete data sets to rapidly form a complete image within 30–40 ms; however, flow and susceptibility phase errors can severely degrade image quality [65]. With the introduction of segmented EPI [36], these phase errors are minimized. For fast breath-hold [67–69] or free-breathing 3D C-MRA [70], two to four excitation pulses are followed by a short EPI readout train, thus, taking advantage of the EPI speed while keeping the echo and acquisition time short to minimize artifacts related to flow and motion [37]. Feasibility of 3D-segmented EPI was first demonstrated by Wielopolski *et al.* [67]. More recently, successful implementation of 3D EPI with 3D-segmented k-space using prospective navigator (Fig. 6.3) [71], GRE using volume coronary angiography with targeted scans [72], and inversion recovery with extrinsic contrast enhancement, [73] has been shown.

Variations of the original EPI approach may have great potential in cardiovascular applications. Interleaved or multishot EPI significantly reduces image artifacts by employing several echoes to cover the data space [36]. Other techniques to more efficiently cover data space and reduce flow artifacts include "partial flyback" and "inside-out" EPI [74]. In "partial flyback" EPI, only the even echoes near the center of k-space are used, reducing artifacts arising from flow in the readout direction. In "inside-out" EPI, data collection begins at the center of k-space, with separate interleaves to acquire the top and bottom halves of k-space, reducing artifacts arising from flow in the phase encoding region. A combination of "partial flyback" and "inside-out" with partial Fourier EPI demonstrates better flow properties and does not require partial k-space reconstruction [74].

Another k-space acquisition strategy for rapid imaging is the spiral acquisition technique adapted to C-MRA by Meyer *et al.* in 1992 [9]. This non-Cartesian acquisition technique generates images by sampling the data space from the center and

(a)

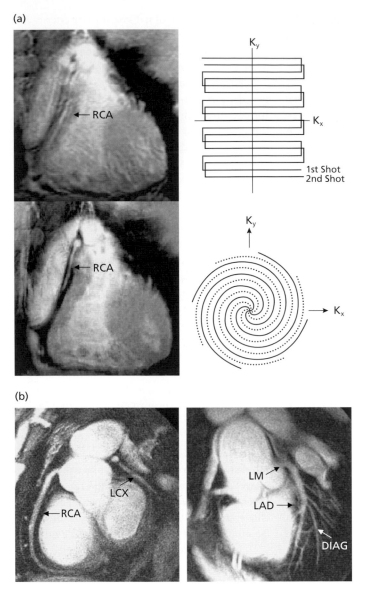

(b)

Fig. 6.4 (a) Coronary MRA of the right coronary artery (RCA) using echo planar imaging and spiral gradient echo (GRE). (b) Two-dimensional breath-hold spiral GRE images of the RCA and the left circumflex (LCX) (left) and left main (LM), left anterior descending artery (LAD) and diagonals (DIAG) (right). (Figure reproduced courtesy of C. Meyer, Stanford University.)

spiraling outward, providing several advantages [65]. Image artifacts are reduced because of lower sensitivity to flow which results from using a short TE [9]. In comparison to EPI, spirals are less sensitive to flow-dependent phase shifts [75]. In addition, spirals achieve higher SNR because fewer excitations per heartbeat are required, allowing application of larger flip angles [9, 76]. Data space coverage of EPI and spiral acquisition techniques with comparative images of the right coronary artery using identical GRE pulse sequence are depicted in Fig. 6.4. Spirals also provide more efficient k-space coverage, resulting in shorter acquisition

time [76]. Thus, blurring from coronary artery motion, often seen in segmented k-space strategies, is reduced. Improved spatial resolution is obtained through full k-space coverage instead of partial k-space coverage as used in the segmented approach. Meyer *et al.* [9] achieved a spatial resolution of 0.5×0.5 mm^2 with an acquisition time of 37 ms using spiral acquisition, compared to a spatial resolution of $1.4–1.9 \times 0.9$ mm with an acquisition time of 78 to 104 ms using 2D segmented GRE [6]. Several studies have confirmed improved temporal and spatial resolution in C-MRA using the spiral k-space acquisitions [76–79]. In 1997, Hu *et al.* introduced a multislice 2D spiral acquisition sequence which imaged 5–15 slices with 3–5 cm in thickness while maintaining acquisition time of 37 ms per slice during a single breath-hold [10, 80]. Sample images using the 2D breath-hold spiral GRE technique with real time localization are shown in Fig. 6.4. However, spiral imaging has its drawbacks, namely, sensitivity to off peak resonance, field inhomogeneity and susceptibility artifacts [76–78].

Intrinsic/extrinsic contrast agents

Both intrinsic and extrinsic contrast agents have been used to differentiate blood and surrounding tissue (myocardial fat and myocardium). The intrinsic contrast between coronary blood pool and surrounding tissue can be altered by using the effect of inflowing blood or by application of prepulses [37]. Because most epicardial arteries are surrounded by fat, fat must be suppressed for coronary visualization. Selective fat suppression is performed using a fat saturation prepulse [25, 49] or a spectral spatial RF pulse [81]. Because fat has a relatively short T_1 with a resultant signal intensity similar to flowing blood, frequency selective fat saturation prepulses are used to minimize fat signal and, thus, allow coronary visualization [25, 49]. Spectral spatial pulse, used in spiral acquisitions, suppresses fat by selectively exciting water [82].

Coronaries are also close to myocardium. T_1 relaxation times between blood and myocardium are similar [37]. Muscle suppression employing magnetization transfer (MT) [25, 81] and T_2 preparation (T_2 prep) improve intrinsic contrast [75, 83]. In magnetization transfer saturation, an off resonance RF pulse is used to saturate bound protons, which in turn, transfer their magnetization to mobile protons in the muscle, thus reducing the signal strength of muscle. Short MT pulses, however, do not affect flowing blood [81]. Li *et al.* [25] adopted this technique in 3D imaging. Improved MT pulse designs using the Shinnar-Le Roux algorithm, adiabatic pulses and off resonance spectral spatial pulses are under investigation [84–86]. Another intrinsic contrast mechanism, T_2 prep, induces T_2-weighted imaging using a train of refocusing 180° excitations. Brittain *et al.* [75] developed and demonstrated this contrast mechanism for coronary imaging. Successful implementation by Botnar *et al.* [55] followed, as shown in Fig. 6.5. Additional RF pulse design work to enhance CNR from T_2 prep has been ongoing,

and has included shorter duration, paired adiabatic pulses, and selective excitation [87]. One shortcoming of intrinsic contrast mechanisms, however, is the compromise in SNR in higher resolution images.

Extrinsic contrast agents may alleviate some of the problems of reduced SNR. The T_1 shortening effects of the agents enhance contrast without significant signal loss. Several sequences have demonstrated significantly improved CNR using gadolinium agents [62, 88] [73, 89, 90]. Gadolinium, however, is an extravascular contrast agent and quickly diffuses into the intracellular space, limiting its clinical utility in C-MRA. Several intravascular pooling agents which have undergone clinical trials include MS-325 (Angiomark: EPIX medical, Cambridge, MA), NC100150 (Clariscan: Nycomed-Amersham, Buckingshire, UK), and B-22956/1 Bracco Imaging Spa, Milano, Italy). While only phase I and II trial results are available, significant improvement in CNR has been observed [71, 91–93], as demonstrated in Fig. 6.5. These agents can also be applied to inversion pulse and/or myocardial nulling sequences and may enable fluoroscopic, projectional imaging of the coronaries if complete myocardial suppression is achieved.

Two-dimensional and three-dimensional imaging

Both bright and black blood techniques may be implemented in 2D and 3D. In 2D techniques, a series of thin, overlapping slices (<2 mm) are obtained sequentially. This technique provides strong blood to background signal in conditions of slow flow. Although 2D techniques are easy to implement, several limitations, including partial volume effects, poor overall SNR, slice mis-registration, and long scan times, exist which can result in image blurring and inadequate coverage of the coronary tree [6].

These limitations, particularly slice misregistration, can be resolved by using 3D [25, 55, 94] or 2D multislice acquisitions [10]. In 3D imaging, a complete volume or single slab is acquired [95] which is then divided into very thin partitions using a second phase encoding gradient. The partitions are reconstructed with slice thickness equal or less than 1 mm, finer than 2D techniques. The 3D technique is effective for relatively fast flow, because blood can be pulsed several times and lose its signal before it traverses the width of the slab [95],

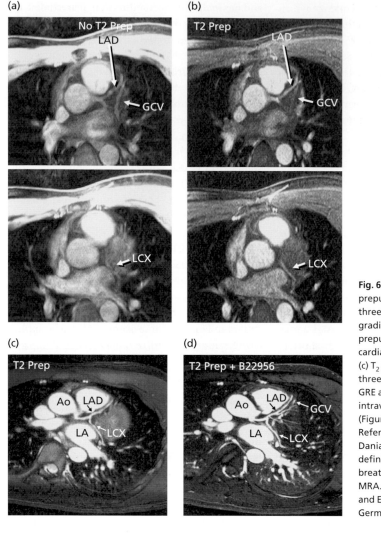

Fig. 6.5 (a) Baseline images and T₂ prepulse enhanced images (b) using a three-dimensional, free-breathing gradient echo (GRE) sequence. T₂ prepulse suppresses signal from the cardiac muscle as well as skeletal muscle. (c) T₂ prep enhanced images using a three-dimensional free-breathing GRE and after administration of an intravascular contrast agent, B22956 (d). (Figure reproduced courtesy of: Reference 55, Botnar R, Stuber M, Danias P *et al.* Improved coronary artery definition with T₂-weighted, free-breathing, three-dimensional coronary MRA. *Circulation* 1999; **99**: 3139–3148, and E. Nagel and I. Paetsch, Cardiology, German Heart Institute, Berlin.)

allowing for extended coverage of anatomical structures, improved SNR, isotropic spatial resolution, and a variety of postprocessing techniques. Small voxels and short TE, which reduce flow and phase dispersion artifacts, are most easily obtained in 3D imaging techniques [95]. Operator dependence is also diminished [37]. Three-dimensional techniques, however, usually result in reduced contrast and require prolonged acquisition, much longer than any patient can hold their breath [37, 96].

These hurdles were removed with the application of suppression pulses and free-breathing navigator techniques, and the recent development of volume coronary angiography with targeted scans (VCATS), which resulted in a widespread adoption of 3D-acquisition techniques [37]. Three-dimen-sional implementation began as early as 1993 when a free-breathing method using averages of multiple acquisitions enabled Li *et al.* [25] to image a 64 mm thick volume using fat saturation and MT. Initial implementation, however, suffered from poor contrast between blood and myocardium. Botnar *et al.* [55] then used T₂ prep to shorten the acquisition window and achieved improved contrast and coronary delineation. Stuber *et al.* [97] then successfully combined a 3D-segmented k-space and EPI acquisition technique with prospective navigator gating to reduce the long acquisition time associated with traditional 3D techniques.

More recently, Wielopolski *et al.* [68] attained high spatial (0.7 × 1 mm) and temporal resolution (38–70 ms acquisition time) using a 3D breath-hold VCATS and segmented EPI with localization by segmented GRE. In this technique a breath-hold 3D-scout data set is loaded into a multiplanar platform to plan subsequent oblique VCATS images of individual coronary segments. Although this approach has lower spatial resolution than free-breathing segmented GRE and acquires data during a longer period from each RR interval, major coronary segments can be acquired in fewer than 13 breath-holds [68], as shown in Fig. 6.3. Comparable results were obtained by Deshpande *et al.* [60] using 3D VCATS and SSFP (spatial resolution 1.7 × 1 mm; acquisition time of 95 ms). In addition to the 3D volume techniques, a different approach, utilizing 2D multislice, was developed using spiral acquisition by Hu *et al.* [10].

Advanced methods

Despite many advances over the past decades, SNR and the speed of data acquisition remain limited. To overcome these limitations, a number of novel strategies have been developed including real time and parallel imaging.

Real time imaging was developed from a rapid acquisition method using EPI [98]. Real time imaging enables continuous image acquisition at high frame rates, providing valuable insights into cardiovascular dynamics and eliminating the need for respiratory and cardiac gating. Data acquisition techniques such as wavelet encoding, sliding reconstruction windows [5], and innovative k-space acquisition techniques [9, 67] have facilitated rapid data acquisition, thereby, allowing frame rates up to 12 frames per sec at 2.0 mm resolution [99]. A clinically robust, reliable RT system has been developed which enables interactive selection of scan planes and provides RT image reconstruction and display for instantaneous image-based feedback [100]. The rapid access to raw data and direct control of reconstruction and display generate interactive images with lag-time of less than 500 ms. Real time localization to acquire high resolution coronary images has been successfully demonstrated [80, 101, 102].

Another innovative RT approach is the implementation of C-MRA using the adaptive RT architecture [103]. This integrated system dynamically reconfigures pulse sequences on a per-acquisition basis and switches between the coil elements in the phased arrays in real time. The conventional MR scanners consist of sequencers that proceed through each acquisition based on downloaded waveforms and timing commands. Utilizing a modern PC, a sequencer that is capable of running selected parameters of different pulse sequences simultaneously has been designed. Utilizing this system, the operator can switch dynamically between spiral real time localization and high resolution imaging in 39 ms, which allows adjustment of scan planes to optimize high resolution image acquisition, as shown in Fig. 6.1. [102]. In addition to RT localization, high resolution RT C-MRA has been achieved at 3T with a spatial resolution of 1.25 mm^2 and a temporal resolution of 190 ms [21, 104].

Another novel approach is parallel imaging, first introduced in 1997 to increase temporal resolution. The two most common parallel imaging methods are simultaneous acquisition of spatial harmonics (SMASH) [104, 105] and spatial sensitivity encoding (SENSE) [106]. These techniques accelerate image acquisition by factors of 2–3 by using spatial encoding information from sensitivity maps of multiple coil arrays, thereby, allowing partial k-space sampling [37]. The remaining lines of k-space are reconstructed using the sensitivity information from individual coil elements. Parallel image encoding can be combined with common MRA approaches [64, 107–109]. The gain in imaging speed may be used for larger volume acquisition without longer acquisition time, resulting in greater anatomic coverage [64, 108]. Parallel imaging has also been combined with RT to increase frame rate [110].

The potential disadvantages of parallel encoding include extended computation power, requirement for prescanning, reduced SNR, and potential artifacts in reconstruction. The SNR reduction is more critical for coronary imaging, given its lower scanning efficiency and need for high resolution, thus potentially limiting its application for C-MRA. Although feasibility was initially demonstrated at 1.5 T, preliminary results have not been satisfactory despite a reported 50% reduction in acquisition time [109, 111]. More encouraging results have been seen at 3 T by Huber *et al.* [112] who demonstrated a two-fold decrease in acquisition time while maintaining equivalent SNR and image quality using 3D navigator-gated segmented GRE. The use of intravascular contrast agents has also improved anatomic coverage in parallel imaging although the loss of SNR and CNR is not fully recovered [113].

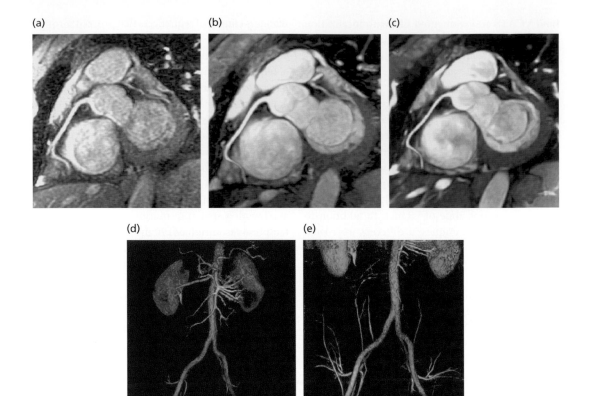

(a)   (b)   (c)

(d)   (e)

Fig. 6.6 Comparison of breath held 3D fiesta images of the right coronary artery (RCA) using 4 channel (a), 8 channel (20% increase in signal-to-noise, ratio (SNR)) (b) and 32 channel parallel imaging arrays (40% increase in SNR) (c). With parallel imaging, the distal RCA is better visualized. (d) Contrast enhanced MRA with parallel imaging of the abdominal aorta in a 22 second breath-hold with spatial resolution of $1.7 \times 1.7 \times 2.2$ mm and acceleration factor of 12. Result corresponding to arterial phase Zoomed view of subsequent acquisition (e). (Figure reproduced courtesy of: Reference 108, Niendorf T, Sodickson D, Hardy CJ *et al*. Towards whole heart coverage in a single breath-hold coronary artery imaging using a true 32 channel phased array MR system. In: Proceedings of the International Society of Magnetic Resonance in Medicine, 12th Annual Scientific Meeting, 2004, Kyoto, Japan, and reference 115, Zhu Y, Hardy CJ, Sodickson DK *et al*. Highly parallel volumetric imaging with a 32-element RF coil array. *Magn Reson Med* 2004; **52**: 869–879.)

Several investigators have recently demonstrated the utility of multi-element array coils with a high intrinsic SNR and spatial encoding capability [114, 115]. A preliminary study by Niendorf *et al.* [108] achieved higher SNR and greater anatomic coverage using a four and eight multichannel array compared to a 32 channel array with the same acquisition time, as shown in Fig. 6.6.

Another potential disadvantage for parallel imaging is the need for a separate scan to determine coil sensitivities. Because coronaries move within the heart, separate coil sensitivities scans can lead to misregistration between the coil and cardiac breath-hold positions, which results in residual aliasing artifacts and random noise in the reconstructed images [64]. Implementation of autocalibration methods such as AUTO-SMASH [116] and generalized autocalibrating partially parallel acquisition (GRAPPA) [117] can enhance spatial resolution by reducing aliasing artifacts. GRAPPA reconstruction provides improved coronary artery definition with up to $0.7–1.0 \times 0.7$ mm in-plane resolution with acceptable artifact suppression and SNR. The use of segmented k-space coil calibration with variable density sampling enables coverage of almost twice the area of k-space along the phase encoding direction compared to that obtained in a conventional 3D breath-hold acquisition [64]. Self calibrating

Table 6.1 MRA methods.

Pulse sequences	
Bright blood	Black blood
Gradient recalled echo	spin echo
Steady state free precession	double inversion recovery
Acquisition strategies	
Contrast enhanced MRA	
Coverage of k-space	
Segmented k-space	
Echo planar imaging	
Spiral acquisition	
2D and 3D acquisitions	
Parallel imaging	
SENSE	
SMASH	
Real time imaging	

parallel imaging has also been performed with non-Cartesian k-space sampling [107].

Comparison studies

A summary of the various techniques developed for C-MRA is shown in Table 6.1. Unfortunately, little information is available regarding the comparative evaluation of MRA techniques in the same subjects. Results from a recent study [118] of six free-breathing, 3D, magnetization prepared sequences has found that the optimal sequence was the Cartesian SSFP followed by the spiral GRE (two shots per heartbeat) and the radial SSFP in terms of visible vessel length and SNR and CNR. Evaluation, however, was performed only in the right coronary artery. The most optimal sequence for C-MRA is yet to be determined.

Technical strategies specific to GV-MRA

Several techniques previously described for C-MRA are also applied in GV-MRA, including the traditional SE and GRE and the more advanced RT and parallel imaging techniques. Unlike for C-MRA where the application of SE is limited, conventional T_1-weighted SE has been the mainstay for great vessel imaging because it provides the best anatomic detail of the great vessel wall [7, 119]. The advent of fast SE has enabled the implementation of T_2-weighted imaging, which may be useful in tissue characterization of the great vessel wall and blood components [7].

In GV-MRA, additional diagnostic information can be provided by cine GRE [120, 121], which displays laminar-moving blood as a bright signal in contrast to stationary tissues [7]. Signal reduction [122, 123] and signal voids [124] suggest anomalous flow disturbance and are associated with specific pathology. One major limitation of cine GRE, however, was a relatively lengthy imaging time per slice location compared with ECG-gated SE [125]. The typical imaging time for images with a 256×128 matrix with conventional cine GRE is 4–5 min (256 heartbeats). Performing cine GRE became more practical with the advent of fast cine GRE with k-space segmentation [46]; imaging time was reduced from 4–5 min to fewer than 16 s and flow and respiratory artifacts were minimized [126].

Additional techniques to reduce scan time, namely RT and parallel imaging, have been recently applied in GV-MRA. Real time application in GV-MRA, however, has been limited. In a recent case series, successful visualization of the aortic arch and extracardiac shunts was demonstrated using real time color flow imaging [127]. More recently, parallel imaging has been applied to GV-MRA to visualize the abdomen [128, 129] and thoracic vasculature [130]. In order to offset the acquisition and reconstruction related SNR losses associated with parallel imaging, several investigators have demonstrated the utility of multi-element array coils with a high intrinsic SNR and spatial encoding capability for GV-MRA [114, 115]. Zhu *et al.* [115] demonstrated successful MRA of the abdominal aorta with up to 16 fold acceleration using a 32 element array, shown in Fig. 6.6. Recent studies have also demonstrated improvement in image quality and acquisition speed with view sharing compared to without view sharing, as shown in Fig. 6.7 [130].

In addition to the techniques common to both C-MRA and GV-MRA, there are several strategies specific to GV-MRA, including multiple overlapping thin slab acquisition (MOTSA), gadolinium-enhanced MRA associated with unique timing techniques, and projectional imaging. Like sequences for C-MRA, GV-MRA techniques can be implemented in 2D or 3D, usually bright blood techniques more commonly referred to as time of flight (TOF). In

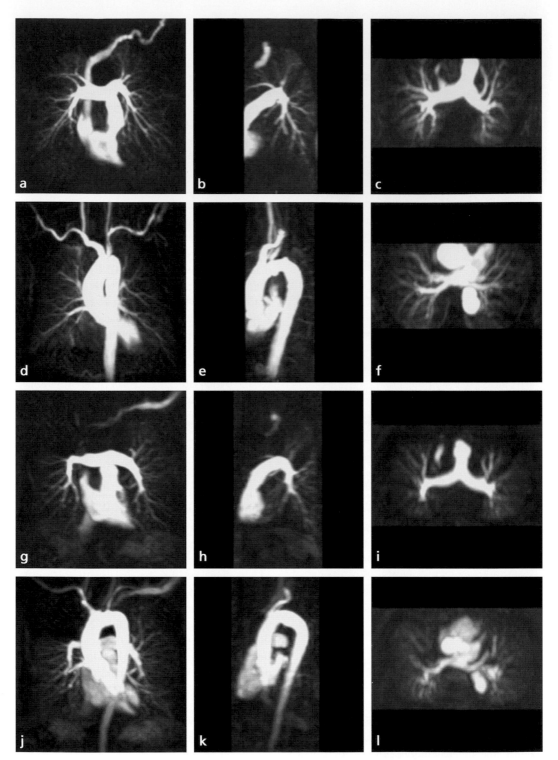

Fig. 6.7 Maximum intensity projections (MIP) of time-resolved MRA acquired with parallel imaging with view sharing (a–f) and conventional parallel-MRA protocol (g–l). MIPs were reconstructed from data sets with a peak-enhancement of the pulmonary artery (a–c; g–i) and aorta (d–f; j–l). Because of the better spatial resolution, images acquired with the parallel imaging with view sharing show a much sharper delineation of the vascular structures. (Figure reproduced courtesy of: Reference 130, Fink C, Ley S, Kroeker R *et al.* Time-resolved contrast-enhanced three-dimensional magnetic resonance angiography of the chest: combination of parallel imaging with view sharing (TREAT). *Invest Radiol* 2005; **40**: 40–48.)

order to provide better flow enhancement than single slab 3D techniques and less dephasing than 2D techniques, while maintaining high resolution [132], Parker *et al.* [133] developed MOTSA, a hybrid of 2D and 3D techniques. In MOTSA, multiple thin 3D slabs are placed orthogonal to the direction of flow and acquired sequentially, as in 2D TOF. Because the slabs are relatively thin, blood can travel through the volume and the signal can be refreshed between RF pulses, resulting in better retention of signal in distal vessels [7, 95]. MOTSA, however, has a number of drawbacks. First, to avoid bands of signal loss at the slab edges where the RF profile trails off, consecutive slabs are overlapped, which increases total scan time. Another disadvantage is that patient motion occurring between slab acquisitions is seen as discontinuity of the luminal edge that can be mistaken for stenosis. Moreover, signal intensity variations within the individual slabs because of saturation effects can cause a "venetian blind" artifact [95].

Instead of relying on blood flow, contrast enhanced MRA (CE-MRA) utilizes gadolinium to create intravascular signal and increase blood signal within the vessel lumen [134–136]. Because imaging is completed within a single breath-hold, CE-MRA eliminates artifacts due to cardiac pulsations and respiration and is more sensitive to in-plane flow, enabling more accurate detection of stenosis [137–139]. In CE-MRA, however, correct timing of injection is important to ensure synchronization between the transit of contrast material and scanning because gadolinium quickly diffuses into the intracellular space [140]. Accurate timing can be achieved by [141] estimating transit time, applying a small test bolus, and using an automated detection of contrast bolus passage or MR fluoroscopy to observe contrast bolus passage [142].

Because distinction between arteries and veins continues to be a challenge in GV-MRA, several innovative strategies have been recently developed to differentiate arterial and venous circulation in 3D CE-MRA, including novel k-space acquisition techniques and ultrafast imaging techniques [95]. Ideally in CE-MRA, the maximal arterial contrast enhancement should coincide with the acquisition of the center of k-space, which contains low spatial frequency information and controls image contrast [141, 142]. In current sequences, the centerlines are

acquired at the midpoint of the acquisition period [143, 144], thus timing of contrast injection can be challenging [142]. A new technique consists of applying a centric phased [145] or an elliptical centric encoding [146, 147] where the lower spatial frequencies are acquired first, during the arterial phase of the contrast enhancement. This provides efficient venous signal suppression when the sequence is manually or automatically triggered at the arrival of contrast material, lessening motion artifact and venous contamination; however, poor timing of contrast injection may be more common.

In addition to novel k-space acquisition strategies, ultrafast imaging techniques, including the time resolved imaging of contrast kinetics (TRICKS) [148], have been developed to differentiate arterial and venous circulation. TRICKS [141, 149] involves sampling low spatial frequency information more frequently than high spatial information to create a 3D data set with the desired temporal window. This allows depiction of the passage of contrast agent, first through arteries then though the veins, similar to x-ray angiography. With this technique, only the center of k-space is acquired every 2–8 s, with the periphery interpolated between consecutive time frames. A precise timing strategy is not needed because the image is updated every 2–8 s. However, depending on the magnitude of undersampling of the peripheral data, the temporal resolution of the edge information may be compromised, resulting in artifacts at the edges of enhancing vessels [150].

Another interesting approach, commonly referred to as time resolved CE-MRA, involves acquiring multiple 2D or 3D data sets using an ultrafast sequence with a temporal resolution between 0.3–0.5 s [151, 152]. Using this method, synchronization between data collection and contrast material injection is not required because the vessels are imaged during different stages of the passage of contrast medium. The main disadvantage of this technique is poorer spatial resolution, which is inadequate for the visualization of small arteries such as the vertebrals [151–153]. Recently, time resolved MRA has been combined with parallel imaging with impressive results, as shown in Fig. 6.7 [130].

The final technique unique to GV-MRA is projection imaging. Although rarely used in C-MRA, projection imaging is standard for GV-MRA. Postprocessing reconstruction techniques [154], such as the maximum intensity projection (MIP) algorithm [95], have enabled display of blood vessels in a projective format similar to x-ray angiography. With the MIP algorithm, the brightest pixels along a user defined direction are extracted to create a projection image. The quality of the MIP can be greatly improved by reduction of pixel size and suppression of signal from stationary tissues, especially in areas of poor flow contrast, (i.e. the edges of blood vessels and small vessels with slow flow) which may be obscured by brighter stationary tissue [155]. Postprocessing can now be performed while the patient is within the magnet and images can be rotated in space [95].

Clinical implementation of C-MRA

While high quality images of the coronary arteries have been obtained with various techniques (Table 6.2) [6, 22, 25, 50–55, 68, 71, 97, 156, 157], clinical implementation has not achieved consistent coronary coverage, image quality, and disease detection. Currently, the only well defined role for C-MRA is in the diagnosis of coronary anomalies [37].

Anomalous coronary arteries

Unlike x-ray angiography, C-MRA provides a 3D spatial relationship to great vessels, allowing evaluation of the origin and course of anomalous coronaries which is helpful in determining risk and advisability of possible surgical intervention [158]. The accuracy of coronary MRA for the identification of coronary anomalies has been shown in several studies. Accurate delineation of the proximal course has been shown with sensitivities of 88–100% and specificity of 100% (Table 6.3) [159–163]. MR can often provide a definitive diagnosis in patients whose x-ray angiography is inconclusive [159, 161].

Coronary artery disease

The role of C-MRA in the diagnosis and management of coronary artery disease (CAD) is still undefined. Clinical trials have produced variable results in the evaluation of native CAD (Table 6.4) [6, 51, 72, 94, 101, 102, 164–175] and bypass grafts [89, 176–184]. Most clinical trials have utilized either 2D or 3D GRE. In GRE, rapidly moving blood with laminar flow appears bright while areas of stagnant flow or flow turbulence appear dark due to local

Table 6.2 Visualization of native coronary arteries.

Reference	n	Technique	Respiratory compensation	RCA %	LM %	LAD %	LCX %
Manning, 1993 [6]	25	2D seg GRE	BH	100	96	100	76
Pennell, 1993 [50]	26	2D seg GRE	BH	95	95	91	76
Duerinchkx, 1994 [51]	20	2D seg GRE	BH	100	95	86	77
Sakuma, 1994 [52]	18	2D seg GRE cine	BH	100	100	100	67
Masui, 1995 [53]	13	2D seg GRE	BH	85	92	100	92
Davis, 1996 [54]	33*	2D seg GRE	BH	100	100	100	100
Yang, 2004 [22]	23	2D spiral GRE (1.5 and 3 T)	BH	100	100	100	100
Nguyen, 2004 [156]	14	2D spiral RT (3 T)	BH	100	100	100	100
Li, 1993 [25]	14	3D seg GRE	mult averages	100	100	86	93
Post, 1996 [94]	20	3D seg GRE	retro nav	100	100	100	100
Botnar, 1999 [55]	32	3D seg GRE	pro nav	97	100	100	97
Stuber, 1999 [97]	15	3D seg, contrast GRE + EPI	pro nav	100	100	100	100
Wielopolski, 1998 [68]	32	3D seg EPI	BH	100	100	100	100
Weber, 2003 [157]	12	3D seg SSFP, whole heart	pro nav	100	100	100	100

* Including 18 heart transplant recipients.

n = number of subjects; RCA = right coronary artery; LM = left main; LAD = left anterior descending artery; LCX = left circumflex; seg GRE = segmented gradient recalled echo; seg EPI = segmented echo planar imaging; RT = real-time; BH = breath-hold; Retro nav = retrospective navigator-gated; pro nav = prospective navigator-gated; SSFP = steady state free precession.

Table 6.3 Anomalous coronary MRA.

Reference	n	Technique	Correctly classified anomalous vessel %
McConnell, 1995 [160]	16	2D seg GRE, BH	14 (93%)
Post, 1995 [163]	19	2D seg GRE, BH	19 (100%)*
Vliegen, 1997 [161]	12	2D seg GRE, BH	11 (92%)**
Taylor, 2000 [162]	16	3D seg GRE, navigator	14 (88%)
Bunce, 2003 [159]	26	3D seg GRE, navigator	26 (100%)***

* Including three misclassified by x-ray angiography.

** Including five patients unable to be classified by angiography and one patient reclassified by MRA.

*** Including one patient unable to be classified by angiography and 11 patients whose course could not be defined by x-ray angiography.

n = number of subjects; seg GRE = segmented GRE; BH = breath-hold.

saturation or dephasing. Amount of signal loss in areas of focal stenosis is thought to be proportionate to the degree of stenosis [165]. However, bright blood coronary MRA methods can sometimes be misleading [37]. Signal loss due to slow flowing blood distal to the lesion can occasionally be mistaken for a stenosis. Moreover, these techniques are insensitive to direction of blood and, therefore, a stenosis will not be detected in a total occlusion that has adequate collateral or retrograde filling.

Initial clinical implementation of C-MRA was performed by Manning *et al.* [6] using a 2D-segmented GRE. In a double-blinded study of 39 patients with suspected coronary artery disease, sensitivity and specificity were 90% and 92%, respectively. Subsequent trials using 2D-segmented GRE [6, 51, 164, 165] generated variable results with sensitivity of 53–90% and specificity of 56–92%. With the advent of free-breathing techniques, several centers have adopted 3D-GRE C-MRA [72, 94, 166–172, 175] for ease of patient acceptance and improved SNR. Data from studies using 3D-segmented k-space have been recently published (Table 6.4) [72, 94, 166–172, 174]. Kim *et al.* [173] performed the first multicenter trial using 3D-segmented GRE with EPI in 109 patients with suspected CAD. Overall sensitivity and specificity was 93 and 42%, respectively in the proximal and mid-segments, with at least diagnostic image quality in 84% of the coronary segments. More recently, spiral acquisition has enabled the detection of distal stenosis as well as proximal and mid-disease. A prospective clinical trial [101] using 2D-multislice spiral GRE of proximal, middle and distal segments in 40 patients generated a sensitivity of 79% and 90%, respectively. Implementation of a new dynamic architecture that allows optimization of scan plane localization in a clinical trial of 45 patients showed improved sensitivity and specificity of 93% and 88%, respectively [102]. Comparative MRI images using 2D-multislice spiral GRE, 3D-VCATS segmented FLASH and 3D-SSFP, along with their corresponding x-ray angiograms, are shown in Fig. 6.8. In comparison with native coronaries, saphenous vein and internal mammary grafts are relatively easier to image because of their larger size and relatively stationary position; thus, relative to native coronaries, C-MRA of bypass grafts has a higher sensitivity, specificity and accuracy [37] (Table 6.5) [89, 176–184]. Today, C-MRA demonstrates the potential to be a routine clinical test for the non-invasive detection of CAD.

Clinical implementation of GV-MRA

Unlike C-MRA, GV-MRA has a proven clinical role [7]. In comparison to other non-invasive modalities, including ultrasound (U/S) and computed tomography (CT), MR provides higher sensitivity and specificity as well as a more comprehensive examination [7, 185–187]. However, because of limited patient access, need for transportation to the scanner, longer examination time, and the question of adequate monitoring while in the scanner,

Table 6.4 Summary of coronary MRA studies for detection of significant coronary artery disease (50% stenosis).

Reference	Technique	n	No. (%) vessels with stenosis	Overall sensitivity % (per vessel)	Overall specificity % (per vessel)
Manning, 1993 [6]	2D seg GRE, BH	39	52 (35)	90 (LM 100, LAD 87, LCX 71, RCA 100)	92 (LM 100, LAD 92, LCX 90, RCA 78)
Duerinckx, 1994 [51]	2D seg GRE, BH	20	27 (34)	63 (LM 50, LAD 73, LCX 0, RCA 62)	56 (LM 56, LAD 84, LCX 37, RCA 82)
Post, 1997 [164]	2D seg GRE, BH	35	35 (28)	n/a (LM 100, LAD 53, LCX 0, RCA 71)	n/a (LM 93, LAD 73, LCX 96, RCA 82)
Pennell, 1996 [165]	2D seg GRE, BH	39	55 (35)	85 (LM, LAD 88, LCX 75, RCA 75–100)	n/a
Yang, 2003 [101]	2D spiral GRE, BH	40	31 (76)	76 (LM n/a, LAD 87, LCX 25, RCA 76)	91 (LM 100, LAD 88, LCX 89, RCA 79)
Yang, 2004 [102]	2D spiral GRE, BH	45	40 (22)	93 (LM 100, LAD 94, LCX 78, RCA 100)	88 (LM 93, LAD 83, LCX 89, RCA 84)
Van Geuns, 2000 [72]	3D GRE, BH	38	39 (34)	68 (LM 77, LAD 77, LCX 50, RCA 64)	97 (LM 97, LAD 97, LCX 100, RCA 94)
Regenfus, 2000 [167]	3D CE-MRA, BH	50	59 (39)	94 (overall result)	57 (overall result)
Woodard, 1998 [167]	3D GRE, navigator	10	10 (30)	70–73 (overall result)	n/a
Kessler, 1997 [168]	3D GRE, navigator	73	87 (33)	65 (overall result)	88 (overall result)
Huber, 1999 [169]	3D GRE, navigator	20	53 (66)	73–79 (LM 75, LAD 62–71, LCX 67–80, RCA 86–89)	50–54 (LM 25–36, LAD 46–50, LCX 58–63, RCA 67–69)
Sandstede, 1999 [170]	3D GRE, navigator	30	37 (31)	81 (overall result)	89 (overall result)
Sardanelli, 2000 [171]	3D GRE, navigator	39	67 (43)	82 (prox segments 90, distal segments 68)	89 (prox segments 90, distal 81)
Post, 1996 [94]	3D GRE, retro navigator	20	21 (27)	63 (overall result)	89 (overall result)
Muller, 1997 [172]	3D GRE, retro navigator	35	54 (31)	83 (overall result)	94 (overall result)
Kim, 2001 [173]	3D, GRE + EPI, free breathing	109*	58 (59)	93 (LM 67, LAD 88, LCX 53, RCA 93)	42 (LM 90, LAD 52, LCX 70, RCA 72)
Sommer, 2005 [174]	3D GRE, RT navigator, 1.5 T + 3 T**	18	17 (16)	82 (overall result)	88 (overall result)
So, 2005 [175]	3D, SSFP, BH + navigator	15	49 (36)	80 (overall result for BH) 75 (overall result for navigator)	100 (overall result for BH) 100 (overall result for navigator)

* Multicenter trial.

** Although SNR and CNR increased for 3 T compared to 1.5 T, image quality and detection of stenosis were comparable.

n = number of subjects; GRE = gradient recalled echo; seg GRE = segmented GRE; EPI = echo planar imaging; SSFP = steady-state free precession; RT = real time; CE-MRA = contrast enhanced magnetic resonance angiography; BH = breath hold; retro navigator = retrospective navigator gated.

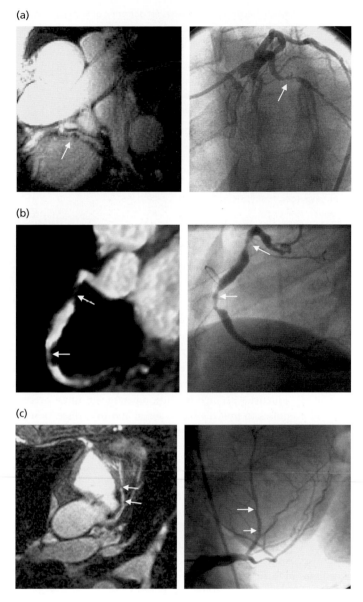

Fig. 6.8 (a) 2D multislice breath-hold spiral GRE of a significant stenosis in the proximal left circumflex artery with corresponding x-ray angiogram. (b) 3D breath-hold (VCATS) segmented GRE of a significant stenosis in the mid right coronary artery with corresponding x-ray angiogram. (c) 3D SSFP of sequential high grade lesions in the mid left anterior descending artery with corresponding x-ray angiogram. (Figure reproduced courtesy of P. Yang, Stanford University; P. Wielopolski, University Hospital, Rotterdam, The Netherlands, and R. McCarthy and D. Li, Northwestern University, Chicago.

MR has been relegated to a secondary role for acute processes [7].

Thoracic and abdominal aorta
Aortic dissection
Aortic dissection is characterized by laceration of the intima and inner layer of the aorta allowing blood to flow through a false lumen. Early and accurate detection of the dissection and its anatomical delineation are critical for successful manage-

ment [188]. The anatomic characteristics of the dissection determine whether medical or surgical management is indicated, and, if surgery is indicated, the type of surgical technique that will provide the greatest long term success [7]. Thus, the imaging modality must be able to clearly delineate the intimal flap and its extension, the entry and re-entry sites, the presence and degree of aortic insufficiency, and the flow in the aortic branches [189]. Moreover, defining involvement of the iliac

Table 6.5 Summary of coronary MRA studies for detection of graft patency.

Reference	Technique	n	No. of grafts	Patency %	Sensitivity %	Specificity %	Accuracy %
White, 1987 [176]	2D spin echo	25	72	69	86	59	78
Rubenstein, 1987 [177]	2D spin echo	20	47	62	90	72	83
Jenkins, 1988 (179)	2D spin echo	16	41	63	89	73	83
Galjee, 1996 [179]	2D spin echo	47	98	74	98	85	89
White, 1988 [180]	2D GRE	28	28	50	93	86	89
Aurigemma, 1989 [181]	2D GRE	45	45	73	88	100	91
Galjee, 1996 [179]	2D GRE	47	98	74	98	88	96
Engelmann, 2000 [182]	2D GRE	40	55	100 (IMA)	100		100
				66 (SVG)	92	85	89
Wintersperger, 1998 [183]	CE-3D GRE	27	76	79	95	81	95
Brenner, 1999 [184]	CE-3D GRE	85	222	95 (IMA)	93.8	50	n/a
Vrachliotis, 1997 [89]	CE-3D GRE	15	45	67	93	97	95

n = number of subjects; GRE = gradient recalled echo; CE = contrast enhanced; IMA = internal mammary artery; SVG = saphenous vein graft.

vessels may be important for the placement of stent grafts [190, 191].

MRI fulfils these necessary requirements for the non-invasive diagnosis of aortic dissection. The initial MR study for suspected aortic dissection begins with an SE sequence with high resolution parameters and prepulses to null the blood signal and to obtain a better definition of the aortic wall [7]. The intimal flap appears as a straight line in the axial plane. The true lumen usually appears as a signal void, whereas, the false lumen has higher signal intensity. Sagittal planes are required to determine the extent of dissection in the thoracic, abdominal and aortic arch branches [192]. Gradient recalled sequences [123, 126] should be performed to identify aortic insufficiency, entry or re-entry sites, and slow flow but is usually reserved for stable patients. If SE images are negative, 3D contrast MRA [193] should be performed to avoid missing a dissection. With SE, artifacts caused by imperfect ECG gating, respiratory motion, or a slow blood pool can result in intraluminal signal simulating or obscuring the intimal flap [7]. In CE-MRA, the intimal flap and the relationship to great vessels is clearly identified. Entry and re-entry sites appear as segmented interruption of the linear intimal flap as shown in Fig. 6.9 [7, 185, 194]. Compared to other imaging modalities, MR is the most accurate modality for detecting aortic dissection with sensitivity and specificity approaching 100% [185–187, 195].

All patients undergoing aortic repair should have imaging surveillance. MR is the imaging modality of choice for postoperative surveillance [196–198]. MR measurement parameters are easily reproduced, which is critical for surveillance because rupture is often preceded by increases in diameter. Residual dissection can be easily seen on SE, and thrombosis is readily detected by GRE [195]. Contrast enhanced MRA is also valuable in assessing postoperative complications, including anastamotic leakage and thrombosis, dissection, and aneurysm of the re-implanted coronaries [7, 199].

Intramural hematoma

Intramural hematoma refers to dissection without intimal tear. The diagnosis of intramural hematoma depends on the visualization of intramural blood, manifested as a locally thickened aortic wall but can be confused with clot or plaque [200]. In comparison with various imaging modalities, MRI demonstrates the best sensitivity for the detection of intramural hematoma [201] and can determine the age of the hematoma [202] based on the different degradation products of hemoglobin. On T_1-weighted SE images, the intramural hematoma appears as a crescent shaped area of abnormal signal within the aortic wall. Acute hematoma (less than seven days of symptom onset) show an intermediate signal intensity due to oxyhemoglobin content, compared to subacute hematoma that show high signal intensity

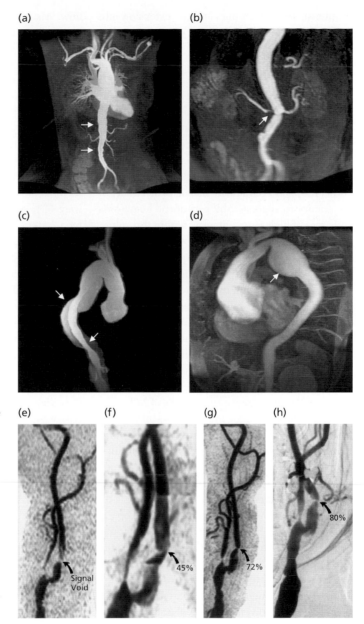

Fig. 6.9 (a) Three-dimensional contrast enhanced MRA showing diffuse atherosclerosis of the thoracic and abdominal aorta. (a), stenosis of the right renal artery (b), dissection of the thoracic aorta extending to the abdominal aorta (c) and aneurysm of the ascending aorta and arch (d). Classic 2D TOF showing signal void (e), followed by MOTSA with 45% measured stenosis (f), and 3D contrast enhanced MRA with 72% measured stenosis in a patient with carotid stenosis (g). The discrepancy was resolved with conventional x-ray angiogram (h), confirming 80% stenosis. (Figure reproduced courtesy of F. Chan, Stanford University, and: Reference 238, De Marco JK, Huston J, Bernstein M *et al.* Evaluation of classic 2D time-of-flight MR angiography in the depiction of severe carotid stenosis. *Am J Roentgenol* 2004; **183**: 787–793.)

due to methemoglobin. Intramural hematoma can be difficult to distinguish from thrombus if signal intensity is medium to low [7]. In those cases, T_2-weighted SE can differentiate hemorrhage, which has a high signal, from thrombus, which has a lower signal. Because of poor sensitivity, TOF and CE-MRA must be combined with SE to detect intramural hematoma or extravascular fluid collections [203].

Aortic ulcers

An aortic ulcer is characterized by rupture of an atheromatous plaque and disruption of the internal elastic lamina. Extension into the media may result in intramural hematoma, dissection or pseudoaneurysm. MR diagnosis of aortic ulcer [204] is based on visualization of a crater-like ulcer in the aortic wall in SE or CE-MRA. Mural thickening with high or intermediate signal may indicate extension into the medium or development of an intramural hematoma [205].

Aortic aneurysms

An aortic aneurysm is a localized or diffuse dilatation (>1.5 times the expected diameter) involving all layers of the aortic wall. MRI is effective in identifying and characterizing thoracic aneurysms [206]. Spin echo sequences can help evaluate alterations in the wall and peri-aortic space in the thoracic aorta [120]. Spin echo easily visualizes instability of the aneurysm suggested by peri-aortic hematoma and areas of high signal intensity within thrombus. Atherosclerotic lesions appear as areas of increased thickness with high signal intensity and irregularity. Accurate measurement of the aneurysm diameter requires fat suppression techniques to differentiate the outer aneurysm wall from peri-adventitial fat [7]. The addition of 3D CE-MRA [203, 207, 208] provides precise topographic information about the extent of the aneurysm and its relationship to aortic branches (Fig. 6.9), important in the preoperative management of these patients.

Unlike thoracic aneurysms, the role of MR in the evaluation of abdominal aneurysms is still yet to be defined [9, 209]. Monitoring of abdominal aneurysms can be easily performed with CT or ultrasound, both of which are capable of accurately determining the size of the aneurysm and its relationship to the iliac and renal arteries. Computed tomography [210] and U/S [211], however, are inadequate for preoperative planning, which requires more precise anatomic detail regarding the vessels of the lower extremities [212]. Moreover, the success of endovascular stenting procedures requires more exquisite detail, including the distance of the aneurysm from the renal arteries, involvement of the iliac arteries, and angle of the aneurysm neck or iliac-femoral axis [213]. In studies using TOF MRA [214–216], often in conjunction with T_1-weighted inversion recovery MRI, accurate classification of aneurysms as suprarenal or infrarenal is sufficient but suffers from inadequate detection of accessory renal arteries, renal artery stenosis and iliac vascular disease [95].

Results with CE-MRA are more promising for imaging the abdominal aorta [213, 217–219]. The use of CE-MRA enables higher resolution and provides high blood signal without the need for fast flow. A study of 27 patients revealed that a combination of CE-MRA, SE and non-contrast 3D TOF detected seven out of nine accessory renal arteries, eight out of 9 renal artery stenosis, all celiac stenosis and all iliac aneurysmal and stenotic disease [213]. MRA correlated with surgical findings as well as x-ray angiography for defining the proximal extent of the aneurysm. A subsequent study in patients with peripheral vascular disease [219] showed that MRA accurately defined the proximal extent of the abdominal aneurysm in 87% of patients. Sensitivities for ileofemoral occlusive and aneurysmal disease were 83% and 79%, respectively. Sensitivities for renal artery stenosis and accessory renal arteries were 71%. In terms of surgical planning, MRA correctly predicted 87% of the cross-clamp sites; 95% of the proximal anastamotic sites; the need for renal revascularization in 91% of the cases, and the use of a bifurcated aortic prosthesis in 75% of the patients. Contrast enhanced MRA, in combination with non-contrast techniques, correctly defined the maximum aneurysm diameter, as well as its proximal and distal extent in all 43 subjects. For the detection of aortic branch artery stenosis involving the celiac, mesenteric, renal or iliac arteries, sensitivity was 94% and specificity 98% [217]. Based on these studies, which demonstrate accurate anatomical delineation, CE-MRA enables surgical decision between the placement of an aortic tube graft or aorto-bifemoral graft [96]. In addition, CE-MRA can determine which patients are candidates for endoluminal repair [220] and may be more sensitive than CT in detecting small endoleaks after surgical or endoluminal repair [221]. Spin echo combined with CE-MRA can also identify inflammatory abdominal aneurysms, which are known to be associated with a higher operative mortality and which require a specialized procedure [7]. Potential limitations include the inability to define the severity of branch vessel stenosis and inadequate visualization of the mesenteric arteries [95]. CE-MRA of the abdominal aorta in a patient with renal artery stenosis is shown in Fig. 6.9.

Aortic rupture

Aortic rupture, which is usually caused by trauma, is a lesion that extends from the intima to the adventitia [222]. In the past, transesophageal echocardiography (TEE) and spiral CT had the advantage over

MR in terms of rapid, timely diagnosis especially in patients with severe hemodynamic compromise. Recent developments have shortened MR imaging time making it a viable option in even the most critically ill patients [7]. A recent study of 24 consecutive patients showed that the diagnostic accuracy of MRI was 100% compared to 84% using angiography (two false negatives) and 69% using CT (two false negatives and two false positives) [223]. The advantage of MR lies in its ability to visualize hemorrhagic components of a lesion. On SE images in the sagittal plane, MR can distinguish a tear limited to the anterior or posterior wall from a lesion encompassing the entire aortic circumference, which is more likely to rupture. Other signs of instability easily identified by MR are the presence of periadventitial hematoma and pleural and mediastinal hemorraghic effusion. MR can also evaluate trauma outside the heart, including lung contusion and edema, pleural effusion, and rib fractures [224].

Aortitis

MRI is the procedure of choice in the diagnosis of inflammatory lesions of the aorta [225]. X-ray angiography can only visualize late changes, including aneurysms and vascular stenosis, and should be avoided because of a high risk for pseudoaneurysm at the puncture site [226]. Computed tomography cannot detect subtle changes during the early phase of aortitis. Using contrast enhanced T_1-weighted and T_2-weighted SE imaging, active inflammation has been demonstrated as mural thickening of the aorta wall which enhances with gadolinium. In chronic stages characterized by fibrosis, lower signal intensity is observed and there is no contrast enhancement [227]. MRA is also useful in diagnosing stenosis and aneurysms and is useful for serial evaluation.

Congenital disease: aortic arch anomalies and aortic coarctation

Several congenital diseases, including aortic arch anomalies, aortic coarctation and aortic pseudo-coarctation, can be diagnosed using MRI [228]. Spin echo and CE-MRA can detect the abnormal vessel, its origin, its relationship to other structures, and any compression of structures in the mediastinum [229, 230]. Because of its ability to provide 3D information, MRI is more effective than x-ray

angiography in the preoperative assessment of patients with congenital arch anomalies.

One of the most common congenital diseases of the aorta is coarctation, which is caused by the formation of a fibrous ridge that protrudes into the aorta and forms a stenosis [231]. The stenosis can be a focal segment (aortic coarctation), diffuse (hypoplastic aortic isthmus) or complete (aortic arch interruption). It is best viewed on sagittal SE images. The severity of the coarctation can be estimated by the length of signal void on cine MRI [7]. Flow mapping can quantify the flow pattern and the volume of collateral flow down the descending aorta [232]. Three-dimensional MRA can also display the extent of the coarctation and its severity [233]. Postoperative complications, including re-stenosis, aortic dissection, aneurysm, and pseudoaneurysms can be readily detected by MR [234, 235]. Compared to U/S, which is the standard for postoperative assessment, MR can provide additional detail, including improved visualization of the arch and proximal portion of the descending aorta, and is not limited by acoustic windows [7].

Carotid and vertebral arteries
Carotid and vertebral artery stenosis

Several MRI techniques are used for imaging the carotid and vertebral arteries, including 2D-TOF [236], 3D-TOF [237], and CEMRA [136, 238]. 2D-TOF provides a strong vascular signal, even when the arterial velocity is low. Two-dimensional TOF should be used to differentiate near and complete internal carotid artery occlusion. Three-dimensional TOF provides superior, submillimeter resolution but at the expense of flow sensitivity. The weak vascular signal of 3D-TOF in slow-flow states can be improved with MOTSA [133]. Three-dimensional TOF acquisition may demonstrate some features of the plaque directly. The area covered by TOF sequences remains limited and complete visualization of both the anterior and posterior circulation from the aortic arch to the skull base is not possible [142]. In addition, scan time is long, leading to frequent image degradation by motion artifacts. Signal loss is also observed in areas of tight stenosis because of turbulent flow.

Contrast enhanced MRA is a quick and robust technique that is not impaired by slow flow but requires appropriate timing of contrast [95]. In

Table 6.6 Summary of TOF MRA studies of the carotid arteries.

Reference	TOF	Comparison	n	Stenosis threshold	Sensitivity %	Specificity %
Anderson , 1994 [242]	2D/3D	XRA/DUS	50	70	92	95
Mittle, 1994 [249]	2D	XRA/DUS	38	70	92	75
Young ,1994 [250]	2D/3D	XRA/DUS	70	70	86	93
Vanninen, 1995 [252]	3D	XRA	55	70	93	88
Kent, 1995 [248]	3D	XRA/DUS	81	70	98	85
Nicholas, 1995 [247]	2D/3D	XRA/DUS	40	70	92	98
Patel, 1995 [246]	2D/3D	XRA/DUS	88	70	94	85
Levi, 1996 [243]	2D/3D	XRA	45	70	95	77
Liberopoulous, 1996 [245]	3D	XRA/DUS/surgery	52	60	100	80
Link, 1992 [119]	3D	XRA	40	70	90	92
Nederkoorn, 2003 [262]	3D	XRA	51	70	86	73
Serfaty, 2001 [259]	3D	XRA/DUS	33	70	88	94

TOF = time of flight; n = number of subjects; XRA = x-ray angiography; DUS = duplex ultrasound.

head and neck imaging, the blood brain barrier prevents the extraction of gadolinium from the intracerebral circulation. This can lead to a rapid enhancement of veins that can hinder visualization of the carotid and vertebral arteries, especially in case of large or duplicated jugular veins. A preliminary study by Slosman *et al.* [239] in 50 patients with atherosclerotic carotid disease using a long scan time of 150 s showed an inability to assess 29 carotid arteries because of venous overlap. Better results were obtained with shorter acquisition time. Levy *et al.* [240], who assessed the bolus timing of a single dose of gadolinium with a 29 s scan time, achieved complete isolation of the arterial phase in about half of patients. Most recent studies [142] show that appropriate timing of gadolinium infusion with selective reconstruction of carotid arteries allowed elimination of overlapping vessels in most cases. A feasibility study [241] of this technique to image supra-aortic vessels in 98 patients showed the carotid bifurcation could be assessed in 95% of cases, whereas the entire lengths of vertebral arteries were visualized in 82%.

Results from recent prospective studies comparing 2D TOF, 3D-TOF, and x-ray angiography for the evaluation of carotid stenosis are shown in Table 6.6 [242–252]. The median sensitivity for a high grade lesion was 93%, whereas median specificity was 88% with 2D and 3D-TOF. An overestimation of stenosis severity can occur, however, in an area of turbulent flow where there is a signal void or

signal loss [253]. The tendency to overestimate stenosis is greatly reduced if interpretation is performed from source or reformatted images rather than projection images [242, 254]. Overestimation is also reduced by 3D acquisitions, because of the additional gradient generation and the use of submillimeter voxels, which results in less phase dispersion. Overestimation is also reduced if a quantitative measure is used rather than a qualitative visual estimate [95].

Compared to TOF, CE-MRA minimizes the problems with overestimation because of the T_1-shortening of gadolinium in areas of turbulent or residual flow. Sardanelli *et al.* [255] demonstrated that CE-MRA overestimated the degree of stenosis in two out of 30 cases; whereas 3D-TOF overestimated the degree of stenosis in nine cases of moderate stenosis. All severe stenoses were correctly detected with 100% sensitivity and specificity using CE MRA. Compared to 3D-TOF, CE-MRA demonstrated better ulcer detection and better depiction of the length of stenosis and slow flow beyond a critical lesion [7, 95]. However, in cases of high grade stenosis, a signal loss and reduced diameter were observed throughout the distal portion of the internal carotid artery despite absence of complete occlusion [256]. Moreover, the SNR of CE-MRA was found to be inferior to non-contrast techniques if peak arterial enhancement was missed because of incorrect timing of acquisition. The combination of CE-MRA and non-contrast techniques has

Table 6.7 Summary of contrast enhanced MRA studies of the carotid arteries.

Reference	CE-MRA	Comparison	n	Stenosis threshold	Sensitivity %	Specificity %
Huston J 3rd, 1999 [146]	3D	XRA	50	70	93.3	85.1
Alvarez-Linera, 2003 [257]	3D	XRA/CT	40	70	97.1	95.2
Borisch, 2003 [258]	3D	XRA/DUS	39	70	94.9	79.1
Serfaty, 2001 [259]	3D	XRA/DUS	33	70	94	85
Randoux B, 2001 [260]	3D	XRA/CT	22	70	93	100
Remonda, 1998 [261]	3D	XRA	120	70	96	95
Nederkoorn, 2003 [262]	3D	XRA	51	70	90	77
Butz, 2004 [263]	2D/3D	XRA	50	70	95.64	90.39
Lenhart, 2002 [264]	3D	XRA	43	70	98	86

CE-MRA = contrast enhanced MR angiography; n = number of subjects; XRA = x-ray angiography; CT = computed tomography; DUS = duplex ultrasound.

resulted, however, in exceptionally high rates of accuracy in comparison with x-ray angiography 95]. Sample images of a patient with carotid stenosis using 2D-TOF, 3D-MOTSA, CE-MRA and x-ray angiography are shown in Fig. 6.9. Results from prospective studies comparing CE-MRA and x-ray angiography for the evaluation of carotid stenosis are shown in Table 6.7 [146, 257–264].

These previous studies used x-ray angiography as the gold standard, which may be problematic [95]. A comparison of x-ray angiography, MRA and U/S [265] with surgical specimens found that both U/S and MRA correlate better with the endarterectomy specimen than does x-ray angiography. The discrepancy may occur because x-ray angiography may not appreciate the smallest diameter in an elliptical or complex lesion [95]. Rotational angiography, a technique that obtains images in many orientations following a single catheter injection, commonly used in coronary angiography, demonstrated that catheter angiography may underestimate the severity of lesions by not viewing it from the most stenotic region [266]. Thus, MRA may not be overestimating lesions but catheter angiography is in fact underestimating lesions [7, 95].

Current recommendations for the evaluation of carotid artery stenosis include initial screening with U/S followed by confirmation with MRA in cases of >70%. X-ray angiography should be performed if U/S and MRA findings are discrepant, in cases of possible hairline patency, or where lesions are so atypical that they can only be understood by an invasive study. MRA is especially advisable when results of U/S are technically limited and include the presence of a shadowing plaque, deep course of the ICA, discordant gray scale, Doppler measurements, and evidence of tandem lesions [95, 267].

For the posterior circulation, the detection of significant vertebral stenosis of greater than 50% in diameter remains difficult on the CE-MRA because of the small diameter of vertebral arteries and frequent anatomic variants [256, 268]. Preliminary studies show that sensitivity and specificity appear lower than for the anterior circulation (268). Randoux et al. [269] reported sensitivity and specificity for VA ostial stenosis was 100% and 85%, respectively, while the positive predictive value was only 58%. This is largely due to overestimation caused by partial volume effect.

Carotid and vertebral dissection

Various techniques have been employed for the detection of dissection. On T_1 and T_2-weighted images [268, 270], a dissection is suggested by an eccentric signal void surrounded by a crescent shaped hyperintensity [271]. Stenosis or complete vascular occlusion may be present but these findings lack specificity for dissection. Time of flight techniques [272, 273] have the advantage of better demonstration of the intramural hematoma than phase contrast techniques. Two-dimensional TOF can image a long segment of artery in a short time but suffers from signal loss in regions of turbulent flow that can simulate stenosis. Three-dimensional

TOF MRA [274] may reveal an "increased" external diameter of the artery due to superimposed intramural hematoma containing methemoglobin. This finding is more useful for the diagnosis of carotid artery dissection, but it is of limited use in vertebral dissection because of the small diameter and marked variation in caliber of the vertebrals [270]. Studies have shown that sensitivity and specificity of MRI and 3D-TOF for carotid dissection are 92% and 99%, respectively [270, 271, 274, 275]. However, the sensitivity and specificity of MRI and 3D-TOF MRA for the detection of vertebrobasilar dissection has been reported as being as low as 20% and 60%, respectively [270]. MRI may also be insufficient to detect pseudoaneurysm, mild stenosis, and fibromuscular displasia, all of which can predispose to dissection. The application of additional sequences may aid in the diagnosis of dissection. Contrast enhanced MRA can help differentiate residual flow from intramural hematoma with greatly improved resolution. The addition of SE T_1-weighted transverse images may also aid in identifying the false lumen [276].

Studies have reported successful serial monitoring of patients with carotid dissection using MRI [273, 277]. Features showing evidence of healing included stenosis and mural hematoma/intimal flap. Persistent luminal irregularities were associated with persistent dissection and late cerebrovascular events [273]. Moreover, two studies [273, 278] have reported encouraging results of combined CE-MRA/MRI for the follow-up of vertebral artery dissection. In one study, [278] contrast enhancement was seen in 71% of vertebrobasilar dissecting aneurysms up to eight weeks after the initial injury when T_1 SE signal of intramural hematoma had disappeared. Enhancement was still present in more than 50% of cases 24 weeks postinjury.

Pulmonary vessels

Pulmonary MRA has been slow in its clinical implementation. Initial approaches used 2D or 3D-TOF with promising results, however, techniques were not reliable for widespread clinical use. Recently, CE-MRA has been applied to the pulmonary arteries, [279] with the entire pulmonary tree covered in one breath-hold. A report of 30 patients showed sensitivities ranging from 75% to 100% plus specificities from 95% to 100% among three readers

with spatial resolution of $1.25 \times 2.5 \times 3.0$ mm. In a prospective study by Oudkerk *et al.* [280], sensitivity of MRA for isolated subsegmental, segmental, and central or lobar pulmonary embolism was 40%, 84%, and 100%, respectively (p < 0.01). Selected visualization of pulmonary arteries and veins has also been demonstrated with high spatial resolution ($1.9 \times 1.4 \times 2$ mm) [281]. Recently, it has been shown, in 61 patients, that 3D CE-MRA can identify pulmonary and systemic venous anomalies as well as catheterization [282].

Future direction

The most significant question in MRA today is how to improve this imaging modality to meet the high standard of routine implementation for the diagnosis of vascular disease. Clearly, impressive technological progress has been made in the past decades. Progress in this direction has enabled a movement toward imaging the entire vasculature. Recently, the global coherent free precession sequence [283] has been developed, which enables dynamic images of vascular morphology and flow, similar to x-ray angiography. Several groups are also developing techniques for whole heart [157, 284, 285] and whole body imaging [286–289].

A promising new technique, called the global coherent free precession (GCPF) [283] has been developed that enables dynamic images of both vascular morphology and blood flow, similar to x-ray angiography. In the GCFP state, excited protons continue to yield signals regardless of where they travel, even in the absence of additional RF excitation. RF excitations can be applied every few milliseconds, creating a continuous outward flow of excited protons. Thus, spatially selective RF pulses produce a continuous stream of coherently excited blood whose spins freely precess as the blood flows through regions of space unaffected by the ongoing excitation.

Another promising approach is whole heart imaging, whose development was supported by recent technological innovations. Whole heart coronary MRA based on 3D free-breathing SSFP [157] with magnetization preparation has shown significantly increased vessel lengths compared to transverse and targeted volumes. Image quality including vessel sharpness, SNR and CNR was at least equal to targeted volumes. Similar results were obtained

(a)

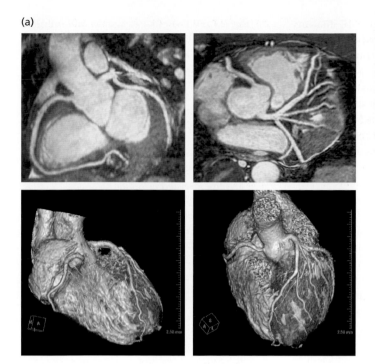

(b)

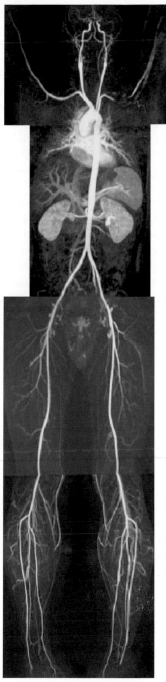

Fig. 6.10 (a) Right coronary artery (RCA) and left circumflex (LCX) (right) and left anterior descending artery (LAD) (right) of a volunteer as imaged using a targeted sequence (top row) and reformatted using the whole heart sequence (bottom row). Note that longer segments of the LAD and LCX are visualized using the whole heart sequence. (b) Whole body MRA images using contrast enhancement and parallel imaging techniques. (Fig. 6.10a reproduced courtesy of H. Sakuma, Mie University, Japan. Figure 6.10b reproduced with permission of: Reference 290, Bernd T. Whole body CE-MRA using gadovist. *Eur Radiol* 2004; **14**: M26–M27.)

with a 3D-free-breathing GRE sequence, as shown in Fig. 6.9 and Fig. 6.10 [285]. Single breath-hold, spiral whole heart imaging at 3T has also been developed with promising results [285].

Similarly, recent advances have enabled the implementation of whole body MRA. Contrast agent dose limitations had initially restricted 3D-MRA to the display of arteries contained in a single 40–48 cm field of view [7]. Before bolus-chase MR imaging, extended coverage could be achieved with separate injections in one examination. Two contiguous areas were studied with separate doses of gadolinium-based contrast agent [286]. Implementation of bolus-chase techniques extended coverage to two or three territories with a single administration of contrast agent. Several studies have demonstrated the feasibility of whole body MRA as demonstrated in Fig. 6.9 and Fig. 6.10 [286–288, 290].

Conclusion

Although clinical implementation of GV-MRA has met with some success, clinical implementation of C-MRA has proven to be challenging. However, active developmental efforts to improve image quality and scan efficiency should enable robust and reliable imaging of vascular pathology. For this imaging modality to become a clinical reality, comparative studies of imaging sequences and multi-center clinical trials need to be conducted to determine the most effective imaging protocol for C-MRA.

References

1. Johnson L, Lozner E, Johnson S et al. Coronary arteriography 1984–1987: A report of the registry of the society for cardiac angiography and interventions. I. Results and complications. *Cathet Cardiovasc Diagn* 1989; **17**: 5–10.

2. Lozner E, Johnson L, Johnson S et al. Coronary arteriography 1984–1987: A report of the registry of the society for cardiac angiography and interventions II. An analysis of 218 deaths related to coronary arteriography. *Cathet Cardiovasc Diagn* 1989; **17**: 11–14.

3. Kunz KM, Skillman JJ, Whittenmore AD et al. Carotid endarterectomy in asymptomatic patients—is contrast angiography necessary? A morbidity analysis. *J Vasc Surg* 1995; **22**: 706–714.

4. Cranney G, Lotan C, Pohost G et al. *Cardiovascular Applications of Magnetic Resonance Imaging*. Little, Brown and Company, Boston, 1991.

5. Blackwell G, Pohost G et al. The evolving role of MRI in the assessment of coronary artery disease. *Am J Cardiol* 1995; **75**: 74D–78D.

6. Manning W, Li W, Edelman R et al. A preliminary report comparing magnetic resonance coronary angiography with conventional angiography. *N Engl J Med* 1993; **328**: 828–32.

7. Higgins C, De Roos A. *Cardiovascular MRI and MRA*. Lippincott Williams and Wilkins, Philadelphia, 2003.

8. Schmitt F, Arz W. An ultra-high performance gradient system for cardio and neuro MR imaging. In: *Proceedings of the International Society of Magnetic Resonance in Medicine,* 7th Annual Meeting, Philadelphia, 1999: 470.

9. Meyer C, Hu B, Nishimura D et al. Fast spiral coronary artery imaging. *Magn Reson Med* 1992; **28**: 202–213.

10. Meyer C, Hu B, Kerr A et al. High-resolution multislice spiral coronary angiography with real-time interactive localization. In: *Proceedings of the International Society of Magnetic Resonance in Medicine,* 5th Annual Meeting, Vancouver, 1997: 439.

11. Fayad Z, Connick T, Axel L et al. An improved quadrature or phased array coil for MR cardiac imaging. *Magn Reson Med* 1995; **34**: 186–193.

12. Bottomley PA, Lugo OC, Giaquinto R et al. What is the optimum phased array coil design for cardiac and torso magnetic resonance? *Magn Reson Med* 1997; **37**: 591–599.

13. Engvall J, Scott G, Santos J et al. MR coronary angiography using a novel 2-element phased array coil: Improved image quality and anatomic coverage. *J Cardiovasc Magn Reson* 2003; **5**: 290–291.

14. Constantinides CD, Westgate C, O'Dell WG et al. A phased array coil for human cardiac imaging. *Magn Reson Med* 1995; **34**: 92–98.

15. Griswold MA, Jakob JP, Edelman RR et al. A multicoil array designed for cardiac smash imaging. *MAGMA*. 2000; **10**: 105–113.

16. Rinck P. *Magnetic Resonance in Medicine* [3rd edn]. Blackwell Scientific Publications, London, 1993.

17. Noll D, Pauly J, Meyer C et al. De-blurring for non-2D Fourier transform magnetic resonance imaging. *Magn Reson Med* 1992; **25**: 319–333.

18. Man L, Pauly J, Macovski A et al. Improved automatic off-resonance correction without a field map in spiral imaging. *Magn Reson Med* 1997; **37**: 906–913.

19. Noeske R, Siefert F, Rhein KH et al. Human cardiac imaging at 3T using phased array coils. *Magn Reson Med* 2000; **44**: 978–982.

20. Singerman RW, Denison TJ, Wen H et al. Simulation of B1 field distribution and intrinsic signal-to-noise in cardiac MRI as a function of static magnetic field. *J Magn Reson* 1997; **125**: 72–83.

21. Nayak K, Cunningham C, Santos J et al. Real-time cardiac MR at 3 Tesla. *Magn Reson Med* 2004; **51**: 655–660.

22. Yang PC, Nguyen P, Shimakawa A et al. Spiral MR coronary angiography at 1.5T and 3T—clinical comparison. *J Cardiovasc Magn Reson* 2004; **6**: 877–884.

23. Stuber M, Botnar R, Larmerichs R et al. A preliminary report on in vivo coronary MRA at 3T in humans. In: *Proceedings of the International Society of Magnetic*

Resonance in Medicine, 10th Annual Meeting, Orlando, 2002: 116.

24. Steenbeck J, Pruessman K. Technical developments in cardiac MRI: 2000 update. *Rays* 2001; **26**: 15–34.

25. Li D, Pascal C, Haacke E *et al.* Coronary arteries: Three-dimensional MR imaging with fat saturation and magnetization transfer contrast. *Radiology* 1993; **187**: 401–406.

26. Sachs T, Meyer C, Irarrazabal P *et al.* The diminishing variance algorithm for real time reduction of motion artifact in MRI. *Magn Reson Med* 1995; **34**: 412–422.

27. Wang Y, Watts R, Mitchell I *et al.* Coronary MR angiography: Selection of acquisition window of minimal cardiac motion with electrocardiography-triggered navigator cardiac motion prescanning—initial results. *Radiology* 2001; **218**: 580–585.

28. Sachs T, Meyer C, Pauly J *et al.* A real-time interactive 3D-DVA for robust coronary MRA. *IEEE Trans Med Imaging* 2000; **19**: 73–79.

29. McConnell MV, Khasgiwala V, Savord BJ *et al.* Prospective adaptive navigator correction for breath hold MR coronary angiography. *Magn Reson Med* 1997; **37**: 148–152.

30. Oshinski JN, Hoffland L, Mukundan S Jr *et al.* Two-dimensional coronary MR angiography without breath-holding. *Radiology* 1996; **3**: 737–743.

31. Hofman MB, Paschal C, Li D *et al.* MRI of coronary arteries: 2D breath-hold vs 3D respiratory-gated acquisition. *J Comput Assist Tomogr* 1995; **1**: 56–62.

32. McConnell M, Khasgiwala V, Savord B *et al.* Comparison of respiratory suppression methods and navigator locations for MR coronary angiography. *Am J Roentgenol* 1997; **168**: 1369–1375.

33. Taylor A, Keegan J, Jhooti P *et al.* Differences between normal subjects and patients with coronary artery disease for three different MR coronary angiography respiratory suppression techniques. *J Magn Reson Imaging* 1999; **9**: 786–793.

34. Larson AC, White RD, Laub G *et al.* Self-gated cardiac cine MRI. *Magn Reson Med* 2004; **51**: 93–102.

35. Larson AC, Kellman P, Arai A *et al.* Preliminary investigation of respiratory self-gating for free-breathing segmented cine MRI. *Magn Reson Med* 2005; **53**: 159–168.

36. McKinnon G. Ultra-fast interleaved gradient-echo planar imaging on a standard scanner. *Magn Reson Med* 1993; **30**: 609–616.

37. Manning W, Pennell D. *Cardiovascular Magnetic Resonance* [1st edn]. Churchill Livingston, Philadelphia, 2002.

38. Lieberman L, Botti R, Nelson A *et al.* Magnetic resonance of the heart. *Radiol Clin North Am* 1984; **22**: 847–858.

39. Paulin S, von Schulthess G, Fossel E *et al.* Magnetic resonance of the heart. *Am J Roentgenol* 1987; **148**: 665–670.

40. Hennig J, Nauerth A, Friedburg H *et al.* Rare imaging: A fast imaging method for clinical MR. *Magn Reson Med* 1986; **3**: 823–833.

41. Simonetti OP, Finn JP, White RD *et al.* "Black blood" T_2-weighted inversion recovery MRA imaging of the heart. *Radiology* 1996; **1**: 49–57.

42. Wang S, Hu B, Macovski A *et al.* Coronary angiography using fast selective inversion recovery. *Magn Reson Med* 1991; **18**: 417–423.

43. Edelman RR, Chien D, Kim D *et al.* Fast selective black blood MR imaging. *Radiology* 1991; **181**: 655–660.

44. Stuber M, Botnar R, Spuentrup E *et al.* Three-dimensional high resolution fast spin echo coronary magnetic resonance angiography. *Magn Reson Med* 2001; **45**: 206–211.

45. Haase A, Frahm J, Matthaei D *et al.* Flash imaging: Rapid NMR imaging using low flip angle pulses. *J Magn Reson* 1986; **67**: 258–266.

46. Atkinson D, Edelman R. Cineangiography of the heart in a single breath-hold with a segmented turbo-flash sequence. *Radiology* 1991; **178**: 357–360.

47. Burstein D. MR imaging of coronary artery flow in isolated and *in vivo* hearts. *J Magn Reson Imaging* 1991; **1**: 337–46.

48. Edelman R, Manning W, Burstein D *et al.* Coronary arteries: Breath-hold MR angiography. *Radiology* 1991; **3**: 641–643.

49. Manning WJ, Li W, Boyle NG *et al.* Fat-suppressed breath-hold magnetic resonance coronary angiography. *Circulation* 1993; **87**: 94–104.

50. Pennell DJ, Keegan J, Firmin DN *et al.* Magnetic resonance imaging of coronary arteries: Technique and preliminary results. *Br Heart J* 1993; **70**: 315–326.

51. Duerinckx AJ, Urman MK. Two-dimensional coronary MR angiography: Analysis of initial clinical results. *Radiology* 1994; **193**: 731–738.

52. Sakuma H, Caputo GR, Steffens JC, *et al.* Breath-hold MR cine angiography of coronary arteries in healthy volunteers: Value of multi-angle oblique imaging planes. *Am J Roentgenol* 1994; **163**: 533–537.

53. Masui T, Isoda H, Mochizuki T *et al.* MR angiography of the coronary arteries. *Radiat Med* 1995; **13**: 47–50.

54. Davis SF, Kannam J, Wielopolski P *et al.* Magnetic resonance coronary angiography in heart transplant recipients. *J Heart Lung Transplant* 1996; **15**: 580–586.

55. Botnar R, Stuber M, Danias P *et al.* Improved coronary artery definition with T_2-weighted, free-breathing, three-dimensional coronary MRA. *Circulation* 1999; **99**: 3139–3148.

56. Oppell A, Graumann R, Berfuss H *et al.* FISP—a new fast MRI sequence. *Electromedica* 1986; **54**: 15–18.

57. Sekihara K. Steady-state magnetization in rapid NRM imaging using small flip angles and short repetition intervals. *IEEE Trans Med Imaging* 1987; **6**: 157–164.

58. Heid O. True FISP cardiac fluoroscopy. In: *Proceedings of the International Society of Magnetic Resonance in Medicine,* 4th Annual Meeting, Berkeley, 1997: 320.

59. Deimling M, Heid O. True FISP imaging with inherent fat cancellation. In: *Proceedings of the International Society of Magnetic Resonance in Medicine*, 7th Annual Meeting, Berkeley, 2000: 1500.

60. Deshpande VS, Shea SM, Laub G et al. 3D magnetization-prepared True-FISP: A new technique for imaging coronary arteries. *Magn Reson Med* 2001; **46**: 494–502.

61. Shea SM, Deshpande VS, Chung YC et al. Three-dimensional True-FISP imaging of the coronary arteries: Improved contrast with T2-preparation. *J Magn Reson Imaging* 2002; **15**: 597–602.

62. Li D, Carr J, Shea S et al. Coronary arteries: Magnetization-prepared contrast-enhanced three-dimensional volume-targeted breath-hold MR angiography. *Radiology* 2001; **219**: 270–277.

63. Deshpande VS, Shea S, Chung YC, et al. Breath-hold three-dimensional TRUE-FISP imaging of coronary arteries using asymmetric sampling. *J Magn Reson Imaging* 2002; **15**: 473–478.

64. Park J, McCarthy R, Debia L et al. Feasibility and performance of breath-hold 3D True-FISP coronary MRA using self calibrating parallel acquisition. *Magn Reson Med* 2004; **52**: 7–13.

65. Nishimura D, Irarrazabal P, Meyer C et al. A velocity k-space analysis of flow effects in echo-planar and spiral imaging. *Magn Reson Med* 1995; **33**: 549–556.

66. Mansfield P. Multiplanar image formation using NMR spin echoes. *J Physics C: Solid State Physics* 1977; **10**: L55–L58.

67. Wielopolski PA, Manning W, Edelman RR et al. Single breath-hold volumetric imaging of the heart using magnetization-prepared 3-dimensional segmented echo planar imaging. *J Magn Reson Imaging* 1995; **5**: 403–409.

68. Wielopolski PA, van Geuns RJ, de Feyter PJ et al. Breath-hold coronary MR angiography with volume targeted imaging. *Radiology* 1998; **209**: 209–219.

69. Slavin GS, Riederer SJ, Ehman RL et al. Two-dimensional multishot echo-planar coronary MR angiography. *Magn Reson Med* 1998; **40**: 883–889.

70. Botnar R, Stuber M, Danias P et al. A fast 3D approach for coronary MRA. *J Magn Reson Imaging* 1999; **10**: 821–825.

71. Stuber M, Botnar R, Danias PG et al. Contrast agent-enhanced, free-breathing, three-dimensional coronary magnetic resonance angiography. *J Magn Reson Imaging* 1999; **10**: 790–799.

72. Van Geuns R, Wielopolski P, de Bruin H et al. MR coronary angiography with breath-hold targeted volumes: Preliminary clinical results. *Radiology* 2000; **217**: 270–277.

73. Deshpande V, Wielopolski P, Shea S et al. Coronary artery imaging using contrast enhanced 3D segmented EPI. *J Magn Reson Imaging* 2001; **13**: 676–681.

74. Luk Pat GT, Meyer C, Pauly JM et al. Reducing flow artifacts in echo-planar imaging. *Magn Reson Med* 1997; **37**: 436–447.

75. Brittain J, Hu B, Wright G et al. Coronary angiography with magnetization prepared T2 contrast. *Magn Reson Med* 1995; **33**: 689–696.

76. Bornert P, Stuber M, Botnar R et al. Direct comparison of 3D spiral vs Cartesian gradient-echo coronary magnetic resonance angiography. *Magn Reson Med* 2001; **46**: 789–794.

77. Taylor A, Keegan J, Jhooti P et al. A comparison between segmented k-space flash and interleaved spiral MR coronary angiography sequences. *J Magn Reson Imaging* 2000; **11**: 394–400.

78. Keegan J, Gatehouse P, Taylor A et al. Coronary artery imaging in 0.5 Tesla scanner: Implementation of real time, navigator echo-controlled segmented k-space flash and interleaved spiral sequences. *Magn Reson Med* 1999; **41**: 392–399.

79. Maintz D, Botnar R, Heindel W et al. Coronary magnetic resonance angiography: An objective quantitative comparison between four different MR techniques. In: *Proceedings of the International Society of Magnetic Resonance in Medicine*, 10th Annual Meeting, Orlando, 2002: 108.

80. Hu B, Meyer C, Macovski A et al. Multslice spiral magnetic resonance coronary angiography. In: *Proceedings of the International Society of Magnetic Resonance in Medicine*, 4th Annual Meeting, Berkeley, 1996: 176.

81. Balaban RS, Ceckler TL. Magnetization transfer contrast in magnetic resonance imaging. *Magn Reson Q* 1992; **8**: 116–137.

82. Meyer C, Pauly J, Macovski A et al. Simultaneous spatial and spectral selective excitation. *Magn Reson Med* 1990; **35**: 521–531.

83. Hu B, Connolly S, Wright G et al. Pulsed saturation transfer contrast. *Magn Reson Med* 1992; **33**: 689–696.

84. Pauly J, Le Roux P, Nishimura D et al. Parameter relations for Shinnar-Le Roux RF pulse design algorithm. *IEEE Trans Med Imaging* 1991; **10**: 53–65.

85. Henkelman R, Stanisz F, Graham S et al. Magnetization transfer in MRI: A review. *NMR Biomed* 2001; **14**: 57–64.

86. Cunningham CH, Wright G, Wood ML et al. High-order multiband encoding in the heart. *Magn Reson Med* 2002; **48**: 689–698.

87. Parrish T, Hu X. A new T_2 preparation technique for ultrafast gradient-echo sequence. *Magn Reson Med* 1994; **32**: 652–657.

88. Bi X, Li D. Coronary arteries at 3.0 T: Contrast enhanced magnetization-prepared three-dimensional breath-hold MR angiography. *J Magn Reson Imaging* 2005; **21**: 133–139.

89. Vrachliotis TG, Bis KG, Aliabadi D *et al.* Contrast enhanced breath-hold MR angiography for evaluating patency of coronary artery bypass grafts. *Am J Roentgenol* 1997; **168**: 1073–1080.

90. Lorenz C, Johansson L. Contrast enhanced coronary MRA. *J Magn Reson Imaging* 1999; **10**: 703–708.

91. Taylor AM, Panting JR, Keegan J *et al.* Safety and preliminary findings with the intravascular contrast agent NC100150 injection for MR coronary angiography. *J Magn Reson Imaging* 1999; **9**: 220–227.

92. Cavagna F, La Noce A, Maggioni F *et al.* MR coronary angiography with the new intravascular contrast agent B-22956/1: First human experience. In: *Proceedings of the International Society of Magnetic Resonance in Medicine,* 10th Annual Meeting, Orlando, 2002: 114.

93. Paetsch I, Huber M, Bornstedt A *et al.* Improved 3D free-breathing coronary MRA using gadocoletic acid (B-22956) for intravascular contrast enhancement. *J Magn Reson Imaging* 2004; **20**: 2288–2293.

94. Post JC, van Rossum A, Bronzwear JG *et al.* Three-dimensional respiratory-gated MR angiography of coronary arteries: Comparison with conventional coronary angiography. *Am J Roentgenol* 1996; **166**: 1399–1404.

95. Yucel AC, Edelman R, Grist T *et al.* Magnetic resonance angiography: Update on applications for extracranial arteries. *Circulation* 1999; **100**: 2284–2301.

96. Wang Y, Grist TM, Korosec FR *et al.* Respiratory blur in 3D coronary MR imaging. *Magn Reson Med* 1995; **33**: 541–548.

97. Stuber M, Botnar R, Danias PG *et al.* Double-oblique free-breathing high resolution three-dimensional coronary magnetic resonance angiography. *J Am Coll Cardiol* 1999; **34**: 524–531.

98. Mansfield P. Real-time echo-planar imaging by NMR. *Br Med Bull* 1984; **40**: 187–189.

99. Nayak K, Yang P, Pauly J *et al.* Real time interactive MRA. *Magn Reson Med* 2001; **46**: 430–435.

100. Kerr A, Pauly J, Hu B *et al.* Real time interactive MRI on a conventional scanner. *Magn Reson Med* 1997; **38**: 355–367.

101. Yang P, Meyer C, Kerr A *et al.* Spiral magnetic resonance coronary angiography with real time localization. *J Am Coll Cardiol* 2003; **41**: 1134–1141.

102. Yang PC, Santos JM, Nguyen PK *et al.* Dynamic real time architecture in magnetic resonance coronary

angiography—a prospective clinical trial. *J Cardiovasc Magn Reson* 2004; **6**: 885–894.

103. Santos J, Wright G, Yang P *et al.* Adaptive architecture of real time imaging systems. In: *Proceedings of the International Society of Magnetic Resonance in Medicine,* 10th Annual Meeting, Orlando, 2002: 468.

104. Sodickson D, Griswold M, Jakob P *et al.* SMASH imaging. *Magn Reson Imaging Clin North Am* 1999; **7**: 237–254.

105. Sodickson D, Manning W. Simultaneous acquisition of spatial harmonics (SMASH): Fast imaging with radio-frequency array coils. *Magn Reson Med* 1999; **38**: 591–603.

106. Pruessmann KP, Wieger M, Scheidegger MB *et al.* SENSE: Sensitivity encoding for fast MRI. *Magn Reson Med* 1999; **42**: 952–962.

107. Yeh E, Botnar R, Leiner T *et al.* Adaptation of coronary imaging pulse sequences for self-calibrated non-Cartesian parallel imaging. In: *Proceedings of the International Society of Magnetic Resonance in Medicine,* 11th Annual Scientific Meeting, Kyoto, Japan, 2003: 1882.

108. Niendorf T, Sodickson D, Hardy CJ *et al.* Towards whole heart coverage in a single breath-hold coronary artery imaging using a true 32 channel phased array MR system. In: *Proceedings of the International Society of Magnetic Resonance in Medicine,* 12th Annual Scientific Meeting, Kyoto, Japan, 2004: 703.

109. Sodickson D, Stuber M, Botnar R *et al.* Accelerated coronary MR angiography in volunteers and patients using double oblique 3D acquisitions combined with SMASH. *J Cardiovasc Magn Reson* 1999; **1**: 260–265.

110. Wieger M, Pruessman KP, Boesiger P *et al.* Cardiac real time imaging using SENSE sensitivity encoding scheme. *Magn Reson Med* 2000; **43**: 177–184.

111. Hong S, Muthupillai R, Smink J *et al.* Accelerated acquisition of free-breathing navigator-guided MR angiography using sensitivity encoding and motion adapted gating (MAG). In: *J Cardiovasc Magn Reson,* 10th Annual Scientific Session, Orlando, 2002: 26.

112. Huber M, Kozerke S, Pruessmann KP *et al.* Sensitivity-encoded coronary MRA at 3T. *Magn Reson Med* 2004; **52**: 221–227.

113. Waltering K, Nassentein K, Massing S *et al.* Coronary magnetic resonance angiography using parallel acquisition techniques and intravascular contrast media. In: *SCMR,* 8th Annual Proceedings, Orlando, 2005: 211.

114. Weiger M, Pruessman K, Leussler C *et al.* Specific coil design for sense: A six-element cardiac array. *Magn Reson Med* 2001; **45**: 495–504.

115. Zhu Y, Hardy CJ, Sodickson DK *et al.* Highly parallel volumetric imaging with a 32-element RF coil array. *Magn Reson Med* 2004; **52**: 869–877.

116. Heidemann RM, Griswold M, Haase A *et al*. VD-AUTO-SMASH imaging. *Magn Reson Med* 2001; **45**: 1066–1074.

117. Griswold MA, Jakob PM, Heidemann RM *et al*. Generalized autocalibrating partial parallel acquisitions (GRAPPA). *Magn Reson Med* 2002; **47**: 1202–1210.

118. Weber O, Pujadas S, Martin A *et al*. Free-breathing, three-dimensional coronary artery magnetic resonance angiography: Comparison of sequences. *J Magn Reson Imaging* 2004; **20**: 395–402.

119. Link KM, Lesko NJ. The role of MR imaging in the evaluation of the thoracic aorta. *Am J Roentgenol* 1992; **158**: 115–112.

120. Hartnell GG, Finn JP, Zenni M *et al*. MR imaging of the thoracic aorta: Comparison of spin echo, angiographic, and breath-hold techniques. *Radiology* 1994; **191**: 697–704.

121. Solomon SL, Brown JJ, Glazer H *et al*. Thoracic aortic dissection: Pitfalls and artifacts in MR imaging. *Radiology* 1990; **177**: 223–228.

122. Seelos KC, Funari M, Higgins CB *et al*. Detection of aortic arch thrombus using MR imaging. *J Comput Assist Tomogr* 1991; **15**: 224–247.

123. Sonnabend SB, Colletti PM, Pentecost M *et al*. Demonstration of aortic lesions via cine magnetic resonance imaging. *Magn Reson Imaging* 1990; **8**: 613–618.

124. Dumoulin CL, Hart HR. Magnetic resonance angiography. *Radiology* 1986; **161**: 717–720.

125. Sechtem U, Pflugfelder P, White RD *et al*. Cine MR imaging: Potential for the evaluation of cardiovascular function. *AJR* 1987; **148**: 239–246.

126. Sakuma H, Bourne M, O'Sullivan M *et al*. Evaluation of thoracic aortic dissection using breath-holding cine MRI. *J Comput Assist Tomogr* 1996; **20**: 45–50.

127. De La Pena E, Nguyen P, Nayak KS *et al*. Real time color-flow MRI in adults with congenital heart disease (manuscript submitted to *J Cardiovasc Magn Reson* 2005).

128. Weiger M, Pruessmann K, Kassner A *et al*. Contrast enhanced 3D MRA using SENSE. *J Magn Reson Imaging* 2000; **12**: 671–677.

129. Sodickson D, McKenzie C, Li W *et al*. Contrast enhanced 3D MR angiography with simultaneous acquisition of spatial harmonics: A pilot study. *Radiology* 2000; **217**: 284–289.

130. Fink C, Ley S, Kroeker R *et al*. Time-resolved contrast enhanced three-dimensional magnetic resonance angiography of the chest: Combination of parallel imaging with view sharing (TREAT). *Invest Radiol* 2005; **40**: 40–48.

131. Wu Y, Goodrich K, Buswell H *et al*. High resolution time-resolved contrast enhanced 3D MRA by combining SENSE with keyhole and SLAM strategies. *Magn Reson Imaging* 2004; **22**: 1161–1168.

132. Davis WL, Blatter DD, Harnsberger HR *et al*. Intracranial MR angiography: Comparison of single-volume three-dimensional time-of-flight and multiple overlapping thin slab acquisition techniques. *Am J Roentgenol* 1994; **163**: 915–920.

133. Parker DL, Yuan C, Blatter DD *et al*. MR acquisition by multiple thin slab 3D acquisition. *Magn Reson Med* 1991; **17**: 434–451.

134. Prince MR, Yucel EK, Kaufman JA *et al*. Dynamic gadolinium enhanced three-dimensional abdominal MR angiography. *J Magn Reson Imaging* 1993; **3**: 877–881.

135. Prince MR. Gadolinium enhanced MR aortography. *Radiology* 1994; **191**: 155–164.

136. Cloft H, Murphy K, Prince M *et al*. 3D gadolinium enhanced MR angiography of the carotid arteries. *Magn Reson Imaging* 1996; **14**: 593–600.

137. Riederer S. Current technical development of magnetic resonance imaging. *IEEE Engineering in Medicine and Biology* 2000; **19**: 34–41.

138. Enochs WS, Ackerman RH, Kaufman JA *et al*. Gadolinium enhanced MR angiography of the carotid arteries. *J Neuroimaging* 1988; **8**: 185–190.

139. Willig DS, Turski PA, Frayne R *et al*. Contrast enhanced 3D MR DSA of the carotid artery bifurcation: Preliminary study of comparison with unenhanced 2D and 3D time-of-flight MR angiography. *Radiology* 1998; **208**: 447–451.

140. Saloner D. Determinants of image appearance in contrast enhanced magnetic resonance angiography. *Investigative Radiology* 1998; **33**: 488–495.

141. Carroll TJ, Grist TM. Technical developments in MR angiography. *Radiology* 2002; **40**: 921–951.

142. Leclerc X, Pruvo J-P. Recent advances in magnetic resonance angiography of carotid and vertebral vessels. *Curr Opin Neurol* 2000; **13**: 75–82.

143. Maki JH, Prince MR, Londy FJ *et al*. The effects of time varying signal intravascular signal intensity and k-space acquisition order on three-dimensional angiography image quality. *J Magn Reson Imaging* 1996; **6**: 642–651.

144. Mezrich R. A perspective on k-space. *Radiology* 1995; **195**: 297–315.

145. Steffens JC, Link J, Gressner J *et al*. Contrast enhanced k-space centered, breath hold MR angiography of the renal arteries and abdominal aorta. *J Magn Reson Imaging* 1997; **7**: 617–622.

146. Huston J 3rd, Fain SB, Riederer SJ *et al*. Carotid arteries: Maximizing arterial to venous contrast in fluoroscopically triggered contrast enhanced MR angiography with elliptic centric view ordering. *Radiology* 1999; **211**: 265–273.

147. Wilman AH, Riederer SJ, Huston J *et al*. Arterial phase carotid and vertebral artery imaging in 3D contrast enhanced MR angiography by combining fluoroscopic

triggering with an elliptical centric acquisition order. *Magn Reson Med* 1998; **40**: 24–35.

148. Korosec FR, Frayne R, Grist TM *et al*. Time-resolved contrast enhanced 3D MR angiography. *Magn Reson Med* 1996; **36**: 345–351.

149. Mistretta CA, Grist TM, Korosec FR *et al*. 3D time-resolved contrast enhanced MR DSA: Advantages and trade offs. *Magn Reson Med* 1998; **40**: 571–581.

150. Naganawa S, Koshikawa T, Fukatsu H *et al*. Contrast enhanced MR angiography of the carotid artery using 3D time-resolved imaging of contrast kinetics: Comparison with real time fluoroscopic triggered 3D-elliptical centric view ordering. *Radiat Med.* 2001; **19**: 185–192.

151. Levy RA, Maki JH. Three-dimensional contrast enhanced MR angiography of the extracranial carotid arteries: Two techniques. *Am J Neuroradiol* 1998; **19**: 688–690.

152. Ramonda L, Heid O, Schroth G *et al*. Carotid artery stenosis, occlusion, and pseudo-occlusion: First pass, gadolinium enhanced, three-dimensional MR angiography: preliminary study. *Radiology* 1998; **209**: 95–102.

153. Wang Y, Donald LJ, Breen JF *et al*. Dynamic MR digital subtraction angiography using contrast enhanced, fast data acquisition, and complex subtraction. *Magn Reson Med* 1996; **36**: 551–556.

154. Laub G. Displays for MR angiography. *Magn Reson Med* 1990; **14**: 222–229.

155. Anderson CM, Saloner D, Tsurada JS *et al*. Artifacts in maximum-intensity-projection display of MR angiograms. *Am J Roentgenol* 1990; **154**: 623–629.

156. Nguyen PK, Nayak K, Cunningham CH *et al*. Real time coronary MR angiography at 3T. In: *Proceedings of the International Society of Magnetic Resonance in Medicine*, 12th Scientific Meeting, Kyoto, Japan, 2004: 1877.

157. Weber O, Alastair J, Higgins C *et al*. Whole-heart steady-state free precession coronary artery magnetic resonance angiography. *Magn Reson Med* 2003; **50**: 1223–1228.

158. Kragel A, Roberts WC. Anomalous origin of either the right or left main coronary artery from the aorta with subsequent coursing between aorta and pulmonary trunk: Analysis of 32 necropsy cases. *Am J Cardiol* 1988; **62**: 771–777.

159. Bunce NH, Lorenz CH, Keegan J *et al*. Coronary artery anomalies: Assessment with free-breathing three-dimensional coronary MR angiography. *Radiology* 2003; **227**: 201–208.

160. McConnell MV, Ganz P, Selwyn AP *et al*. Identification of anomalous coronary arteries and their anatomic course by magnetic resonance coronary angiography. *Circulation* 1995; **92**: 3158–3162.

161. Vliegen HW, Doornbos J, de Roos A *et al*. Value of fast gradient echo magnetic resonance angiography as an adjunct to coronary angiography in detecting and con-firming the course of clinically significant coronary artery anomalies. *Am J Cardiol* 1997; **79**: 773–776.

162. Taylor AM, Thorne SA, Rubens MB *et al*. Coronary artery imaging in grown up congenital heart disease: Complementary role of magnetic resonance and x-ray coronary angiography. *Circulation* 2000; **101**: 1670–1678.

163. Post JC, van Rossum A, Bronzwaer JG *et al*. Magnetic resonance angiography of anomalous coronary arteries. A new gold standard for delineating the proximal course? *Circulation* 1995; **92**: 3163–3171.

164. Post JC, van Rossum A, Hofman MB *et al*. Clinical utility of two-dimensional magnetic resonance angiography in detecting coronary artery disease. *Eur Heart J* 1997; **18**: 426–433.

165. Pennell D, Bogren H, Keegan J *et al*. Assessment of coronary artery stenosis by magnetic resonance imaging. *Heart* 1996; **75**: 127–133.

166. Regenfus M, Ropers D, Achenbach S *et al*. Non-invasive detection of coronary artery stenosis using contrast enhanced three-dimensional breath-hold magnetic resonance coronary angiography. *J Am Coll Cardiol* 2000; **36**: 44–50.

167. Woodard PK, Li D, Haacke EM *et al*. Detection of coronary stenoses on source and projection images using three-dimensional MR angiography with retrospective respiratory gating: Preliminary experience. *Am J Roentgenol* 1998; **170**: 883–888.

168. Kessler W, Achenbach S, Moshage W *et al*. Usefulness of respiratory gated magnetic resonance coronary angiography in assessing narrowings > or = 50% in diameter in native coronary arteries and in aortocoronary bypass conduits. *Am J Cardiol* 1997; **80**: 989–993.

169. Huber M, Nikalaou K, Gonschior P *et al*. Navigator echo-based respiratory gating for three-dimensional MR coronary angiography: Results from healthy volunteers and patients with coronary artery stenosis. *Am J Roentgenol* 1999; **173**: 95–101.

170. Sandstede JJ, Pabst T, Beer M *et al*. Three-dimensional MR coronary angiography using the navigator technique compared with conventional coronary angiography. *Am J Roentgenol* 1999; **172**: 135–139.

171. Sardanelli F, Molinari G, Zandrino F *et al*. Three-dimensional, navigator-echo MR coronary angiography in detecting stenosis of the major epicardial vessels, with conventional coronary angiography as the standard of reference. *Radiology* 2000; **214**: 808–814.

172. Muller MF, Fleisch M, Kroeker R *et al*. Proximal coronary artery stenosis: Three-dimensional MRI with fat saturation and navigator echo. *J Magn Reson Imaging* 1997; **7**: 644–651.

173. Kim W, Danias P, Stuber M *et al*. Coronary magnetic resonance angiography for the detection of coronary stenoses. *N Engl J Med* 2001; **345**: 1863–1869.

174. Sommer T, Hackenbroch M, Hofer U *et al.* Coronary MR angiography at 3.0 T versus that at 1.5 T: Initial results in patients suspected of having coronary artery disease. *Radiology* 2005; **234**: 718–725.

175. So NM, Lam W, Li D *et al.* Magnetic resonance coronary angiography with 3D TRUE FISP: Breath-hold versus respiratory gated imaging. *Br J Radiol* 2005; **78**: 116–121.

176. White RD, Caputo GR, Mark AS *et al.* Coronary artery bypass graft patency: Non-invasive evaluation with MR imaging. *Radiology* 1987; **164**: 681–686.

177. Rubenstein RI, Akenase AD, Thickman D *et al.* Magnetic resonance imaging to evaluate patency of aortocoronary bypass grafts. *Circulation* 1987; **76**: 786–791.

178. Jenkins JP, Love H, Foster CJ *et al.* Detection of coronary artery bypass graft patency as assessed by magnetic resonance imaging. *Br J Radiol* 1988; **61**: 2–4.

179. Galjee MA, van Rossum A, Doesburg T *et al.* Value of magnetic resonance imaging in assessing patency and function of coronary artery bypass grafts. An angiographically controlled study. *Circulation* 1996; **93**: 660–666.

180. White RD, Pflugfelder P, Lipton MJ *et al.* Coronary artery bypass grafts: Evaluation of patency with cine MR imaging. *Am J Roentgenol* 1988; **150**: 1271–1274.

181. Aurigemma GP, Riechek N, Axel L *et al.* Non-invasive determination of coronary artery bypass graft patency by cine magnetic resonance imaging. *Circulation* 1989; **80**: 1595–1602.

182. Engelmann G, Knez A, von Smekal A *et al.* Non-invasive coronary bypass graft imaging after multivessel revascularization. *Int J Cardiol* 2000; **76**: 65–74.

183. Wintersperger BJ, Engellman MG, von Smekal A *et al.* Patency of coronary bypass grafts: Assessment with breath-hold contrast enhanced MR angiography—value of a non-electrocardiographically triggered technique. *Radiology* 1998; **208**: 345–351.

184. Brenner P, Wintersperger BJ, von Smekal A *et al.* Detection of coronary artery bypass graft patency by contrast enhanced magnetic resonance angiography. *Eur J Cardiothorac Surg* 1999; **15**: 389–393.

185. Bogaert J, Meyns B, Rademakers FE *et al.* Follow-up of aortic dissection: Contribution of MR angiography for the evaluation of the abdominal aorta and its branches. *Eur Radiol* 1997; **7**: 695–702.

186. Nienaber CA, von Kodolitsch Y, Nikolas V *et al.* The diagnosis of thoracic aortic dissection by non-invasive imaging procedures. *N Engl J Med* 1993; **328**: 1–9.

187. Sommer T, Fehski W, Holzknecht N *et al.* Aortic dissection: A comparative study of diagnosis with spiral CT, multiplanar transesophageal echocardiography and MR imaging. *Radiology* 1996; **199**: 347–352.

188. Coady MA, Rizzo JA, Goldstein LJ *et al.* Natural history, pathogenesis and etiology of thoracic aneurysms and dissection. *Cardiol Clin* 1999; **17**: 615–633.

189. Cigarroa JE, Isselbacher E, De Sanctis RW *et al.* Diagnostic imaging in the evaluation of suspected aortic dissection. Old standards and new directions. *N Engl J Med* 1993; **328**: 35–43.

190. Nienaber CA, von Kodolitsch Y, Nikolas V *et al.* Nonsurgical reconstruction of thoracic aortic dissection by stent-graft placement. *N Eng J Med* 1999; **140**: 1338–1345.

191. Dake MD, Kato N, Mitchell RS *et al.* Endovascular stent-graft placement for the treatment of acute aortic dissection. *N Engl J Med* 1999; **140**: 1546–1552.

192. Kersting-Somerhoff BA, Higgins CB, White RD *et al.* Aortic dissection: Sensitivity and specificity of MR imaging. *Radiology* 1988; **166**: 651–655.

193. Fernandez GC, Tardaguila F, Duran D *et al.* Dynamic 3-dimensional contrast enhanced magnetic resonance angiography in acute aortic dissection. *Curr Probl Diagn Radiol* 2002; **31**: 134–145.

194. Kunz RP, Oberholzer K, Kuroczynski W *et al.* Assessment of chronic aortic dissection: Contribution of different ECG-gated breath-hold MRI techniques. *Am J Roentgenol* 2004; **182**: 1319–1326.

195. Fisher U, Vossherich R, Kopka L *et al.* Dissection of the thoracic aorta: Pre- and postoperative findings of TURBO-FLASH MR images in the plane of the aortic arch. *Am J Roentgenol* 1994; **163**: 1069–1072.

196. Moore NR, Parry AJ, Trottman-Dickenson B *et al.* Fate of the native aorta after repair of acute type a dissection: A magnetic resonance imaging study. *Heart* 1996; **75**: 62–66.

197. Mesana TG, Caus T, Gaubert J *et al.* Late complications after prosthetic replacement of the ascending aorta: What did we learn from routine magnetic resonance imaging follow-up? *Eur J Cardiothorac Surg* 2000; **18**: 313–320.

198. Gaubert J, Moulin G, Mesana T *et al.* Type A dissection of the thoracic aorta. Use of MR imaging for long term follow-up. *Radiology* 1995; **196**: 363–369.

199. Cesare ED, Giordano A, Cerone G *et al.* Comparative evaluation of tee, conventional MRI and contrast enhanced 3D breath-hold MRA in the post-operative follow-up of dissecting aneurysms. *Int J Card Imaging* 2000; **16**: 135–147.

200. Nienaber CA, von Kodolitsch Y, Petersen B *et al.* Intramural hemorrhage of the thoracic aorta: Diagnostic and therapeutic implications. *Circulation* 1995; **92**: 1465–1472.

201. Moore A, Oh J, Bruckman D *et al.* Transesophageal echocardiography in the diagnosis and management of aortic dissection. An analysis of data from the international registry of aortic dissection (IRAD). *J Am Coll Cardiol* 1999; **1999**: 470A.

202. Murray JG, Manisali M, Flamm SD *et al.* Intramural hematoma of the thoracic aorta: MR imaging findings and their prognostic implications. *Radiology* 1997; **204**: 349–355.

203. Krinsky G, Rofsky N, de Corato DR *et al*. Thoracic aorta: Comparison of gadolinium-enhanced three-dimensional angiography with conventional MR imaging. *Radiology* 1997; **202**: 183–193.

204. Yucel EK, Steinberg FL, Egglin TK *et al*. Penetrating aortic ulcers: Diagnosis with MR imaging. *Radiology* 1990; **177**: 779–781.

205. Hayeshi H, Matsuoka Y, Sakamoto I *et al*. Penetrating atherosclerotic ulcer of the aorta: Imaging features and disease concept. *Radiographics* 2000; **20**: 995–1005.

206. Hartnell GG. Imaging of aortic aneurysms and dissection: CT and MRI. *J Thorac Imaging* 2001; **16**: 35–46.

207. Neimatallah MA, Ho VB, Dong Q *et al*. Gadolinium-enhanced 3D magnetic resonance angiography of the thoracic vessels. *Magn Reson Imaging* 1999; **10**: 758–770.

208. Prince MR, Narasimham DL, Jacoby WT *et al*. Three-dimensional gadolinium-enhanced MR angiography of the thoracic aorta. *Am J Roentgenol* 1996; **166**: 1387–1397.

209. Nasim A, Thompson MM, Sayers RD *et al*. Role of magnetic resonance angiography for assessment of abdominal aortic aneurysm before endoluminal repair. *Br J Surg* 1998; **85**: 641–644.

210. Papanicolaou N, Wittenberg J, Ferrucci JT Jr *et al*. Preoperative evaluation of abdominal aortic aneurysms by computed tomography. *Am J Roentgenol* 1986; **146**: 711–715.

211. Pavone P, Di Cesare E, Di Renzi P *et al*. Abdominal aortic aneurysm evaluation: Comparison of US, CT, MRI, and angiography. *Magn Reson Imaging* 1990; **8**: 199–204.

212. Gomes MN, Choyke P. Pre-operative evaluation of abdominal aortic aneurysms: Ultrasound or computed tomography? *J Cardiovasc Surg (Torino)*. 1987; **28**: 159–166.

213. Kaufman JA, Geller SC, Petersen MJ *et al*. MR imaging (including MR angiography) of abdominal aortic aneurysms: Comparison with conventional angiography. *Am J Roentgenol* 1994; **163**: 203–210.

214. Kaufman JA, Yucel EK, Waltman AC *et al*. MR angiography in the preoperative evaluation of abdominal aortic aneurysms: A preliminary study. *J Vasc Interv Radiol* 1994; **5**: 489–496.

215. Durham JR, Hackworth CA, Tober JC *et al*. Magnetic resonance angiography in the preoperative evaluation of abdominal aortic aneurysms. *AM J Surg* 1993; **166**: 173–177.

216. Ecklund K, Hartnell GG, Hughes LA *et al*. MR angiography as the sole method of evaluating abdominal aortic aneurysms: Correlation with conventional techniques and surgery. *Radiology* 1994; **192**: 345–350.

217. Prince MR, Narasimham DL, Stanley JC *et al*. Gadolinium-enhanced magnetic resonance angiography of abdominal aortic aneurysms. *J Vasc Surg* 1995; **21**: 656–669.

218. Liassy JP, Soyer P, Tebboune D *et al*. Abdominal aortic aneurysms: Assessment with gadolinium-enhanced time of flight coronal MR angiography (MRA). *Eur J Radiol* 1995; **20**: 1–8.

219. Petersen MJ, Cambria RP, Kaufman JA *et al*. Magnetic resonance angiography in the preoperative evaluation of abdominal aortic aneurysms. *J Vasc Surg* 1995; **21**: 891–898.

220. Lookstein RA, Goldman J, Pukin L *et al*. Time-resolved magnetic resonance angiography as a non-invasive method to characterize endoleaks: Initial results compared with conventional angiography. *J Vasc Surg* 2004; **39**: 27–33.

221. Insko E, Kulzer L, Fairman R *et al*. MR imaging for the detection of endoleaks in recipients of abdominal aortic stent-grafts with low magnetic susceptibility. *Acad Radiol* 2003; **10**: 509–513.

222. Pate JW, Fabian TC, Walker W *et al*. Traumatic rupture of the aortic isthmus: An emergency? *World J Surg* 1995; **19**: 119–126.

223. Fattori R, Celleti F, Bertraccini P *et al*. Delayed surgery of traumatic aortic rupture: Role of magnetic resonance imaging. *Circulation* 1996; **94**: 2865–2870.

224. Fattori R Celleti F, Descovich B *et al*. Evolution of post-traumatic aneurysm in the subacute phase: Magnetic resonance imaging follow-up as a support of the surgical timing. *Eur J Cardiothorac Surg* 1998; **13**: 582–587.

225. Yamada I, Nakagawa T, Himeno Y *et al*. Takayasu arteritis: Diagnosis with breath-hold contrast enhanced three-dimensional MR angiography. *J Magn Reson Imaging* 2000; **11**: 481–487.

226. Kissin EY, Merkel PA. Diagnostic imaging in Takayasu arteritis. *Curr Opin Rheumatol* 2004; **16**: 31–37.

227. Choe YH, Kim DK, Koh EM *et al*. Takayasu arteritis: Diagnosis with MR imaging and MR angiography in acute and chronic stages. *J Magn Reson Imaging* 1999; **10**: 751–757.

228. Thiene G, Frescura C. Etiology and pathology of aortic arch malformations. In: Nienaber CA FR, ed. *Diagnosis of Aortic Diseases*. Kluwer Academic Publishers, New York, 1999.

229. Kersting-Somerhoff BA, Sechtem V, Fisher MR *et al*. MR imaging of congenital anomalies of the aortic arch. *Am J Roentgenol* 1987; **149**: 9–13.

230. Carpenter JP, Holland GA, Golden MA *et al*. Magnetic resonance angiography of the aortic arch. *J Vasc Surg* 1997; **25**: 145–151.

231. Fixler DE. Coarctation of the aorta. *Cardiol Clin* 1988; **6**: 561–571.

232. Julsrud PR, Breen JF, Felmlee JP *et al*. Coarctation of the aorta: Collateral flow assessment with phase-contrast MR angiography. *Am J Roentgenol* 1997; **169**: 1735–1742.

233. Godart F, Labrot G, Devos P *et al.* Coarctation of the aorta: Comparison of aortic dimensions between conventional MR imaging, 3D MR angiography, and conventional angiography. *Eur Radiol* 2002; **12**: 2034–2039.

234. Paddon AJ, Nicholson AA, Ettles DF *et al.* Long term follow-up of percutaneous balloon angioplasty in adult aortic coarctation. *Cardiovasc Intervent Radiol* 2000; **23**: 364–367.

235. Bogaert J, Kuzo R, Dymor K *et al.* Follow-up of patients with previous treatment for coarctation of the thoracic aorta: Comparison between contrast enhanced MR angiography and fast spin echo. *Eur Radiol* 2000; **10**: 1047–1054.

236. Keller PJ, Drayer BP, Fram EK *et al.* MR angiography with two-dimensional acquisition and three-dimensional display. *Radiology* 1989; **173**: 527–532.

237. Masaryk TJ, Modic MT, Ruggieri PM *et al.* Three-dimensional (volume) gradient echo imaging of the carotid bifurcation: Preliminary clinical experience. *Radiology* 1989; **171**: 801–806.

238. De Marco JK, Huston J, Bernstein M *et al.* Evaluation of classic 2D time-of-flight MR angiography in the depiction of severe carotid stenosis. *Am J Roentgenol* 2004; **183**: 787–793.

239. Slosman F, Stolpen A, Lexa FJ *et al.* Extracranial atherosclerotic carotid artery disease: Evaluation of non-breath-hold three-dimensional gadolinium-enhanced MR angiography. *Am J Roentgenol* 1998; **170**: 489–495.

240. Levy RA, Prince MR. Arterial-phase three-dimensional contrast enhanced MR angiography of the carotid arteries. *Am J Roentgenol* 1996; **167**: 211–215.

241. Leclerc X, Gauvrit J, Nicol L *et al.* Gadolinium-enhanced fast three-dimensional angiography of the neck: Technical aspect. *Invest Radiol* 1999; **34**: 204–210.

242. Anderson CM, Lee RE, Levin DL *et al.* Measurement of internal carotid stenosis from source MR angiograms. *Radiology* 1994; **193**: 219–226.

243. Levi CR, Mitchell A, Fitt G *et al.* The accuracy of magnetic resonance angiography in the assessment of extracranial carotid occlusive disease: A comparison with digital subtraction angiography using NASCET criteria for stenosis measurement. *Cerebrovasc Dis* 1996; **6**: 231–236.

244. Korogi Y, Takahashi M, Mabuchi N *et al.* Intracranial vascular stenosis and occlusion: Diagnostic accuracy of three-dimensional, Fourier transform, time-of-flight MR angiography. *Radiology* 1994; **193**: 187–193.

245. Liberopoulous K, Kaponis A, Kokkins K *et al.* Comparative study of magnetic resonance angiography, digital subtraction angiography, duplex ultrasound examination with surgical and histological findings of atheros-clerotic carotid bifurcation disease. *Int Angiol* 1996; **15**: 131–137.

246. Patel MR, Kuntz KM, Klufas RA *et al.* Preoperative assessment of carotid bifurcation: Can magnetic resonance angiography and duplex ultrasonography replace contrast angiography? *Stroke* 1995; **26**: 1753–1758.

247. Nicholas GG, Osborne MA, Jaffe JW *et al.* Carotid stenosis: Preoperative non-invasive evaluation in a community hospital. *J Vasc Surg* 1995; **22**: 9–16.

248. Kent KC, Kuntz KM, Patel MR *et al.* Peri-operative imaging strategies for carotid endarterectomy: An analysis of morbidity and cost effectiveness. *JAMA* 1995; **274**: 888–893.

249. Mittle RL Jr, Broderick M, Carpenter JP *et al.* Blinder-reader comparison of magnetic resonance angiography and duplex ultrasonography for carotid artery bifurcation stenosis. *Stroke* 1994; **25**: 4–10.

250. Young GR, Humphrey PR, Shaw MD *et al.* Comparison of magnetic resonance angiography, duplex ultrasound and digital subtraction angiography in the assessment of extracranial internal carotid artery stenosis. *J Neurol Neurosurg Psychiatry* 1994; **57**: 1466–1478.

251. Young GR, Sandercock PA, Slattery J *et al.* Observer variation in the interpretation of intra-arterial angiograms and the risk of inappropriate decisions about carotid endarterectomy. *J Neurol Neurosurg Psychiatry* 1996; **60**: 152–157.

252. Vanninen R, Manninen H, Soimakallio S *et al.* Imaging of carotid artery stenosis: Clinical efficacy and cost effectiveness. *Am J Neuroradiol* 1995; **16**: 1875–1883.

253. Urchuk SN, Plewes D. Mechanisms of flow-induced signal loss in MR angiography. *J Magn Reson Imaging* 1992; **2**: 453–462.

254. De Marco JK, Nesbit GM, Wesbey GE *et al.* Prospective evaluation of extracranial carotid stenosis: MR angiography with maximum-intensity projections and multiplanar reformation compared with conventional angiography. *Am J Roentgenol* 1994; **163**: 1205–1212.

255. Sardanelli F, Zandrino F, Parodi RC *et al.* MR angiography of internal carotid arteries: Breath-hold GD-enhanced 3D fast imaging with steady-state free precession versus unenhanced 2D and 3D time of flight techniques. *J Comput Assist Tomogr* 1999; **23**: 208–215.

256. Leclerc X, Martinat P, Goldefroy O *et al.* Contrast enhanced three-dimensional with steady state (FISP) MR angiography of supra-aortic vessels: Preliminary study. *Am J Neuroradiol* 1998; **19**: 1405–1413.

257. Alvarez-Linera J, Benito-Leon J, Escribano J *et al.* Prospective evaluation of carotid artery stenosis: Elliptic centric contrast enhanced MR angiography and spiral CT angiography compared with digital subtraction angiography. *Am J Neuroradiol* 2003; **24**: 1012–1019.

258. Borisch I, Horn M, Butz B *et al.* Pre-operative evaluation of carotid artery stenosis: Comparison of contrast-enhanced MR angiography and duplex sonography with digital subtraction angiography. *Am J Neuroradiol* 2003; **24**: 1117–1122.

259. Serfaty JM, Chirossel P, Chevallier JM *et al.* Accuracy of three-dimensional gadolinium-enhanced MR angiography in the assessment of extracranial carotid artery disease. *Am J Roentgenol* 2001; **175**: 455–463.

260. Randoux B, Marro B, Koskas F *et al.* Carotid artery stenosis: Prospective comparison of CT, three-dimensional gadolinium-enhanced MR, and conventional angiography. *Radiology* 2001; **220**: 179–185.

261. Remonda L, Senn P, Barth A *et al.* Contrast-enhanced 3D MR angiography of the carotid artery: Comparison with conventional digital subtraction angiography. *Am J Neuroradiol* 2002; **23**: 213–219.

262. Nederkoorn PJ, Elgersma OE, van der Graaf Y *et al.* Carotid artery stenosis: Accuracy of contrast-enhanced MR angiography for diagnosis. *Radiology* 2003; **228**: 677–682.

263. Butz B, Dorenbeck U, Borisch I *et al.* High-resolution contrast enhanced magnetic resonance angiography of the carotid arteries using fluoroscopic monitoring of contrast arrival: Diagnostic accuracy and interobserver variability. *Acta Radiol* 2004; **45**: 164–170.

264. Lenhart M, Framme N, Volk M *et al.* Time-resolved contrast enhanced magnetic resonance angiography of the carotid arteries: Diagnostic accuracy and inter-observer variability compared with selective catheter angiography. *Invest Radiol* 2002; **37**: 535–541.

265. Pan XM, Saloner D, Reilly LM *et al.* Assessment of carotid artery stenosis by ultrasonography, conventional angiography, and magnetic resonance angiography: Correlation with *ex vivo* measurement of plaque stenosis. *J Vasc Surg* 1995; **21**: 82–88.

266. Elgersma OE, Wust AF, Buijs PC *et al.* Multidirectional depiction of internal carotid artery stenosis: Three-dimensional time-of-flight MR angiography versus rotational and conventional digital subtraction angiography. *Radiology* 2000; **216**: 511–516.

267. Culebras A, Kase CS, Masdeu JC *et al.* Practice guidelines for the use of imaging in transient ischemic attacks and acute stroke. A report of the stroke council, American Heart Association. *Stroke* 1997; **7**: 1480–1497.

268. Tay K, U-King Im J, Trivedi R *et al.* Imaging the vertebral artery. *Eur Radiol* 2005; **15**: 1–28.

269. Randoux B, Marro B, Koskas F *et al.* Proximal great vessels of the aortic arch: Comparison of three-dimensional gadolinium-enhanced MR angiography and digital subtraction angiography. *Radiology* 2003; **229**: 697–702.

270. Levy C, Laissy JP, Raveau V *et al.* Carotid and vertebral artery dissections: Three-dimensional time-of-flight MR angiography and MR imaging versus conventional angiography. *Radiology* 1994; **190**: 97–103.

271. Goldberg HI, Grossman RI, Gomori JM *et al.* Cervical internal carotid dissection hemorrhage: Diagnosing using MR. *Radiology* 1986; **158**: 157–161.

272. Oelerich M, Stogbauer F, Kurlemann G *et al.* Craniocervical artery dissection: MR imaging and MR angiographic findings. *Eur Radiol* 1999; **9**: 1385–1391.

273. Kasner S, Hankins L, Bratina P *et al.* Magnetic resonance angiography demonstrates vascular healing of carotid and vertebral artery dissections. *Stroke* 1997; **28**: 1993–1997.

274. Stringaris K, Liberopoulous K, Giaka E *et al.* Three-dimensional time-of-flight MR angiography and MR imaging versus conventional angiography in carotid artery dissections. *Int Angiol* 1996; **15**: 20–25.

275. Klufas RA, Hsu L, Barnes PD *et al.* Dissection of the carotid and vertebral arteries: Imaging with MR angiography. *Am J Roentgenol* 1995; **164**: 673–677.

276. Provenzale JM. Dissection of the internal carotid and vertebral arteries: Imaging features. *Am J Roentgenol* 1995; **165**: 1099–1104.

277. Jacobs A, Lanfermann H, Szelies B *et al.* MRI- and MRA-guided therapy of carotid and vertebral artery dissections. *Cerebrovasc Dis* 1996; **6**: 80–87.

278. Nagahiro S, Hamada J, Sakamoto Y *et al.* Follow-up evaluation of dissecting aneurysms of the vertebrobasilar circulation by using gadolinium-enhanced magnetic resonance imaging. *J Neurosurg* 1997; **87**: 385–390.

279. Meaney JF, Weg JG, Chenevert TL *et al.* Diagnosis of pulmonary embolism with magnetic resonance angiography. *N Engl J Med* 1997; **336**: 1422–1427.

280. Oudkerk M, van Beek EJ, Wielopolski P *et al.* Comparison of contrast enhanced magnetic resonance angiography and conventional pulmonary angiography for the diagnosis of pulmonary embolism: A prospective study. *Lancet* 2002; **359**: 1643–1647.

281. Schoenberg SO, Bock M, Floemer F *et al.* High-resolution pulmonary arterio- and venography using multiple-bolus multiphase 3D-GD-MRA. *J Magn Reson Imaging* 1999; **3**: 339–346.

282. Greil G, Powell A, Gildein H *et al.* Gadolinium-enhanced three-dimensional magnetic resonance angiography of pulmonary and systemic vein anomalies. *J Am Coll Cardiol* 2002; **39**: 335–341.

283. Rehwald W, Klem I, Wagner A *et al.* GCFP—a new non-invasive non-contrast cine angiography technique using selective excitation and global coherent free precession. In: *International Society of Magnetic Resonance in Medicine*, 11th Annual Proceedings, Kyoto, Japan, 2004: 4.

284. Santos JM, Cunningham C, Hargreaves B *et al.* Single breath-hold whole-heart MRCA with variable density spirals at 3 T. In: *J Cardiovasc Magn Reson* 12th Annual Scientific Session, San Francisco, 2005: 188.

285. Maintz D, Ozgun M, Hofmeier A *et al.* Initial results of free-breathing balanced fast field echo whole heart MR angiography. In: *Proceedings of the International Society of Magnetic Resonance in Medicine*, 12th Annual Scientific Meeting, Kyoto, Japan, 2004: 706.

286. Earls JP, Patel NH, Smith PA *et al.* Gadolinium-enhanced three-dimensional MR angiography of the aorta and peripheral arteries: Evaluation of a multi-station examination using two gadopentetate dimeglumine infusions. *Am J Roentgenol* 1998; **171**: 599–604.

287. Goyen M, Herborn C, Kruger K *et al.* Detection of atherosclerosis: Systemic imaging for systemic disease with whole body three-dimensional angiography—initial experience. *Radiology* 2003; **227**: 277–282.

288. Meaney JF, Ridgeway JP, Chakraverty S *et al.* Stepping-table gadolinium-enhanced digital subtraction MR angiography of the aorta and lower extremity arteries: Preliminary experience. *Radiology* 1999; **211**: 59–67.

289. Goyen M, Quick H, Debatin J *et al.* Whole-body three-dimensional MR angiography with a rolling table platform: Initial clinical experience. *Radiology* 2002; **224**: 270–277.

290. Bernd T. Whole body CE-MRA using gadovist. *Eur Radiol* 2004; **14**: M26–M27.

CHAPTER 7

Cardiovascular magnetic resonance: Evaluation of myocardial function, perfusion and viability

Padmini Varadarajan, Karam Souibri, Krishna S. Nayak,
& Gerald M. Pohost

Introduction

Felix Bloch [1] at Stanford and Edward Purcell [2] at Harvard first reported the phenomenon of nuclear magnetic resonance (NMR) in 1946. Since then, substantial advances have been made in the clinical application of NMR to assess chemical composition (spectroscopy) and morphology and function (imaging) of biological tissue. In the late 1970s, NMR was adapted for the clinical evaluation of the cardiovascular system. Imaging was made possible through the introduction of gradients as suggested by Paul Lauterbur, PhD [3] and by Peter Mansfield, PhD [4]. Richard Ernst, PhD used the mathematical operation of Fourier transformation to generate a spectrum from the information contained after radiofrequency excitation, in a domain known as "k-space" [5]. Because of the importance of these discoveries, Purcell, Bloch, Ernst, Lauterbur and Mansfield have all received Nobel prizes, far more than have been awarded for any other medical imaging modality. Another early contributor to the field was Raymond Demadian.

It is now possible to generate images of the heart and blood vessels, a technique now called cardiovascular magnetic resonance (CMR), with high resolution and in real time. The evolution of CMR has been made possible by the advances in computer technology and higher field and magnetically homogeneous superconducting magnets [7, 8]. With its high spatial and contrast resolution, CMR has become widely regarded as the "gold standard" for the assessment of the morphology and function of the heart. Furthermore, decades of experience have shown it to be safe for biologic tissues, without ionization such as that produced by x-rays or radionuclides. Additionally, when used with gadolinium chelate-based paramagnetic contrast agents, there is no nephrotoxicity as there can be with iodinated x-ray contrast agents. Perhaps its major advantage is that it possesses the ability to provide the most comprehensive evaluation of the cardiovascular system. CMR can generate high resolution images of morphology and function; it can assess myocardial perfusion; it can define myocardial necrosis and scar, and it can assess myocardial metabolism, (e.g. that of the high energy phosphates, ATP and phosphocreatine).

With such advantages, one may ask why CMR has not become more widely applied. There are a few reasons for this. First, CMR is the most complex of the imaging modalities. In addition to the physical complexity of CMR, there is also a functional complexity inherent in this technique. This stems from the ability to generate considerable information about the heart. Specifically, CMR allows for the evaluation of cardiac morphology and ventricular function; myocardial perfusion and viability;

coronary artery status, and myocardial metabolism, using high energy phosphates. Second, the magnetic and radiofrequency fields of CMR can have deleterious effects on implantable devices, such as the pacemaker and implantable defibrillator.

CMR principles and techniques

CMR is the newest of the non-invasive cardiovascular imaging modalities and has become the modality of choice for the evaluation of ventricular function and volumes. It is preferred to catheter-based left ventriculography, which is invasive, requires radioopaque iodinated contrast medium, and is two dimensional. CMR of cardiac function requires an elaborate array of equipment including radiofrequency coils; instrumentation that allows the generation of radio-frequency pulses of varying durations and strengths; a homogeneous magnetic field; hardware to allow selection of tomographic slices in any plane orientation; phase encoding and readout gradients, and the software and hardware needed to differentiate between cardiac and respiratory motion. Understanding the physical basis of CMR can be challenging, since, as has been said, it is the most complex of all of the imaging modalities. Briefly, CMR images result from a mathematical transformation, a Fourier transformation, of the signal released in a uniform magnetic field by the sensitive nuclei contained within the organ(s) to be imaged after pulsing with the appropriate radiofrequency (known as the Larmor frequency) for the magnetic field. For imaging the sensitive nucleus is the proton, i.e. the hydrogen nucleus. The uniform magnetic field generally has a field strength of 1.5 (1.0 to 3.0) Tesla. A Tesla is the unit of magnetic field equivalent to 2×10^4 fold greater than the earth's magnetic field. A second (weaker) unit of magnetic field is the Gauss. The earth's magnetic field is ~0.5 Gauss. A Tesla is 10,000 Gauss.

After excitation of the magnetic field with a radiofrequency (RF) field, restitution of the magnetic field occurs in two planes and is determined by the longitudinal (T_1) and the transverse (T_2) relaxation times. Intensity of tissue on a CMR image depends on the number of hydrogen nuclei (or other sensitive nuclei), and the relaxation times, which depend on the strength of the interaction between these nuclei and the surrounding molecu-

Table 7.1 Approximate values of T1 and T2 relaxation times at 1.5 T.

Tissue	T1 (milliseconds)	T2 (milliseconds)
Myocardium	880	75
Blood	1200	360
Fat	260	110

lar environment [9, 10]. Table 7.1 provides T_1 and T_2 values for different tissues in a commonly used 1.5 T magnet [11].

CMR evaluation of structure and function

Radiofrequency pulse sequences used to generated CMR images are spin-echo and gradient-echo sequences, and other more complex sequences such as steady state free precession, echo-planar, velocity encoded imaging and radiofrequency tagging. Spin-echo sequences were among the first pulse sequences to be used to generate cardiovascular images, consisting of a single 90° pulse (rotating the net magnetization vector **B** within the tissue to be imaged by 90°) followed by a 180° pulse (inverting the net magnetization or **B** vector). Spin-echo images depict the ventricular cavity or blood pool as being darker, i.e. "black blood images". The spin-echo images can be acquired more rapidly (fast spin-echo imaging) using multiple echoes generated by a train of 180° refocusing pulses that increase the signal-to-noise ratio. Spin-echo sequences are frequently used to assess morphology.

The gradient-echo pulse sequence uses a second gradient with opposite polarity that increases MR signal as it leads to the restitution of spin phase coherence. The gradient echo pulse sequence has been used to assess ventricular function and wall motion, as well as flow patterns in valvular disease, shunts and great vessels. This pulse sequence depicts the blood pool with a high signal, resulting in bright blood images. Infusion of paramagnetic contrast agents such as gadolinium chelates can further increase the signal-to-noise ratio and highlight differences between various tissues or in pathology within a given tissue (e.g. normal myocardium, reperfused viable myocardium or infarcted myocardium). In addition, these agents can highlight differences between edematous and non-edematous tissue as well as other differences in the molecular environment within the tissue that affect T_1 and T_2 or the relaxitivity of the excited protons (e.g. an increase in both T_1 and T_2 is observed in the presence of myocardial edema) [12]. Gadolinium chelate distributes into the interstitium of all water-containing tissue. Because of their molecular size, however, these chelates do not enter the intracellular space of viable cells [13]. This means that a contrast agent related increase in signal intensity on delayed imaging provides evidence of infarcted or scarred myocardium [14–18]. The chelates accumulate in the extracellular volumes about 10 min after the first pass of the contrast agent [19].

Each of the pulse sequences described above can be applied in conjunction with a pulse sequence designed to suppress or to null the underlying tissue (myocardial) intensity. A pulse sequence that affects image contrast by nulling the myocardium is the inversion recovery (IR). In addition, another pulse sequence can lead to suppression of the signal generated by fat or lipid. This removes the confounding effects of the lipid signal that can obscure the bright appearance of contrast agent accumulation in necrotic or scarred myocardium.

The use of the steady state free precession (SSFP) pulse sequence in cine CMR imaging results in a substantial improvement in the quality of images compared with those obtained with conventional fast gradient-echo sequences [20, 21]. SSFP requires high speed gradients with extremely short repetition times of 3–5 ms. The steady state is achieved and maintained between the transverse and longitudinal magnetization while the magnetic field is exposed to a train of equally spaced radiofrequency pulses. With the use of SSFP, acquisition is less dependent on the inflow of fresh spins than it is with fast gradient-echo sequences, and signal intensity is related mainly to inherent properties of the tissue (the ratio between T_2 and T_1). Thus, the use of SSFP-based pulse sequences has found widespread application in cardiac imaging because of the excellent contrast between blood and myocardium in addition to its excellent signal-to-noise characteristics.

Since the magnetic properties of fluids are influenced by motion, flow can be described in terms of absolute velocity using echo-planar imaging (EPI), the fastest MR imaging technique. In EPI, the acquisition is made after a single or multiple (multishot EPI) pulse using rapid switching of gradients. This technique can be used to evaluate ventricular function and myocardial perfusion, and allows measurement of, for example, cardiac outputs, shunts, and pressure gradients across stenotic valves. Phase contrast, phase shift or velocity encoded (VEC) imaging are flow quantification techniques that use a pulse sequence specifically designed to produce a phase angle within a pixel where signal is proportional to velocity. Once pixel by pixel velocity is known, flow in a vessel or through a valve can be determined by multiplying the pixel area by the pixel velocity. Summation of the pixels within the region of interest determines the flow volume. This technique can accurately assess flow and has a wide dynamic range, allowing encoding of a wide range of velocities from several millimeters per second to at least 10 meters per second [22, 23].

Since the late 1980s, it has been possible to visualize intrinsic myocardial contractile patterns using RF tagging. These patterns are produced by a combination of restricted presaturation localized radiofrequency pulses and conventional radiofrequency "spoiled" gradient-echo (SPGR) readout gradients [24]. The changes in shape and size of the cardiac chambers throughout the cardiac cycle reflect the function of the atria and ventricles in three dimensions. Such parameters as ventricular eccentricity can be readily determined. The increasing availability of fast automated postprocessing software provides a means for rapid generation of more information about function than is available with any other methodology. RF tag lines have provided CMR images of the heart, which are useful for assessing the detailed contractile function of the myocardium. [25] This includes the ability to measure left ventricular circumferential fiber shortening, wall thickening as an indicator of the radial strain, and changes in systolic torsion in patients at baseline and after medical or surgical therapy [26–30]. Fig. 7.1 shows a HARmonic Phase image (HARP) analysis of short axis tagged CMR images.

Although successfully used in clinical studies, conventional SPGR tagging has intrinsic disadvantages resulting from the fading of the tag lines during the cardiac cycle (related to repeated

(a)

(b)

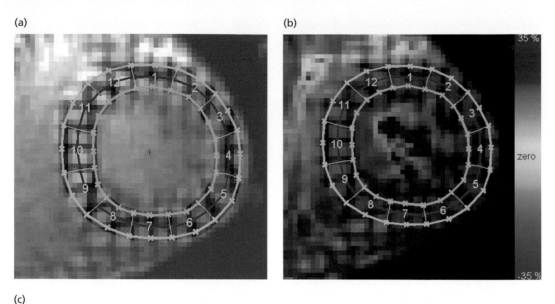

(c)

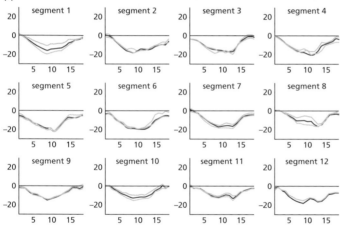

Fig. 7.1 HARmonic Phase image (HARP) analysis of short axis tagged CMR images. (a) A circular grid that contains a variable number of chords of equal size is defined by the user to represent the region of measurement within the left ventricular wall, where the green line represents the subendocardial layer, the red line the mid-wall portion and the blue line the subepicardium. Points on the grid are then automatically tracked through all the image sections in the data set, and strain values are calculated from the trajectory of each point. (b) Calculated strain values are displayed as a color-coded map superimposed on the tagged images. (c) Strain plots showing circumferential shortening in every segment and in all three layers. The x axis represents the number of imaged phases of the cardiac cycle, and the y axis is the percentage of change in circumferential shortening. (Figure reproduced with permission from and courtesy of: Castillo E, Lima JAC, Bluemke DA. Regional myocardial function: advances in MR imaging and analysis techniques. *RadioGraphics* 2003; **23**: 5127–5140.)

radiofrequency excitation and T_1 relaxation). Using higher field magnets such as 3 T allows the tag lines to persist for practically the entire cardiac cycle. Pulse sequences use the combination of partial modulation of magnetization (SPAMM) tagging preparation and a fully balanced SSFP pulse sequence [31, 32]. Table 7.2 provides an overview of the terminology of these pulse sequences from the three major manufacturers of CMR instruments and software.

Table 7.2 Pulse sequence nomenclature for each of the companies.

	General Electric	Philips	Siemens
Generic			
Spin echo (black blood)			
Standard	SE	SE	SE
Fast breath-hold	FSE	TSE	TSE
Ultrafast (single heartbeat)	SSFSE	single shot TSE	HASTE
Gradient echo (bright blood)			
Standard non-breath-hold	GRASS, GRE	FFE	GRE
Fast breath-hold segmented k-space	Fast GRE	TFE	Turbo FLASH
Steady state free precession (breath-hold segmented k-space, high SNR/CNR, real time)	FIESTA	balanced FFP	true FISP
Angiographic option			
Velocity encoding imaging	phase contrast	phase contrast	phase contrast
Suppression techniques			
Inversion recovery	STIR, fseSTIR, fastFLAIR	STIR, tseSTIR, tseFLAIR	IR, STIR, IR-TSE
Fat suppression	fatSAT	SPIR	fatSAT

Global and regional systolic myocardial function

Cardiac oriented planes start with breath-hold scout images in the coronal plane, followed by the transverse plane. A line drawn between the left ventricular apex and the middle of the mitral annulus defines the vertical long axis or two-chamber view. The horizontal long axis or four-chamber view is then obtained using a comparable cutting line and, followed by the short axis, can be used to generate the left ventricular outflow tract view. Images from planes within the principal axes of the body are particularly useful in the evaluation of the anterior right ventricular wall, but are also useful in the assessment of pericardial thickening or effusion, paracardiac masses, and the aorta.

The management of cardiovascular disease is critically dependent on the assessment of left and right ventricular function. It is widely demonstrated that CMR offers the reference standard for the non-invasive assessment of cardiac mass and global function [33–39]. It is accurate and reproducible in both normal [40–42] and deformed or asymmetrically contracting ventricles. Such asymmetrical contraction can be caused by a broad spectrum of conditions, including ischemia, [43, 44]

hypertrophy and dilatation, [45–48] and pulmonary hypertension, [49] or after surgical repair [50]. Simpson's rule is the most commonly used method to measure volume and thereby function. Short axis cine MR images using gradient-echo pulse sequence are obtained, spanning the whole left ventricle and the volume in each slice is measured and summed over the ventricle. The volumes obtained by this method are independent of geometric assumption and are dimensionally accurate whether or not the papillary and trabecular volumes are subtracted [51]. Left ventricular volumes can also be determined by the simplified Simpson formula $V = L/2$ (AMV + 2/3 APM) in which the area of the ventricle (V) is measured on two short axis views (the initial section is obtained just below the mitral valve, (AMV) the second at the level of the papillary muscles, (APM) and the length of the cavities (L) is measured on a four-chamber view. Subtraction of the end-systolic from the end-diastolic volume gives the stroke volume. Multiplying the stroke volume by the heart rate yields the cardiac output, which demonstrates a close correlation with thermodilution catheter methods [52–55]. The right ventricle's function is also known to be an important determinant of prognosis in coronary artery disease, [56] in congenital heart disease and in pulmonary hypertension [49]. The same Simpson's rule approach can be readily applied to the determination of the volume of the right ventricle since no standard geometric model has readily fit this chamber [57].

Furthermore, right and left ventricular volume measurements using Simpson's equation allow the calculation of the regurgitant fraction, i.e. the ratio of the regurgitant volume (difference in stroke volume between the regurgitant ventricle and the normal ventricle) and the stroke volume of the regurgitant ventricle, and this calculation correlates well with the severity of regurgitant valvular disease: regurgitation of 15–20%, 20–40% and greater than 40% represents mild, moderate and severe regurgitation respectively [58]. Moreover, gradient-echo sequences that depict normally circulating blood as a bright signal depict regurgitant or stenotic valvular high-velocity flow patterns as a signal loss or void [59]. Although the area and maximum length of the void vary greatly depending on scanning variables and "echo time" (TE) in particular [60] these sequences provide specificity, sensitivity and diagnostic accuracy greater than 93%, 89%, and 92% respectively for severity of aortic and mitral regurgitation [23]. There is also significant correlation with Doppler echocardiography and catheter determined pressure gradients in aortic and mitral stenosis [61–63].

Right and left ventricular stroke volumes can also be calculated by using velocity encoded (VEC) MR imaging to measure flow in the ascending aorta and pulmonary artery in planes either perpendicular to (through-plane velocity measurement) or parallel to (in-plane velocity measurement) the direction of flow [64–65]. This pulse sequence is specifically designed so that the phase angle in each pixel of the selected region of interest on each of the sixteen time frames constituting the cardiac cycle is proportional to the velocity. The product of the cross-sectional area and the average per pixel velocity within a given region of interest yields the instantaneous flow volume and an estimated flow volume per heartbeat when integrated [66, 67]. Since valvular disease is likely to decrease myocardial compliance and contractile function, MR imaging provides a non-invasive and accurate means

of quantifying related pathological states such as compliance. The severity of shunt size can be reliably expressed as the ratio of pulmonic to systemic flow ratio [68, 69]. VEC MR imaging quantifies the degree of pulmonary [70], tricuspid, [71] aortic, [72, 73] or mitral [74, 75] regurgitation by measuring maximum velocity in the flow jet. This too shows a strong correlation with Doppler echocardiography and angiographic data [72–75]. Thus, the best way to quantify the volume of mitral regurgitation is to combine ventricular volume measurements obtained from the left and right ventricular stroke volumes.

Systolic global and regional myocardial function

CMR imaging allows the most precise evaluation of myocardial dysfunction. It provides high quality display of ventricular volumes, mass and function, but also allows assessment of valvular function, myocardial necrosis, fibrosis and infiltration. CMR imaging has profound implications for clinical diagnosis and prognosis, which are partly attributable to its tissue contrast, its large field of view and the lack of limitation of cardiac scanning planes oriented with respect to the axes of the heart or the axial planes of the body. In order to optimally evaluate function and relevant other parameters, defined scan planes still must be well defined, standardized via cine gradient-echo sequences with measurements of forward flow into the aorta obtained via VEC MR imaging. This approach maximizes intra and inter-observer agreement (±4.8% and ±7.7%) and has the advantages of being independent of the effects of tricuspid and pulmonary regurgitation and allowing correction for the presence of aortic regurgitation [76]. Similarly, pressure gradients across a stenotic valve estimated by VEC MRI vs Doppler echocardiography are closely related for aortic, [77–79] mitral [80, 81] and pulmonary stenosis when measured either in the main, right or left pulmonary artery [82].

Regional left ventricular function can be assessed both qualitatively, as with echocardiography, [83] or quantitatively. CMR images, especially those acquired in the short axis, have been shown to effectively determine left ventricular regional wall parameters [29, 84, 85]. Their excellent depiction of endocardial and epicardial borders of the myocardium allows the assessment of not only the wall motion but also the wall thinning and thickening. Wall thickening has been shown to be more sensitive for the detection of abnormal myocardium than wall motion analysis [86]. Regional wall thickness can be derived using acquisitions from manually or automatically defined endocardial and epicardial boundaries in each short axis image which rely on an approximately circular shape of the myocardium and the selected center point in the left ventricle. Alternatively, the centerline method [87, 88] relies on a path between the endo- and the epicardial contours. Equally spaced perpendicular chords are constructed starting at a clearly visible anatomical reference and spanning the whole circumference of the short axis ventricular slice. The length of such a chord represents the local wall thickness, and the ratio between the end-systolic and end-diastolic chord length equals the local end-systolic wall thickening. Subsequently, the size, extent, and severity of a wall thickening abnormality can be quantified [89] (Fig. 7.2). The use of CMR tag lines and grids in multiple short and long axis slices provides a means for measurement of 3D myocardial strain [90] at different points during the cardiac cycle and reflects regional ventricular performance. Thus, the systolic clockwise rotation at the base and counter clockwise rotation at the apex is significantly reduced during chronic heart failure and improves at the base with appropriate treatment [91]. In hypertrophic cardiomyopathy, the regional dysfunction combines a reduction of both the rotational pattern, mainly in the posterior ventricular wall, and the septal radial strain [26]. In ischemic heart disease, left ventricular circumferential shortening has a strong correlation with ejection fraction by ventriculography [65] and has proved to be very accurate for the quantitation of the recovery of the segmental left ventricular function after revascularization [28, 92].

Diastolic function

These three imaging sequences have also been used to accurately describe myocardial relaxation [65]. Gradient-echo imaging provides a means to generate reproducible measurements of ventricular volumes throughout the cardiac cycle. From the

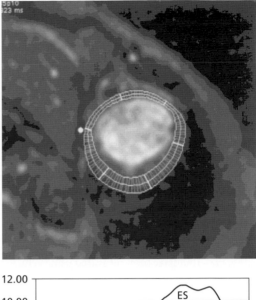

(a)

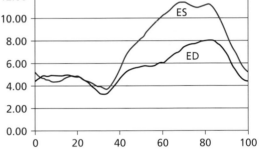

(b)

Fig. 7.2 (a) Application of the centerline method for the calculation of regional wall thickness in an end-systolic short axis MR image. The centerline chords, which are constructed at evenly spaced intervals perpendicular to the centerline, are numbered in a clockwise fashion starting at the white dot. (b) The graph depicts the lengths of the centerline chords. The lack of wall thickening in the region defined by chords 2–35 corresponds to the region of myocardial infarction. ES = end-systolic, ED = end-diastolic. (Figure reproduced with permission from: Reference 87, Van der Geest RJ, Reiber JH. Quantification in cardiac MRI. *J Magn Reson Imaging* 1999; **10**: 602–608.)

contours describing the endocardial and epicardial borders of the myocardium, ventricular volumes and mass can be calculated. Additionally, peak (ventricular) filling rate (PFR) and the time to PFR can be determined using the maximal change during the rapid filling phase [93–95]. Prolongation of the time-to-peak during the early filling phase and the time-to-peak wall thickness/thinning rate indicate impaired relaxation. Such information indicates segments with extensive fibrosis. It also correlates with decreased perfusion in hypertrophic cardiomyopathy [96]. The ratio between early-to-late filling (i.e. the peak early rate divided by the peak late rate) and early filling percentage (i.e. the volume increase from the end of systole to the diastolic midpoint divided by the stroke volume multiplied by 100) can be demonstrated before changes in the classical mitral Doppler pattern in patients with left ventricular hypertrophy occur [97]. Since flow measurements are obtained at high temporal resolution over the complete cardiac cycle, VEC is especially useful for the evaluation of left and right ventricular diastolic function parameters. Peak velocity and volume flow of the early (E) and atrial filling waves (A) through both mitral and tricuspid valves [98–100] have been measured using velocity encoding in a reproducible and accurate manner regardless of jet orientation [101]. These measurements show close agreement with Doppler-derived indices in normal [101], hypertrophic [102] and ischemic myocardium [103]. Left ventricular deformation during diastole can be determined by cardiac tagging. Such assessment of the time for ventricular "untwisting" [104] was reported to be prolonged in myocardial infarction [105] and to be normalized after reperfusion [106]. More recently, the time to peak "untwisting" was found to be an accurate parameter for identifying patients with coronary artery disease (CAD) when evaluated during low dose dobutamine administration [107].

Specific CMR findings in ischemic, dilated, hypertrophic and restrictive cardiomyopathies

Ischemic heart disease

Comprehensive assessment of ischemic heart disease is made possible by the plethora of information provided by CMR, and specifically by its ability to evaluate function, perfusion and viability. Such information allows determination of prognosis. Protocols lasting less than one hour can combine multiphase cine gradient-echo imaging for function, myocardial perfusion imaging using the first pass of paramagnetic contrast agent at rest and during stress, and delayed contrast enhancement for assessment of myocardial viability [108, 109]. Such imaging has been applied in the emergency room to allow diagnosis and risk stratification in patients

presenting with chest pain with sensitivity and specificity of 85% for diagnosis of myocardial infarction [110, 111]. CMR imaging provides a means of determining the total size rather than just the presence of a transmural myocardial infarction (as indicated by the presence of the Q waves by electrocardiography) [112, 113]. The superior spatial resolution of CMR imaging allows detection of the extent of transmural involvement of myocardial infarction [114] and adds temporal information to conventional imaging analysis because of its ability to differentiate between acute (< two weeks old) and chronic (> four weeks old) myocardial infarction. Whereas both acute and chronic myocardial infarction exhibit delayed enhancement, [115, 116] T_2 weighted CMR imaging allows sensitive detection of infarct associated myocardial edema and the extent of the acute damaged tissue [117]. In combination with delayed enhancement CMR imaging of acute and chronic myocardial infarction (MI) can be differentiated with a specificity of 96% [118]. The reproducibility of CMR imaging has significant cost and time implications in cardiovascular research, as illustrated by the small sample size required to show the efficiency of beta-blockers [119] and angiotensin-converting enzyme inhibitors in reducing left ventricular volumes and improving function by decreasing infarct segment extent, expansion and mass-to-volume ratio [120, 121]. Furthermore, using velocity encoded techniques; CMR imaging can evaluate the physiologic significance of a native or stented coronary artery stenosis by measuring coronary artery blood flow before and after pharmacologically induced hyperemia [122–125]. The signal-intensity-time curves using first-pass contrast enhanced imaging have been reported to detect significant coronary artery stenosis (>75%) with sensitivity, specificity and accuracy of 90%, 83% and 87% respectively, [126, 127] and to improve after revascularization procedures [85, 128].

Ischemic heart disease is the leading cause of both myocardial diastolic and systolic dysfunction. The underlying cause, i.e. CAD frequently can be detected using cardiovascular magnetic resonance angiography of the coronary arteries [129–144]. This topic has been the focus of several two and three-dimensional technical advances in the past few years which have improved the ability of CMR for assessing CAD severity and extent. Furthermore the role of CMR for characterizing plaque is promising, but still under investigation [145–148]. Approximately, 72% of patients have been accurately diagnosed as having any CAD and 87% as having left main or three vessel coronary disease [149]. For saphenous vein coronary artery bypass grafts that are typically of larger diameter and more fixed in position than native coronary arteries, the sensitivity and specificity for detection of occlusion or of stenosis of 70% or greater were 83% and 99% (for occlusion), and 73% and 83% (for stenosis) [150]. The current method of choice for coronary artery imaging uses fat-saturated ECG-triggered steady state free precession (SSFP) imaging with or without gadolinium contrast agent administration or respiratory gating. Coronary imaging with CMR requires further refinement to improve its ability to provide consistent visualization of more than the proximal and mid-portions of the major coronary artery branches with a resolution higher than 1.5 mm^3. Several approaches have improved the visualization of the normal and diseased coronary arteries. One approach uses a spin-echo or dark blood approach with a dual-inversion magnetization preparation scheme to suppress the signal of the blood that moves into the imaging plane between the preparation pulses and data acquisition [151–153]. Others include: accelerated imaging speed with a multicomponent detection array and parallel data acquisition; [154–155] development of blood pool contrast agents with greater T$_1$ shortening effect than the conventional extracellular agents; [156, 157] 3 Tesla platform, and [158, 159] radial [160, 161] and spiral sampling of the k-space with their expected superior SNR, CNR and image quality [162–163]. CMR coronary angiography is not yet adequate for routine diagnosis of CAD, since its spatial resolution is inferior to that of catheter coronary angiography, but its application is regarded as good for identification of the origin and the initial course of anomalous coronary arteries, which frequently present with angina pectoris and may be difficult to delineate by conventional coronary angiography [164–166].

Myocarditis

Delayed enhancement is by no means specific for myocardial infarction. It detects necrotic or scarred myocardium in a number of other conditions. Examples include myocarditis and cardiomyopathies that can affect myocardial function and thus prognosis. Acute myocarditis is a life-threatening inflammatory disease process [167, 168] most frequently resulting from Coxsackie B or adenovirus infection [169]. It may progress to an autoimmune phase, then to progressive cardiac dilatation and may lead to the development of dilated cardiomyopathy. CMR with gadolinium induced signal enhancement provides a marker of inflammation associated with myocardial necrosis. The inflammatory process spreads from a focal to a disseminated involvement of the myocardium within the first two weeks of the onset of the symptoms [170]. The extent of delayed enhancement correlates with left ventricular dysfunction in the very early stages of myocarditis and to clinical status in the longer term since the presence of symptoms after three months seems to be accompanied by a sustained elevation of global myocardial enhancement after gadolinium diethyltriaminetetraacetic acid (Gd-DTPA) [171]. In terms of sensitivity, this technique is more effective than radionuclide techniques using gallium-67 to visualize white blood cells or radiolabeled antimyosin antibody to visualize myocardial necrosis [172, 173]. The standard for diagnosis of myocarditis is endomyocardial biopsy which also serves when performed serially to evaluate the progression or regression of disease [165–167, 174].

Left ventricular non-compaction cardiomyopathy

Left ventricular non-compaction (LVNC) is a unique unclassified congenital disorder of endomyocardial morphogenesis with a pattern of inheritance suggesting genetic heterogeneity [156–167]. This form of cardiomyopathy is more frequently associated with complications of congestive heart failure, thromboembolism and malignant ventricular arrhythmias, [168–169] both in the adult and pediatric populations [170]. The morphological features inconsistently identified by 2D echocardiography include prominent trabeculations and deep intertrabecular recesses in hypertrophied and hypokinetic segments affecting most commonly apical and mid-ventricular segments of both the inferior and lateral wall in more than 80% of patients, [168] with or without concomitant right

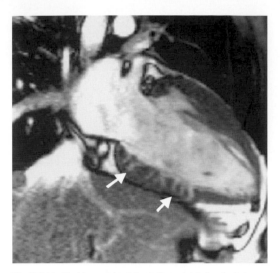

Fig. 7.3 Vertical long axis of the left ventricle in diastole using SSFP sequence showing multiple inferior wall intertrabecular recesses in communication with the left ventricular cavity (arrows). (Figure adapted with permission from: Reference 179, McCrohon JA, Richmond DR, Pennell DJ *et al.* Isolated non-compaction of the myocardium. A rarity or missed diagnosis? *Circulation* 2002; **106**: e22–e23.)

ventricular involvement [171–173]. Indeed, a high prevalence of anomalous images (47%) as false tendons (75%), trabeculations (23%), or thrombi (2%) of the left ventricle were reported by Tamborini *et al.* [174] for patients with or without pathologic hearts, suggesting the need to update the imaging tools for this misdiagnosed disease [175]. CMR imaging is to be considered the diagnostic modality of choice for patients in whom LVNC is suspected. Cine CMR using a SSFP pulse sequence shows the numerous trabeculations and intertrabecular recesses in communication with the left ventricular cavity (Fig. 7.3) and the hypokinesis of the non-compacted ventricular wall during the cardiac cycle [176]. It also allows estimation of left ventricular mass both with and without the incorporation of trabeculations from a contiguous stack of short axis images. When expressed as a percentage of total mass, trabecular mass of greater than 20% of the total mass suggested the diagnosis of LVNC [177]. After gadolinium injection, analysis of first-pass perfusion suggested reduced trabecular perfusion without demonstration of either LV thrombus on the early inversion-recovery images

or myocardial fibrosis on the later images using the same sequence [177, 178].

Familial hypertrophic cardiomyopathy

Familial hypertrophic cardiomyopathy (HCM) is a cardiac autosomal-dominant disorder characterized by left ventricular hypertrophy, myofibrillar disarray and a high prevalence of sudden death [180–184] due to ventricular tachycardia and fibrillation in most patients [184, 185]. Although no single test can reliably predict risk in HCM, most investigators and physicians have found that CMR provides excellent morphological definition and accurate non-invasive tissue characterization. These data may contribute to risk stratification. Septal thickness of at least 15 mm at end-diastole in the four-chamber or the short axis view [186–188] is commonly observed in HCM. CMR allows longitudinal follow-up [189] of both right and left ventricular systolic and diastolic dimensions and volumes, and calculation of left ventricular systolic function and mass. Thus CMR provides a comprehensive evaluation of the three-dimensional distribution [190, 191] of myocardial mass. CMR can also demonstrate, using [26, 192] transmural tagging, enhanced left ventricular torsion, myocardial perfusion abnormalities [193] and myocardial transmural wall motion and, using contrast enhancement techniques, [194, 195] in patients with varying clinical courses. An important anatomic component of the arrhythmogenic substrate has been postulated to be the plexiform fibrosis depots [183] that have been shown to occur in hypertrophied regions, predominantly in the junction of the septum and the right ventricular free wall in a patchy manner [194]. A positive correlation between the magnitude of septal hypertrophy and the extent of replacement scarring in young patients with HCM experiencing ventricular tachycardia and sudden death has been described [195, 196]. This underlies the important role of CMR imaging in diagnosis and risk stratification of HCM. Finally, the abnormal systolic anterior motion of the anterior mitral leaflet and the related eccentric mitral regurgitation are easily detected in this condition.

Arrhythmogenic right ventricular dysplasia

The right ventricle is the most challenging portion of the heart for imaging and function studies, [41] and CMR imaging is the ideal approach for its evaluation. The right ventricle is involved in diseases such as arrhythmogenic right ventricular dysplasia (ARVD), an autosomal dominant familial cardiomyopathy [197, 198] that can lead to sudden death in the young due to ventricular arrhythmias [199–201]. Unfortunately, CMR, as a solitary diagnostic technique, is not as helpful for this disease as physicians had hoped. None the less, using up-to-date scanners and imaging sequences, as well as defined imaging protocols, CMR information is abundant and can potentially provide findings that can contribute to the accurate diagnosis of this disease. CMR has the potential to demonstrate fibro-fatty infiltration of the right ventricle free wall growing from the epicardial region of the myocardium to the endocardial region, with high intensity signal on T_1 weighted images [199–202]. As an isolated finding, intramyocardial fat is neither specific nor relevant for the diagnosis of ARVD and may be a source of false positive diagnosis [203]. Other anatomic features associated with this disease include dilatation of the RV and its outflow tract, [204, 205] and variable size aneurysms that are assessed using a multisection inversion-recovery segmented fast-spin-echo pulse sequence [206]. Global and regional systolic function is generally best assessed by a steady state free precession pulse sequence. Several studies have addressed the presence of right ventricular diastolic dysfunction as an early marker of disease, even when systolic function is still preserved, [207, 208] and this might be considered by some as an additional feature or criterion for ARVD [209].

Infiltrative myocardial diseases

The clinical and hemodynamic features of restrictive cardiomyopathy can overlap with those of constrictive pericarditis. CMR imaging provides a means to differentiate between these two conditions. Although Talreja *et al.* reported normal pericardial thickness in 18% of constrictive pericarditis patients, [210] the CMR measurement of pericardial thickness provides help in the diagnosis of constrictive pericarditis. When spin-echo CMR imaging showed a pericardial thickness that exceeded 4 mm, the sensitivity, specificity and accuracy for the presence of constrictive pericarditis were 88%, 100% and 93% respectively [211]. Early posterior

movement of the ventricular septum during inspiration provides a means for diagnosis of pericardial constriction. This abnormal septal motion can be detected using spin-echo imaging or even more effectively using real time CMR imaging.

Certain infiltrative diseases of the myocardium can cause typical signal changes. In amyloid involvement of the myocardium, restrictive physiology is associated with increased right atrial volume, right atrial wall thickness and right ventricular free wall thickness and reduced wall motion and ejection fraction. These measurements differentiate amyloid cardiomyopathy from hypertrophic cardiomyopathy. Furthermore, CMR imaging can differentiate amyloid involvement of the myocardium in patients with hypertrophic cardiomyopathy from that in a group of healthy volunteers. Myocardial signal intensity in cardiac amyloidosis is significantly lower both at an echo delay (TE) of 20 ms and a TE of 60 ms [212].

Cardiac involvement in patients with sarcoidosis can precede, follow or, occur concurrently with the sarcoid involvement of other organs. It has no specific clinical signs. Two-dimensional echocardiography can miss structural or functional changes due to granuloma formation and fibrosis [186]. Thallium-201 (^{201}Tl) myocardial imaging findings have no prognostic value when positive [213] and when absent do not exclude the presence of cardiac involvement with saracoidosis if normal [214]. Furthermore, the sensitivity of myocardial biopsy is as low as 20% [215]. The ability of CMR imaging to diagnose sarcoid heart disease has been demonstrated in several case reports [216–219]. CMR imaging results were recently shown to correlate with clinical findings and immunosuppressive treatment responses during follow-up [220]. The patchy sarcoid infiltrate progresses through three successive histologic stages: granulomatous, exudative, and fibrotic. All are visible on CMR images as zones of increased intramyocardial signal intensity that are more pronounced on T_2 weighted images (Fig. 7.4) because of the edema associated with inflammation and enhanced after gadolinium injection [221]. Early aggressive treatment of sarcoidosis diagnosed with CMR imaging can avoid the serious consequences of myocardial involvement, mainly sudden death due to conduction system involvement or ventricular arrhythmias.

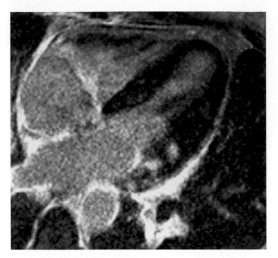

Fig. 7.4 Delayed enhancement CMR images in a four-chamber view showing patchy infiltration of the left ventricular lateral wall (multiple foci with increased intensity) due to sarcoid involvement. (Figure adapted with permission from: Reference 219, Nemeth MA, Muthupillai R, Wilson JM *et al.* Cardiac sarcoidosis detected by delayed hyperenhancement magnetic resonance imaging. *Tex Heart Inst J* 2004; **31**: 99–102.)

Unfortunately, patients with older pacemakers or automated implantable cardioverter defibrillator are unable to receive CMR imaging, [222] and still need to undergo ^{201}T1 scanning to assess the extent of myocardial damage.

Conclusions (morphology and function)

Cardiovascular magnetic resonance provides complete and reliable morphologic and functional information about the cardiac chambers. It is harmless to myocardium and other biologic tissue using the magnetic field strengths of 3 Tesla or less. It is a superb high resolution diagnostic tool that can be used to assess risk. It can reliably measure ejection fraction, ventricular volumes, cardiac outputs, myocardial mass, myocardial wall thickening and even differences in wall motion between the subendo and subepicardium using RF tagging. With the use of non-magnetic implantable devices and the increasing safety of CMR used with electrical devices such as pacemakers and ICDs and the increase in magnetic field strength, CMR is becoming more involved as an integral diagnostic technique and is becoming the gold standard for imaging of ventricular function.

Cardiovascular magnetic resonance myocardial perfusion imaging

Decisions regarding revascularization in CAD are based not only on the anatomic severity of arterial stenoses, but also on their physiological significance [223]. The extent and severity of perfusion abnormalities are directly related to outcomes [224, 225]. Radionuclide methods, especially single photon emission computed tomography (SPECT) has been the most widely employed test to evaluate regional myocardial perfusion. Radionuclide methods, though widely employed, have their limitations, including limited resolution and, more importantly, the confounding effect of attenuation artifacts [226, 227]. In addition, SPECT exposes patients to ionizing radiation. In recent times, methods to assess myocardial perfusion and coronary artery blood flow using cardiovascular magnetic resonance imaging have been developed. CMR imaging has high resolution and has no ionizing radiation. While CMR perfusion methods involve the use of paramagnetic contrast agents, they are more suitable for serial studies to evaluate the progression or regression of CAD.

In CAD myocardial perfusion is frequently normal at rest but as with radionuclide approaches abnormal perfusion patterns are induced by physical exercise (treadmill stress testing) or pharmacological vasodilator agents (adenosine or related agents). While physical stress induces perfusion abnormalities in parallel with other evidence of myocardial ischemia (angina pectoris, ST segment depression and wall motion abnormalities), vasodilators generally induce perfusion abnormalities without concomitant myocardial ischemia unless stenoses are severe enough to induce a steal phenomenon. In a study by Gould *et al.*, it was shown that coronary artery stenoses with a greater than 50% reduction in diameter limit hyperemic flow during vasodilation, leading to perfusion deficit [228]. Accordingly, coronary lesions which are angiographically determined to be greater than 50% are considered significant, and are typically treated by percutaneous coronary intervention or bypass graft surgery when clinical circumstances are appropriate. Data from studies such as the coronary artery surgical study or CASS have shown that vessels with significant stenosis are associated with myocardial infarction

[229, 230]. Iskandrian *et al.* have shown that the extent and severity of myocardial perfusion defects were strong predictors of future cardiac events [224]. Perfusion imaging with SPECT, positron emission tomography (PET) and CMR imaging are all used for evaluating both myocardial perfusion and viability. In contrast to the radionuclide approaches, CMR uses a method known as delayed contrast enhancement to assess myocardial viability and rather than labeling viable myocardium the technique labels myocardial infarction and scar [231]. Briefly, CMR perfusion/viability imaging works as follows. After administration of the paramagnetic contrast agent, generally a gadolinium chelate, (e.g. Gd-DTPA) intravenously administered using a non-magnetic power injector, high speed CMR imaging allows assessment of perfusion during the first pass of the contrast agent through the myocardium. After approximately ten minutes, repeat imaging shows contrast agent localization in myocardial infarct or scar territory.

In conjunction with CMR myocardial perfusion imaging it is possible to compare resting and vasodilated imaging studies to determine coronary flow reserve (CFR): hyperemic flow divided by resting flow. CFR is impaired in patients with cardiac risk factors but anatomically normal coronary arteries (less than 50% diameter stenosis) [232]. PET has been used to estimate CFR. Studies using PET have demonstrated that hyperemic flow data correlated strongly with both the severity of stenosis by coronary angiography and CFR [233–235].

CMR perfusion imaging using first pass of contrast agent

Myocardial perfusion is observed by rapid imaging after the peripheral injection of an extracellular contrast agent (typically Gd-DTPA), which have a T_1-lowering effect. The contrast agent passes from the blood pool via the coronary circulation into the myocardium substantially reducing the T_1 (spin-lattice relaxation time) from 1500 ms for blood and 1100 for myocardium [236] to 50 and 0 ms respectively depending on the concentration of the Gd-DTPA. The reduction in tissue T_1 depends on the baseline T_1 of the blood or tissue, the concentration of Gd-DTPA and the tissue parameters relating to water exchange. During the first pass of contrast agent, CMR pulse sequences are used that

produce strong T_1 contrast (making short T_1s in the tissue with the contrast agent bright and the longer T_1s of tissue with less contrast agent dark). Accordingly, during the wash-in of paramagnetic contrast agent, the myocardium gets brighter, and during wash-out, the myocardium gets darker (Fig. 7.5).

Qualitative assessment of hypoperfused areas using CMR is accomplished by visually estimating the wash-in rates of extracellular contrast agent into the myocardium supplied by normal or insignificantly stenotic coronary arteries compared with coronary arteries with significant stenoses [101, 237–239]. Signal intensity time curves can be used to calculate parameters such as peak signal intensity; [240–242] signal change over time (slope), [119, 237, 242–246] arrival time; time to peak signal; mean transit time, [242, 247] and area under the signal intensity time curve [248]. Signal intensity is a simple function of T_1 (and the pulse sequence), and T_1 is a simple function of contrast agent concentration, baseline T_1 and water exchange rate. In animal models a close correlation has been shown between microsphere measurements and upslope of the intensity time curve; [246] the upslope is used as a semiquantitative measure of perfusion. The upslope method uses the initial portion of the signal intensity time curve, which lasts up to 20 seconds. In view of the need for a 20 second acquisition time the sensitivity of the measurement can be affected due to motion, since the breath-holding required for high quality imaging is not readily accomplished by all patients. Myocardial upslope data are divided by the upslope data of the signal in the left ventricular blood pool to obtain a measure of input [119, 237, 243–247].

$$\nu = \gamma B/2\pi$$
Lar

Where ν is the precession frequency in cycles per second
Where B is the applied magnetic field and
Where γ is the gyromagnetic constant

This method of correction is not optimal as the value may change based on homodynamic status in patients, as in vasodilator studies. In a recent study, upslope of signal intensity during hyperemia divided by the upslope in the left ventricular blood pool was calculated in 32 sectors per heart (eight sectors per

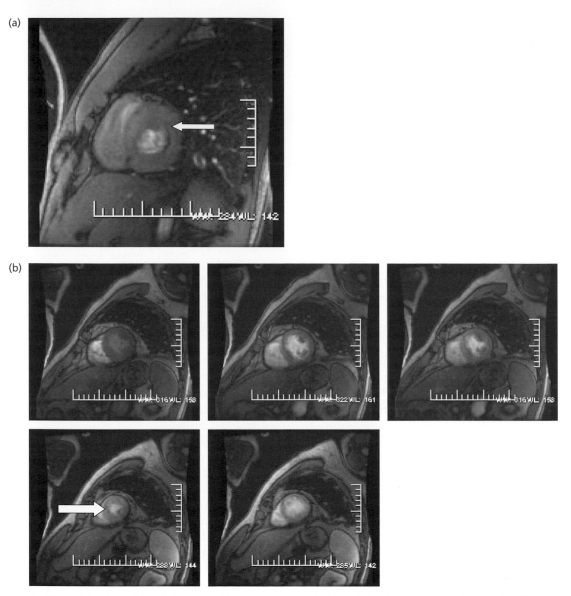

Fig. 7.5 (a) Subendocardial perfusion defect. Short axis tomograph during the myocardial phase of the first-pass of the gadolinium chelate. The white arrow points to a subendocardial perfusion defect. (b) Subendocardial perfusion defect in a patient with CAD. First-pass gadolinium chelate from the upper left image (RV blood pool) through the upper right image (biventricular blood pool). Myocardial phase is seen in the lower two images. Above the arrow in the lower left image is a subendocardial perfusion defect.

slice) and was compared to a normal database of upslope values [237]. This method allowed color coding of the "wash-in" of contrast agent, producing a parametric map and allowing the identification of hypoperfused areas.

Perfusion imaging during the "first pass" is particularly demanding, since whole heart coverage is necessary. One must be able to resolve the first 20 seconds of "wash-in" with high tem-poral resolution in order to determine rates of perfusion.

During CMR perfusion imaging, artifacts are also observed. These artifacts must be eliminated or corrected in order to reliably image regional myocardial perfusion. Otherwise, regions that have reduced signal intensity due to artifact might be confused with regions that have reduced signal intensity due to reduced myocardial perfusion, as is the case with attenuation artifacts with radionuclide imaging. Artifacts can occur because of the sensitivity of the receiver coil (the coil which detects the signal from the body after a transmitted pulse). Signal intensity decreases with increasing coil distance. This means that the signal intensity during the "first pass" of contrast agent can be reduced in posterior myocardium compared with anterior myocardium. Cardiovascular magnetic resonance imaging can correct for this reduced signal with increasing coil distance by computing the relative change in signal. Dividing the absolute signal change by the baseline precontrast signal intensities can be used to determine the relative value. In addition, the perfusion data should be corrected for motion artifacts either due to diaphragmatic drift or breathing prior to generating a signal intensity time curve [249–251].

Techniques used in clinical studies

Inversion recovery has been the most widely used pulse sequence to evaluate perfusion in animals. By appropriate setting of the time between the inversion and the read pulse, signal can be markedly reduced or nulled. Contrast agent then produces the greatest impact on myocardium during its first pass. In human studies, several methods, including inversion recovery; [119, 122, 238, 242, 244, 246, 252–254] saturation recovery; [237, 243, 247, 255, 256] notched saturation recovery, [257] and T_2^* preparation, have been employed [41, 42]. Most of these initial studies only examined feasibility of CMR perfusion imaging. They were performed in healthy human volunteers [256, 258–260] or in patients with knowledge of their angiographically determined coronary anatomy and disease [122, 257, 261]. Perfusion was evaluated in the 1990s, using a multislice approach, but the sensitivity and specificity were low. This was in part because of hardware limitations and in part because of artifacts. Al-Saadi and colleagues [119] tried to evalu-

ate perfusion with data acquisition limited to a single slice, using contrast injected into the right atrium. Recent improvements in hardware with fast echoplanar readout and the use of saturation recovery sequences have made it possible to evaluate perfusion in multiple slices [237, 247] during a single-injection first-pass experiment. Today, the most widely used protocol (which is supported by the major manufacturers) is based on multislice saturation recovery followed by fast gradient-echo acquisitions. Image acquisition time is on the order of 150–200 ms, allowing imaging of three slices per R-R interval. Typically, six parallel short axis slices are acquired with a temporal resolution of two R-R intervals. A typical non-selective saturation pulse is used before each slice acquisition, resulting in very short saturation recovery times.

CMR myocardial perfusion imaging: the future

Scanner hardware, receiver coils, and pulse sequences are constantly improving. Speed and SNR improvement can be expected with the adoption of parallel imaging [142, 262] and steady state free precession techniques [248]. The availability and prevalence of commercial 3 T systems with high speed gradients are advantageous in evaluating perfusion; these systems also improve SNR and provide longer myocardial T_1s. Robust myocardial perfusion imaging is an actively researched and emerging area of CMR.

Myocardial viability using cardiovascular magnetic resonance imaging

Heart failure is a common consequence of many diseases that affect the myocardium. The leading cause of heart failure in the Western world is CAD [263]. Knowledge of structure, metabolism and function is crucial to understanding myocardial response to injury such as ischemia. Detection of viable myocardium in patients with left ventricular dysfunction in the setting of CAD is important in deciding between medical and surgical management. Revascularization of dysfunctional yet viable myocardium can improve ventricular function and long term survival [264–266].

Non-contractile but viable myocardium may result from acute, subacute or chronic reduction in myocardial perfusion and is frequently described as stunning or hibernation. In the 1970s, patients with regional wall motion abnormalities recovered contractile function after coronary artery bypass graft surgery (CABG) [267, 268]. Inotropic stimulation, for example involving ventricular contraction after a ventricular premature beat, demonstrated improved wall motion in viable territories. Such postextrasystolic improvement in wall motion was used to identify viable myocardium and thus patients whose abnormal wall motion would benefit from CABG [269, 270]. The term "hibernating myocardium" was used to refer to patients with reduced myocardial contractile function at rest in the presence of severe coronary artery stenoses, presumably associated with reduced blood supply [271, 272]. Hibernation is a chronic condition of resting left ventricular (LV) dysfunction due to reduced coronary blood flow. It can be partially or completely reversed by revascularization. Chronically reduced perfusion is thought to down regulate metabolism, decreasing energy demand and limiting necrosis. Myocardial stunning is characterized by prolonged mechanical dysfunction after coronary reflow and resumption of perfusion without evidence of permanent tissue damage [273, 274]. Stunning seems to be related to alterations in contractile proteins in response to ischemic insult [275–277]. Myocardial stunning can occur in conjunction with various conditions, such as unstable angina or exercise-induced ischemia, as well as in other situations, such as following cardiac surgery or early successful reperfusion of acute myocardial infarction.

Myocardial viability has great influence on patient outcome in terms of mortality and morbidity. Several studies have shown that in the setting of acute LV dysfunction, prognosis is worse in the presence of myocardial necrosis compared to reversible myocardial dysfunction [278, 279]. The extent of viable (or non-viable) myocardium dictates the need for and type of further patient management. The detection of stunned myocardium following reperfusion therapy [278, 280] and the demonstration of viability in a dysfunctional area may determine the need for early revascularization.

The prognosis in a patient with chronic LV dysfunction may be improved by revascularization, provided there is sufficient viable myocardium to permit recovery of contractile function. Revascularization in the presence of non-viable myocardium may be detrimental to patient outcomes and may be associated with an increase in mortality [281]. The extent of myocardial viability, in addition to its presence, is also useful in selecting patients who are likely to benefit from therapy (Fig. 7.6).

Non-invasive methods to assess viability

Techniques currently available to assess myocardial viability include PET using ^{18}F-fluorodeoxyglucose

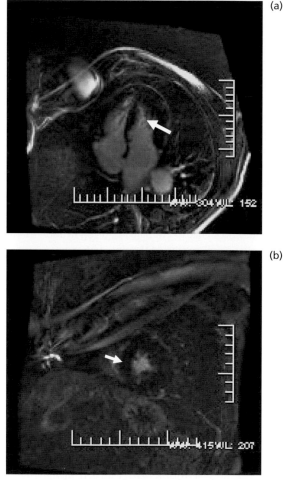

(a)

(b)

Fig. 7.6 No delayed enhancement in a patient with angina but without previous MI. The patient received gadolinium contrast agent 10 to 15 minutes prior to acquisition of the images. (a) Four-chamber long axis image. The arrow is pointing to the LV blood pool. (b) Short axis image. The arrow is pointing to the interventricular septum.

(FDG); SPECT with either ^{201}Tl or technetium-99m (^{99m}Tc), and low dose dobutamine echocardiography (DobE). Each of these imaging approaches defines myocardial viability in different ways: FDG-PET images the distribution of myocardial glucose metabolic activity or evidence of anaerobic glycolysis, ^{201}Tl-SPECT images sarcolemmal cell membrane integrity, ^{99m}Tc-SPECT images mitochondrial membrane integrity, and dobutamine echocardiography (DobE) assesses the presence of myocardial contractile reserve. Dobutamine echocardiography (DobE), PET, and SPECT have similar predictive accuracy, however, dobutamine CMR is significantly better for detecting myocardial ischemia compared with DE, because of the improved ability of CMR to visualize the left ventricle in 3D.

PET, SPECT, and DobE (or dobutamine CMR) assess different markers of viability. Using dobutamine stimulation, the presence of contractile reserve in hibernating myocardium is demonstrated in the presence of viable myocardium [282].

All of these tests have inherent limitations. DobE is limited by adequacy of the acoustic window or suboptimal images in 15% of patients [283]. Additionally, DobE is operator-dependent, endocardial definition in the posterolateral segment is poor, the apical segments may be foreshortened, and the approach is presently inherently two-dimensional. An additional problem is the long period of training necessary to acquire the skills for optimum image display and interpretation [284]. The accuracy of SPECT studies is confounded by attenuation artifacts and poor spatial resolution. PET is limited by the expense of radionuclide tracer production (using either an on-site cyclotron to produce ^{13}N-ammonia and FDG or a generator to produce Rubidium-82 ([82]Rb)). ^{13}N-ammonia or [82]Rb are used to image myocardial perfusion while FDG is used to image anaerobic myocardial glucose utilization. The ^{13}N-ammonia or [82]Rb are used to image perfusion and the ^{18}F is used to image anaerobic metabolism. When perfusion is reduced or absent the involved territory may be viable or non-viable. When FDG is present in a region of perfusion deficit, metabolic activity and thus viability has been defined. Like SPECT, PET procedures are also limited by low spatial resolution compared to CMR, with SPECT substantially worse than PET. This section concentrates on the imaging techniques of CMR that allow assessment of myocardial viability. CMR provides several approaches to defining viability, including dobutamine stimulation of asynergic ventricular wall segments, delayed enhancement by paramagnetic contrast agent, and abnormal myocardial high energy phosphate metabolism.

Viability assessment using cine CMR to determine regional function

As noted in the section on function, cine CMR imaging allows high resolution visualization of myocardial wall motion, wall thickness, and wall thickening. Scarred myocardium is associated with loss of myocardial mass, leading to wall thinning. Previous studies have shown that the total thickness of scarred myocardium is usually ≤5 mm [285]. This assumption of thinned and akinetic myocardium representing scar has been studied by comparing CMR with PET and SPECT [286, 287]. Observation of morphology and function of the LV at rest cannot detect viability, per se. The presence of even a small amount of wall thickening with low dose dobutamine in an area of asynergy suggests myocardial contractile function and hence some degree of viable myocardium.

Dobutamine CMR to assess viability

The question of viability arises in myocardium with regional or global contractile dysfunction. When such dysfunction is associated with heart failure, successful treatment depends on whether or not the dysfunction is associated with ischemic but viable or non-viable myocardium (or scar). Viable myocardium demonstrates improvement in contractile function with infusion of low dose dobutamine. This method of assessing residual function is the same as that used in dobutamine echocardiography. A low dose infusion of dobutamine (5–10 μg/kg/min) is used and two or three sets of cine images are acquired, one before and the other during infusion at each level of dobutamine. The sets of cine images are examined side by side to detect changes in regional wall thickening. Improvement of contractile function compared to resting images indicates viable myocardium. If there is wall motion improvement at the lowest dobutamine dose, testing can be stopped, since viability has been demonstrated.

Newer approaches use fast gradient-echo and high speed steady state free precession such as fast low angle shot (FLASH), fast imaging with steady-state precession (True-FISP), balanced fast field echo (FFE), and fast imaging employing steady-STAte excitation (FIESTA). These newer approaches have greater temporal resolution, permitting the acquisition of cine loops of the beating heart. These sequences make it possible to acquire studies during multiple breath-holds, resulting in high quality short and long axis views of the myocardium, both at rest and with the infusion of dobutamine. Image sequences require a breath-hold of about 20 seconds. Images are displayed in cine mode, pairing short axis cuts in comparable locations. Resolution is high and still frames from end-systole and end-diastole can be displayed with well defined epicardial and endocardial borders. These images allow precise quantification of myocardial volumes, mass, and thickness, as well as assessment of regional wall motion and wall thickening in the cine mode.

Dendale and colleagues [288] were the first to report the use of low dose dobutamine CMR in assessing viability. They studied 25 patients early after acute myocardial infarction with low dose dobutamine CMR and echocardiography, and quantitative assessment of wall motion was performed using both modalities. Concordance between these two modalities for identifying viable from non-viable segments was 81%. The "gold standard" was recovery of function after revascularization. The positive and negative predictive values for dobutamine CMR ranged from 89–100% and 73–94%, respectively, [289, 290] significantly better than dobutamine echocardiography.

Baer *et al.* [291] compared dobutamine CMR, dobutamine transesophageal echocardiography (TEE), and FDG uptake on PET imaging to detect viable myocardium. The sensitivity and specificity for dobutamine TEE compared to dobutamine CMR were 77% and 94% vs 81% and 100% respectively.

The use of dobutamine CMR was suboptimal until recently because of the lack of availability of fast imaging sequences. Another disadvantage of dobutamine CMR (and echocardiographic studies) is the risk involved in administering dobutamine. The infusion of a positive inotropic agent in a patient with CAD can elicit an ischemic or arrhyth-

mic event. The physical distance between physician and patient while in the scanner precludes optimum patient-physician interaction. In addition, the ECG waveform cannot be utilized to assess ST segment changes due to its alteration by the magnetic field. Considering this problem, i.e. the difficulty in using ST segment depression as a means of detecting ischemia, a number of groups have reported using low dose dobutamine CMR for successfully assessing viability. A few other groups have also reported the use of higher doses of dobutamine to detect ischemia [283, 292].

Potential disadvantages of dobutamine CMR also include underestimation of the extent of viable myocardium and inability to estimate the transmural extent of myocardial ischemia. Several manuscripts in the literature regarding dobutamine echocardiography have shown that compared to ^{201}Tl-SPECT, the use of contractile reserve to assess viability will result in higher specificity but lower sensitivity [293–295]. This reduced sensitivity may be due to the development of ischemia at even low levels of inotropic stimulation or the nature of hibernating myocardium, which may cause myofibrillar dropout. In these two situations, myocardium will not be able to respond to inotropic stimulation [296].

Delayed contrast enhancement and viability

Relaxation agents such as gadolinium chelates are large molecules that rapidly diffuse from the intravascular space into the interstitial space and tend to remain in the extracellular compartment. The presence of these contrast agents decreases both the longitudinal (T_1) and the transverse (T_2) relaxation times of the protons (of water and fat). At clinical doses of these agents the effect on T_1 relaxation time is greater, resulting in increased signal intensities on T_1-weighted images. As a direct effect, the CMR pulse sequences used to elucidate contrast are designed to generate image patterns with intensities that are strongly T_1-weighted.

ECG-gated spin-echo images were used earlier to assess viability, in which one k-space line was acquired for each cardiac cycle. Since the duration of cardiac cycle (800 ms) was comparable to myocardial T_1 relaxation time, T_1 weighted images were obtained. Using these approaches myocardial infarction was first detected in animal and human studies, [297, 298] and Dendale *et al.* [290] and Yokota *et al.* [299] visualized non-transmural infarction.

Improvement in CMR techniques

In recent years there have been a number of technical improvements in CMR, one of the most important being the use of k-space segmentation. This has enabled the acquisition of multiple k-space lines of data during each cardiac cycle, [300] leading to a reduction in imaging times, even to the point of acquiring images in a single breath-hold. This has translated into improved breath-hold tolerance by patients, improved image quality, and wider application of CMR in clinical practice.

Advances in imaging pulse sequences to allow increased T_1 weighting have been crucial for imaging myocardial viability. The preparation of magnetization prior to image acquisition by the use of an inversion recovery pulse sequence significantly increases the degree of T_1-weighting. When compared to other pulse sequences, a segmented inversion recovery sequence resulted in improved visualization of viable myocardium [301]. A much higher contrast between necrotic or scarred myocardium and normal myocardium was achieved with this sequence, with the inversion time set to substantially reduce (or null) the signal from myocardium prior to administration of contrast agent. This sequence has shown a difference in the intensities between normal and enhanced myocardium on the order of 1000% in animals, [301] translating to a 10 fold increase in the degree of image contrast compared with older, previously used spin-echo sequences.

Images are acquired in end-diastole to reduce cardiac motion. A non-selective 180 degree pulse is used to prepare the magnetization of the heart to increase T_1 weighting. The inversion time (TI) is defined as the time between this 180 degree pulse and the center of acquisition of the segmented k-space lines. This time is chosen so that the magnetization of normal and non-contrast enhanced myocardium is near its zero-crossing, ensuring that normal myocardium will appear as dark as possible (Fig. 7.7).

Contrast enhanced CMR with spin-echo pulse sequences was able to detect the transmural and overall extent of acute myocardial infarction in

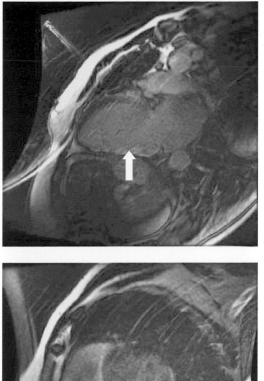

(a)

(b)

Fig. 7.7 A patient with an extensive inferoposterior myocardial infarction, six months prior to these imaging studies, demonstrating delayed enhancement. (a) Two-chamber long axis view depicting inferior wall delayed enhancement (DE) (arrow). (b) Short axis view depicting inferoapical and posterior wall (arrow) DE.

patients with medium to larger infarcts. The transmural extent of smaller infarcts was not measurable because of the low resolution of spin-echo sequences [298, 302–304]. Dendale and colleagues [290] used spin-echo techniques to assess viability and differentiate between transmural and subendocardial infarcts. Non-transmural involvement was visualized, but in 15 (27%) of the 56 infarcted segments no visible enhancement was seen. Similarly, Yokota *et al.* [299] did not visualize enhancement in six (13%) of the 44 patients with documented infarctions. The infarcts that were missed were generally small with normal wall motion at rest [290] and had lower peak creatine levels [299]. This inability to detect smaller infarcts is due to the limitations of the spin-echo sequence with image acquisition over several minutes during free breathing. Other factors that decrease the ability to detect smaller infarcts include partial volume effects due to motion averaging over the respiratory cycle, image artifacts caused by respiratory motion, and lower T_1 weighting that limits repetition time. With the advent of newer inversion recovery sequences, smaller subendocardial infarcts can be easily visualized [231, 305].

Acute and chronic myocardial infarction and delayed contrast enhancement

Both acute (myocardial necrosis) and chronic (myocardial scar) infarction show delayed contrast enhancement in laboratory animal and patient studies. Kim and colleagues scanned dogs between one and three days following reperfused or non-reperfused coronary artery occlusion, and demonstrated enhancement in histologically confirmed infarction [231]. Similar enhancement was shown by Simonetti *et al.* in a study of 18 consecutive patients after documented myocardial infarction. In each of these patients, enhancement correlated with the appropriate infarct related artery territory [301].

Kim *et al.* have shown that both acute and chronic infarcts enhance even given the difference between the tissue characteristics of acute and chronic infarcts [231]. In their study, dogs were scanned eight weeks after myocardial infarction. Using high resolution *ex vivo* imaging, the regions of enhancement observed in chronic infarcts appeared to occur in the same regions as those defined by histology.

Wu and colleagues [305] used segmented inversion recovery pulse sequences to systematically evaluate if chronic infarcts enhanced. Patients were enrolled at the time of acute infarction and underwent CMR several months later. At the same time, healthy volunteers and patients with non-ischemic cardiomyopathy were also studied. The researchers found a wide variety of enhanced areas, ranging from full transmural enhanced areas to small sub-

endocardial areas of delayed contrast enhancement. In all instances these areas of enhancement correlated with the IRA. Delayed enhancement was not seen in the healthy volunteers or in patients with non-ischemic dilated cardiomyopathy, resulting in a specificity of 100%. The sensitivity for detection of old infarcts was 91% in three-month-old and 100% in 14-month-old infarcts.

Mechanism of delayed contrast enhancement

The mechanism of late enhancement is not fully understood. The fluid volume of normal myocardial tissue is predominantly intracellular. The volume of distribution of the extracellular contrast agents (e.g. gadolinium chelate) in normal myocardium is quite low, suggesting that viable myocardial cells exclude contrast agents. In myocardial infarction, the myocyte membranes rupture, allowing the passage of the contrast agent into the intracellular space and giving rise to a higher level of contrast agent. Cell death is thought to be closely related to loss of sarcolemmal membrane integrity, and this correlates with delayed enhancement [306, 307]. This also explains the relationship between the spatial distribution of delayed CMR enhancement and histologically observed necrosis [231]. Extracellular contrast agents such as Gd-DTPA are excluded from the myocyte's intracellular space by an intact sarcolemmal membrane [13, 308]. Viable myocardium has an intact sarcolemmal membrane which excludes the chelate and helps explain the lack of delayed contrast enhancement.

Chronic infarction or scar, on the other hand, is characterized by dense collagen. The interstitial space between the collagenous scar tissue may be greater than the interstitial space between the densely packed living myocardial cells. Rehwald and associates [123] have shown a greater volume of distribution of contrast agent in a scar compared to viable myocardium.

In the setting of reversible ischemic injury, myocardium is viable and the cell membrane is intact. Thus, delayed enhancement of contrast agent is not seen. This is because the sarcolemmal membrane is intact and the contrast agent is excluded from the intracellular space [306]. Here the volume of distribution of the contrast agent in the reversible ischemic areas will be similar to that of normal myocardium, resulting in no enhancement of these areas.

Technical considerations

Partial volume effects can occur whenever the spatial resolution is low. Even with adequate spatial resolution, partial volume effects can occur when the imaging time is long due to either respiratory or patient motion.

Areas of hypo-enhancement or deficits in the distribution of the contrast agent are often observed in the central areas of myocardial infarcts surrounded by areas of delayed enhancement. The area of hypo-enhancement has been related to the phenomenon of no-reflow [309, 310]. This no-reflow territory, characterized by markedly reduced perfusion, is thought to be due to damage or destruction at the microvascular level, impeding the presence of blood flow and the penetration of the MR contrast agent. Since flow in these areas is low but not absolutely zero, they initially appear dark, but slowly enhance as contrast agent accumulates. Accordingly, these hypo-enhanced or darker areas should be included in the quantification of infarct size (Fig. 7.8).

Clinical applications

CMR assessment of wall motion, perfusion and contrast enhancement allows accurate high resolution evaluation of normal, ischemic viable and ischemic non-viable myocardium. When wall motion and thickening are normal, perfusion is normal and there is no delayed contrast enhancement, normal myocardium has been defined. When wall motion and thickening are normal, perfusion is abnormal and there is no delayed contrast enhancement, early myocardial ischemia is present. When wall motion and thickening are reduced, perfusion is abnormal and there is no contrast enhancement, a higher level of myocardial ischemia has been defined. When wall motion is akinetic and thickening is absent, perfusion is abnormal and there is no delayed enhancement, myocardium is most likely viable and ischemia severe. Finally, when wall motion is akinetic or dyskinetic, wall thickening is absent or wall thinning is present, when perfusion is absent, and when there is delayed contrast enhancement, myocardium is non-viable. The rela-

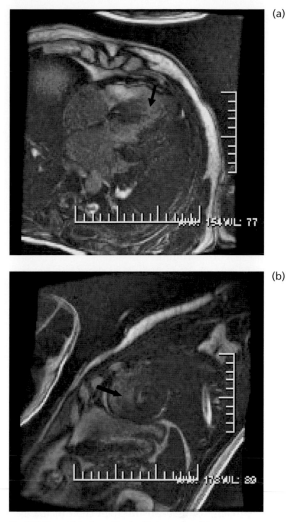

(a)

(b)

Fig. 7.8 Example of a patient with hypertrophic cardiomyopathy who demonstrates a non-ischemic etiology for delayed enhancement (DE). (a) Four-chamber long axis view depicting DE in the apical interventricular septum (arrow). (b) Short axis view showing DE.

tionship between ventricular function (wall motion and wall thickening), perfusion pattern (subendocardial and transmural), and contrast enhancement pattern is complex. Ventricular function, perfusion and contrast enhancement all reflect different physiological processes and therefore, combinations of the three are useful for evaluation of the level of myocardial ischemic process. In the clinical setting of acute myocardial infarction CMR can fully characterize the ischemic process (delayed enhancement determines the presence and extent of the infarct, perfusion imaging determines the presence and extent of the ischemic plus infarcted territory, and the cine study determines the function of the involved myocardial segment). In the case of myocardial stunning after reperfusion wall motion is reduced (stunned), perfusion is normal or can show non-transmural or transmural deficits, and enhancement pattern is generally absent or subendocardial. The combined observation of these three imaging characteristics defines the resulting reperfusion. Likewise, the combined assessment of function, perfusion and enhancement can be applied in the chronic setting to distinguish between scarred, hibernating and normal myocardium.

In an animal study by Hillenbrand and associates, [311] the relationship between the transmural extent of contrast enhancement and myocardial salvage after reperfusion treatment for acute myocardial infarction was examined. In this study the transmural extent of delayed contrast enhancement on post MI day three predicted improvement in contractile function.

Viability assessment weeks or longer after acute MI is also essential to determine the optimal therapeutic strategy. The involved myocardium could be scar or it could have reduced wall motion but still be viable, such as is the case in hibernation. Myocardial dysfunction associated with viable myocardium is usually reversible, but the treatment also depends on the extent of the dysfunction. A very small region of viability and a substantial amount of scar may not be worth an interventional PCI or bypass graft procedure. The total extent of involvement is evaluated by assessment of ventricular function, while the extent of scar (irreversible by revascularization) is identifiable by the extent of delayed contrast enhancement. In a study conducted by Kim *et al.*, [128] cine and contrast CMR were performed in 50 consecutive patients before they underwent revascularization by PCI or CABG. Cine CMR was repeated at 11 weeks after revascularization to assess changes in regional wall motion. The likelihood of improvement was related to the extent of transmural enhancement in this study. Seventy eight per cent with no enhancement improved after revascularization whereas only one out of 58 seg-

ments with greater than 75% delayed enhancement showed improvement. The relationship between delayed enhancement and contractile dysfunction was the same for severe hypokinesis, akinesis or dyskinesis at baseline. It was also shown that the greater the extent of dysfunctional but viable myocardium the greater the improvement in wall motion (p < 0.001) and ejection fraction (p < 0.001) after revascularization.

Contrast CMR has advantages over other imaging modalities used to assess viability. Detection of the transmural extent of delayed enhancement or DE is helpful in predicting functional improvement. Kim *et al.* showed that the mean extent of DE was 10% ± 7% in patients who improved versus 41% ± 14% in patients with no improvement (p < 0.001). Previous studies have shown that significant viability can exist without functional improvement. This underscores the importance of combining the high resolution assessment of myocardial function, perfusion pattern and delayed contrast enhancement by CMR in the assessment of viability.

Future applications of contrast enhanced CMR

Contrast enhanced CMR now allows routine detection of the transmural extent of infarcted or scarred myocardium and even the presence of less extensive subendocardial defects. Cine CMR and contrast CMR allow evaluation of the intricate relationship between infarction and contractile function. The application of the method of delayed enhancement to the assessment of viability in patients with suspected CAD will provide an understanding of the incidence of myocardial damage even when wall motion appears normal. Of course, the dynamic importance of such an observation may not be of much clinical importance, but the presence of such findings may have a bearing on outcomes in CAD.

Delayed CMR contrast enhancement and normal wall motion

Traditionally it has been assumed that MI is associated with contractile dysfunction. It has been shown by Lieberman and colleagues [312] that contractile dysfunction when used alone results in overestimation of the infarct size. Though the infarct may be small, the extent of the contractile dysfunction itself may be large [313–315]. Recently, Wu *et al.* [305] have shown that the area of contractile dysfunction may be smaller than the infarct itself. In their study of patients with chronic infarction, 25% of segments with subendocardial infarction had normal wall motion. The relationship between transmural infarct and wall thickening is mainly based on studies conducted in patients with acute myocardial infarction. Mahrholdt and colleagues [316] studied patients with chronic enzyme-positive myocardial infarction and single vessel CAD. They showed that in a setting of reperfused chronic MI, contractile dysfunction occurs when thickness of the transmural infarction approaches 50% of normal. Hence, contractile function alone cannot be used to rule out chronic MI. These studies suggest that the relationship of contractile function and infarct size are complex. They also show that infarct size can be overestimated in the acute setting and underestimated in the chronic setting. Magnetic resonance imaging techniques cannot evaluate the presence and size of infarction based only on contractile dysfunction. Chronic subendocardial infarcts with normal wall motion may be missed by imaging techniques in the absence of biochemical evidence of infarction or wall thinning.

Performance of CMR when infarcts are missed by SPECT

SPECT has lower resolution compared to CMR. An inversion recovery CMR pulse sequence provides a voxel size of 1.4 mm × 1.9 mm × 6.0 mm (0.016 cm^3). SPECT has a resolution of approximately 10 mm × 10 mm × 10 mm (1 cm^3) [317, 318]. The resolution is almost 50 fold greater for CMR compared with SPECT. Wagner *et al.* [107] conducted a study of 91 patients to determine whether CMR is capable of detecting infarcts that are missed by SPECT. Both CMR and SPECT were analyzed and scored for the presence, location and extent of infarcts. At the same time, they also conducted delayed contrast enhanced CMR in 12 animals with MI and three without MI. The presence of MI was determined by histochemical staining.

Both CMR and SPECT detected nearly all transmural infarctions. CMR was able to detect sub-

endocardial infarcts in 100 of 109 segments (92%), compared to SPECT which identified infarcts in only 31 (28%) segments. Both SPECT and CMR had high specificity for the detection of infarction: 97% vs 98% respectively. In the nine patients, all transmural infarcts identified by CMR were also detected by SPECT. But of the 181 segments with subendocardial infarction (less than 50% of the transmural thickness of the LV wall), 85 were not detected by SPECT. This means that while six (13%) of the patients whose subendocardial infarction was visible by CMR, their infarctions were undetected by SPECT.

In conclusion, it can be said that while both CMR and SPECT detect infarction equally, CMR is superior for detecting subendocardial infarcts.

CMR delayed enhancement in the absence of a history of MI

Myocardial infarcts occur without patient or physician knowledge in 30–40% of cases. This estimate is based on the detection of new Q waves by ECG, and does not include some subendocardial infarcts which may not be detectable by routine ECG [319–321].

Delayed CMR contrast enhancement that has been performed for routine evaluation has been positive in patients without ECG or historical evidence of MI. Kim and associates [322] studied 100 patients who were referred for coronary angiography, with no prior history of MI or revascularization. They detected delayed contrast enhancement in 57% with Q waves on ECG present in only 14%. CMR detection of infarction is four-fold higher than that of routine 12 lead ECG. The prognostic significance of such silent, clinically unrecognized, delayed enhancement needs further investigation.

High energy phosphate metabolism to assess ischemia and viability

Introduction to myocardial CMR spectroscopy

Another unique aspect of CMR is its ability to evaluate metabolism using its capacity to detect sensitive nuclei that comprise important molecular species within the myocardium. These nuclei include the proton or hydrogen nucleus (H$^+$), and the nuclei of carbon-13, fluorine-19, sodium-23, and phosphorus-31. Within the myocardium (and all viable tissue), all function depends on the use of the presence of the high energy phosphates, including adenosine triphosphate (ATP), adenosine diphosphate (ADP), adenosine monophosphate (AMP) and phosphocreatine (PCr). Using a surface coil placed over the myocardium to generate the radio-frequency specific for ^{31}P at the magnetic field used, (e.g. 1.5 Tesla, 3.0 Tesla, etc), spectra of the myocardium can be generated which allow visualization of ATP, PCr and inorganic phosphates. Spectra are generated using methods which define a region of interest within the myocardium. While these regions are relatively large, making imaging difficult, the sample of myocardium interrogated provides a means, like a biopsy, of assessing global myocardial concentrations of the phosphates. As the magnetic field increases, the ability to resolve the various molecular peaks is improved, since signal to noise increases. At a higher field than the 1.5 Tesla that is present in the most widely available CMR systems, i.e. 3.0 Tesla, the myocardial inorganic phosphate can be resolved. This peak is capable of assessing the pH within the myocardium using the so called chemical shift. Chemical shift is the term given to the process that leads to the relocation of the Pi as a function of pH. When the pH decreases, as is the case in association with the acidosis associated with myocardial ischemia, the Pi peak shifts to the left or downfield. The converse is true with an increase in pH.

Myocardial ^{31}P spectroscopy and ischemic insult

When the myocardium becomes ischemic, as for example during stress, the PCr and PCr/ATP ratio decrease. If the Pi can be resolved, that peak will move downfield consistent with a decrease in pH. Accordingly, this approach allows the definition of myocardial ischemia by directly interrogating the myocardium. No contrast agent is used and stress is commonly induced using a handgrip. Intracellular metabolic markers such as PCr and ATP provide a direct means of assessing ischemia and infarction. PCr is a labile molecule that is the first to decrease and does so rapidly when blood supply decreases and/or when work increases, leading to a reduction in PCr/ATP. As the ischemic insult progresses ATP begins to decrease. By the time of cell death, ATP has decreased substantially and there is little if any PCr. Concomitantly, during the early phase of

myocardial ischemia, there is a shift in Pi downfield consistent with acidosis. Accordingly, while PCr/ATP provides an excellent definition for myocardial ischemia, it is a less effective means for determination of loss of viability, since the level of ATP that portends cell death is not well defined.

Clinical applications of ^{31}P myocardial spectroscopy

The most important study describing the use of PCr/ATP with handgrip stress to define myocardial ischemia was that of Weiss et al. [323]. Two groups of patients were compared: those with no significant CAD and those with significant CAD. The normal PCr/ATP is between 1.3 and 1.7. In patients with significant CAD the PCr/ATP decreased from 1.45 ± 0.31 to 0.91 ± 0.24 (p < 0.001). In five patients measurements were made before and after revascularization. After revascularization the PCr/ATP at rest was 1.60 ± 0.20, while the PCr/ATP with handgrip stress was 1.62 ± 0.18 (p = NS). Such direct evaluation of intracellular myocardial metabolism has been considered as the "gold standard" to define ischemia clinically.

Another important study that applied ^{31}P spectroscopy is that of Neubauer et al., which used PCr/ATP to prognosticate in patients after acute MI. Mortality rate after five years increased significantly from 5% when the PCr/ATP was ≥1.60 to 40% when the PCr/ATP was < 1.60 (p < 0.02). A third interesting study [324] using ^{31}P myocardial spectroscopy evaluated women as part of the United States National Heart Lung and Blood Institute (NHLBI) supported Women's Ischemia Syndrome Evaluation (WISE). Selected women with chest pain who were referred for coronary angiography, but without significant CAD, also underwent ^{31}P myocardial spectroscopy. The study included two control groups, one group of healthy, but age matched volunteers, and one with significant left anterior descending CAD. The volunteer control group was used to define the abnormal change with handgrip stress in PCr/ATP or mean minus-2SD as the threshold for abnormality. Twenty per cent of the 35 women in the WISE group had an abnormal change in PCr/ATP (below 2SD less than the mean value) with a significant change minus-6.6%. Thirty five per cent of the 20 patients with ≥70% stenosis of the LAD had a significant change of minus-19.6%. These data suggest that a moderate percentage of WISE patients with chest pain but without evidence of angiographically demonstrable significant CAD had an abnormal fall in PCr/ATP, suggesting myocardial ischemia. The change was more dramatic in patients with significant LAD disease. It is likely that the WISE patients had microvascular disease which led to myocardial ischemia in 20%, with a modest level of myocardial stress associated with microvascular disease. In a follow-up study by Johnson *et al.*, [325] the WISE patients with the greater fall in PCr/ATP had more frequent hospital admissions and more coronary angiograms, but no increase in morbidity and mortality.

Conclusions

Myocardial viability can be routinely assessed by CMR either by evaluation of the response of abnormal wall motion using cine CMR to low dose dobutamine or by the use of delayed contrast enhancement. Low dose dobutamine cine CMR provides information in a manner similar to that of low dose dobutamine echocardiography but with greater sensitivity and specificity. The definition of viability in this instance is the documentation of improved contractile function with low dose dobutamine providing indirect evidence of myocardial contractile reserve. Delayed contrast enhanced myocardial segments provides evidence of acute and/or chronic myocardial infarction, and has correlated well with histochemical staining in laboratory animal studies. The absence of delayed contrast enhancement detected by CMR is indicative of viable myocardium. In both the acute and chronic settings, regions of myocardium with contractile dysfunction, but without evidence of delayed enhancement are likely to recover function with revascularization. In routine practice, delayed contrast enhanced CMR is preferable to low dose dobutamine CMR as the former is safer and gives direct evidence of viability.

Contrast enhanced CMR is able to detect infarcts or scar in regions of normal wall motion, subendocardial infarcts not detected by SPECT, and infarcts that are not clinically recognized. The prognostic significance of such delayed enhancement requires further investigation.

Finally, another unique aspect of CMR, the ability to assess metabolism using ^{31}P spectroscopy, provides a specific way to assess myocardial ischemia, but is less useful to define viability.

References

1. Bloch F. Nuclear induction. *Physical Review (Physics)*. 1946; **70**: 460–473.
2. Purcell E, Torrey H, Pound R. Resonance adsorption by nuclear magnetic moments in a solid. *Physical Review (Physics)*. 1946; **69**: 37–38.
3. Lauterbur P. Image formation by induced local interactions: Examples employing nuclear magnetic resonance. *Nature* 1973; **242**: 190–191.
4. Mansfield P. Multiplanar image formation using NMR spin echoes. *J Phys* 1977; **10**: L55–L58.
5. Kumar A, Welti D, Ernst RR. NMR Fourier zeugmatography. *J Magn Reson* 1975; **18**: 69–83.
6. Damadian RV. Tumor detection by nuclear magnetic resonance. *Science* 1971; **171**: 1151–1153.
7. Goldman MR, Pohost GM, Ingwall JS *et al.* Nuclear magnetic resonance imaging: Potential cardiac applications. *Am J Cardiol* 1980; **46**: 1278–1283.
8. Blackwell G, Doyle M, Cranney G. Cardiovascular MRI techniques. In: Blackwell GG, Cranney GB, Pohost GM, eds. *MRI: Cardiovascular System*. Gower Medical Publishing, New York, 1992.
9. McRobbie DW, Moore EA, Graves MJ *et al. MRI from Picture to Proton*. Cambridge University Press, Cambridge, 2003.
10. Elster AD, Burdette JH. *Questions and Answers in MRI*. Mosby, London, 2001.
11. Bottomley PA, Foster TH, Argersinger RE *et al.* A review of normal tissue hydrogen NMR relaxation times and mechanisms from 1–100 mHz: Dependence on tissue type, NMR frequency, temperature, species, excision and age. *Med Phys* 1984; **11**: 425–448.
12. Donahue KM, Weisskoff RM, Burnstein D. Water diffusion and exchange as they influence contrast enhancement. *J Magn Reson Imaging* 1997; **7**: 102–110.
13. Weinmann HJ, Brasch RC, Press WR *et al.* Characteristics of gadolinium-DTPA complex: A potential NMR contrast agent. *Am J Roentgenol* 1984; **142**: 619–624.
14. Saeed M, Wagner S, Wendland MF *et al.* Occlusive and reperfused myocardial infarcts: Differentiation with Mn-DPDP enhanced MR imaging. *Radiology* 1989; **172**: 59–64.
15. Saeed M, Wendland MF, Takehara Y *et al.* Reversible and irreversible injury in the reperfused myocardium: Differentiation with contrast material-enhanced MR imaging. *Radiology* 1990; **175**: 633–637.

16. Saeed M, Wendland MF, Takehara Y *et al.* Reperfusion and irreversible myocardial injury: identification with a non-ionic MR imaging contrast medium. *Radiology* 1992; **182**: 675–683.

17. Saeed M, Wendland MF, Masui T *et al.* Reperfused myocardial infarctions on T1- and susceptibility-enhanced MRI: Evidence for loss of compartmentalization of contrast media. *Magn Res Med* 1994; **31**: 31–39.

18. Geschwind JF, Wendland MF, Saeed M *et al.* Identification of myocardial cell death in reperfused myocardial injury using dual mechanisms of contrast enhanced magnetic resonance imaging. *Acad Radiol* 1994; **1**: 319–325.

19. Adzamli IK, Jolesz FA, Bleier AR *et al.* The effect of gadolinium DTPA on tissue water compartments in slow- and fast-twitch rabbit muscles. *Magn Reson Med* 1989; **11**: 172–181.

20. Barkhausen J, Ruehm SG, Goyen M *et al.* MR evaluation of ventricular function: True fast imaging with steady-state precession versus fast low-angle shot cine MR imaging-feasibility study. *Radiology* 2001; **219**: 264–269.

21. Plein S, Bloomer TN, Ridgway JP *et al.* Steady-state free precession magnetic resonance imaging of the heart: Comparison with segmented k-space gradient-echo imaging. *J Magn Reson Imaging* 2001; **14**: 230–236.

22. Pettigrew RI, Oshinski JN, Chatzimavroudis G *et al.* MRI techniques for cardiovascular imaging. *J Magn Reson Imaging* 1999; **10**: 590–601.

23. Szolar DH, Sakuma H, Higgins CB. Cardiovascular applications of magnetic resonance flow and velocity measurements. *J Magn Reson Imaging* 1996; **1**: 78–89.

24. Zerhouni EA, Parish DM, Rogers WJ *et al.* Human heart tagging with MR imaging—a method for non-invasive assessment of myocardial motion. *Radiology* 1988; **169**: 59–63.

25. Garot J, Bluemke DA, Osman NF *et al.* Fast determination of regional myocardial strain fields from tagged cardiac MR images using harmonic phase (HARP) MRI. *Circulation* 2000; **101**: 981–988.

26. Maier SE, Fischer SE, McKinnon GC *et al.* Evaluation of left ventricular segmental wall motion in hypertrophic cardiomyopathy with myocardial tagging. *Circulation* 1992; **86**: 1919–1928.

27. Bogaert J, Maes A, van de Werf F *et al.* Functional recovery of subepicardial myocardial tissue in transmural myocardial infarction after successful perfusion: An important contribution to the improvement of regional and global left ventricular function. *Circulation* 1999; **99**: 36–43.

28. Maniar HS, Cupps BP, Potter DD *et al.* Ventricular function after coronary artery bypass grafting: Evaluation by magnetic resonance imaging and myocardial strain analysis. *J Thorac Cardiovasc Surg* 2004; **128**: 76–82.

29. Fuchs E, Muller MF, Oswald H *et al.* Cardiac rotation and relaxation in patients with chronic heart failure. *Eur J Heart Fail* 2004; **6**: 715–722.

30. Dubach P, Myers J, Bonetti P *et al.* Effects of bisoprolol fumarate on left ventricle size, function, and exercise capacity in patients with heart failure: Analysis with magnetic resonance myocardial tagging. *Am Heart J* 2002; **143**: 676–683.

31. Scheffler K, Heid O, Henning J. Magnetization preparation during the steady state: Fat saturated 3D TrueFISP. *Magn Reson Med* 2001; **45**: 1075–1080.

32. Markl M, Reeder SB, Chan FP *et al.* Steady state free precession MR imaging improved myocardial tag persistence and signal-to-noise ratio for analysis of myocardial motion *Radiology* 2004; **230**: 852–861.

33. Semelka RC, Tomei E, Wagner S *et al.* Normal left ventricular dimensions and function: Interstudy reproducibility of measurements with cine MR imaging. *Radiology* 1990; **174**: 763–768.

34. Germain P, Roul G, Kastler B *et al.* Interstudy variability in left ventricular mass measurement. Comparison between M-mode echography and MRI. *Eur Heart J* 1992; **13**: 1011–1019.

35. Lorenz CH, Walker ES, Morgan VL *et al.* Normal human right and left ventricular mass, systolic function and gender differences by cine-magnetic resonance imaging. *J Cardiovasc Magn Reson* 1999; **1**: 7–21.

36. Longmore DB, Klipstein RH, Underwood SR *et al.* Dimensional accuracy of magnetic resonance in studies of the heart. *Lancet* 1985; **1**: 1360–1362.

37. Shapiro EP, Rogers WJ, Beyar R *et al.* Determination of left ventricular mass by MRI in hearts deformed by acute infarction. *Circulation* 1989; **79**: 706–711.

38. Semelka RC, Tomei E, Wagner S *et al.* Interstudy reproducibility of dimensional and functional measurements between cine-magnetic resonance studies in the morphologically abnormal left ventricle. *Am Heart J* 1990; **119**: 1367–1373.

39. Chuang ML, Hibberd MG, Salton CJ *et al.* Importance of imaging method over imaging modality in non-invasive determination of left ventricular volumes and ejection fraction: Assessment by two- and three-dimensional echocardiography and magnetic resonance imaging. *J Am Coll Cardiol* 2000; **35**: 447–487.

40. Doherty NE 3rd, Fujita N, Caputo GR *et al.* Measurement of right ventricular mass in normal and dilated cardiomyopathic ventricles using cine-magnetic resonance imaging. *Am J Cardiol* 1992; **69**: 1223–1228.

41. Grothues F, Moon JC, Bellenger NG *et al.* Interstudy reproducibility of right ventricular volumes, function, and mass with cardiovascular magnetic resonance. *Am Heart J* 2004; **147**: 218–223.

42. Katz J, Whang J, Boxt LM *et al.* Estimation of right ventricular mass in normal subjects and in patients with primary pulmonary hypertension by nuclear magnetic resonance imaging. *J Am Coll Cardiol* 1993; **21**: 1475–1481.

43. Lorenz CH, Walker ES, Graham TP Jr *et al.* Right ventricular performance and mass by use of cine MRI late after atrial repair of transposition of the great arteries. *Circulation* 1995; **92** (Suppl II): II233–II239.

44. Sievers B, Kirchberg S, Bakan A *et al.* Impact of papillary muscles in ventricular volume and ejection fraction assessment by cardiovascular magnetic resonance. *J Cardiovasc Magn Reson* 2004; **6**: 9–16.

45. Utz JA, Herfkens RJ, Heinsimer JA *et al.* Cine MR determination of left ventricular ejection fraction. *Am J Roentgenol* 1987; **148**: 839–843.

46. Culham JA, Vince DJ. Cardiac output by MR imaging: An experimental study comparing right ventricle and left ventricle with thermodilution. *Can Assoc Radiol J* 1988; **39**: 247–249.

47. Hunter GJ, Hamberg LM, Weisskoff RM *et al.* Measurement of stroke volume and cardiac output within a single breath-hold with echoplanar MR imaging. *J Magn Reson Imaging* 1994; **4**: 51–58.

48. Hundley WG, Li HF, Hillis LD *et al.* Quantitation of cardiac output with velocity encoded, phase-difference magnetic resonance imaging: Validation with invasive measurements. *Am J Cardiol* 1995; **75**: 1250–1255.

49. Zehender M, Kasper W, Kauder E *et al.* Right ventricular infarction as an independent predictor of prognosis after acute inferior myocardial infarction. *N Engl J Med* 1993; **328**: 981–988.

50. Rominger MB, Bachmann GF, Pabst W *et al.* Right ventricular volumes and ejection fraction with fast cine MR imaging in breath-hold technique: Applicability, normal values from 52 volunteers, and evaluation of 325 adult cardiac patients. *J Magn Reson Imaging* 1999; **10**: 908–918.

51. Sechtem U, Pflugfelder PW, Cassidy MM *et al.* Mitral or aortic regurgitation: Quantification of regurgitant volumes with cine MR imaging. *Radiology* 1988; **167**: 425–430.

52. Didier D, Ratib O, Friedli B *et al.* Cine gradient-echo MR imaging in the evaluation of cardiovascular disease. *RadioGraphics* 1993; **13**: 561–573.

53. Suzuki J, Caputo GR, Kondo C *et al.* Cine MR imaging of valvular heart disease: Display and imaging parameters affect the size of the signal void caused by valvular regurgitation. *Am J Roentgenol* 1990; **155**: 723–727.

54. Higgins CB, Wagner S, Kondo C *et al.* Evaluation of valvular heart disease with cine gradient echo magnetic resonance imaging. *Circulation* 1991; **84** (3 Suppl): I198–I207.

55. Mitchell L, Jenkins JP, Watson Y *et al.* Diagnosis and assessment of mitral and aortic disease by cine flow magnetic resonance imaging. *Magn Reson Med* 1989; **12**: 181–197.

56. De Roos A, Reichek N, Axel L *et al.* Cine MR imaging in aortic stenosis. *J Comput Assist Tomogr* 1989; **13**: 421–425.

57. Cosolo GC, Zampa V, Rega L *et al.* Evaluation of mitral stenosis by cine-magnetic resonance imaging. *Am Heart J* 1992; **123**: 1252–1260.

58. Kondo C, Caputo GR, Semelka R *et al.* Right and left ventricular stroke volume measurements with velocity encoded cine NMR imaging: *In vitro* and *in vivo* evaluation. *Am J Roentgenol* 1991; **157**: 9–16.

59. Mohiaddin RH, Pennell DJ. MR blood flow measurement: Clinical application in the heart and circulation. *Cardiol Clin* 1998; **16**: 161–187.

60. Honda N, Machida K, Hashimoto M *et al.* Aortic regurgitation: Quantification with MR imaging velocity mapping. *Radiology* 1993; **186**: 189–194.

61. Wang ZJ, Reddy GP, Gotway MB *et al.* Cardiovascular shunts: MR imaging evaluation. *RadioGraphics* 2003; **23** Spec No: S181–S194.

62. Hundley WG, Li HF, Lange RA *et al.* Assessment of left-to-right intracardiac shunting by velocity encoded, phase-difference magnetic resonance imaging. *Circulation* 1995; **91**: 2955–2960.

63. Rebergen SA, Niezen RA, Helbing WA *et al.* Cine gradient echo MR imaging and MR velocity mapping in the evaluation of congenital heart disease. *RadioGraphics* 1996; **16**: 467–481.

64. Kayser HV, Stoel BC, van der Wall EE *et al.* MR velocity mapping of tricuspid flow: Correction for through-plane motion. *J Magn Reson Imaging* 1997; **7**: 669–673.

65. Sondergaard L, Lindvig K, Hildebrandt P *et al.* Quantification of aortic regurgitation by magnetic resonance imaging mapping. *Am Heart J* 1993; **125**: 1081–1090.

66. Dulce MC, Mostbeck GH, O'Sullivan M *et al.* Severity of aortic regurgitation: Interstudy reproducibility of measurements with velocity encoded cine MR imaging. *Radiology* 1992; **185**: 235–240.

67. Hundley WG, Li HF, Willard JE *et al.* Magnetic resonance imaging assessment of the severity of mitral regurgitation: Comparison with invasive techniques. *Circulation* 1995; **92**: 1151–1158.

68. Fujita N, Chaouilleres AF, Hartiala MM *et al.* Quantification of mitral regurgitation by velocity encoded cine nuclear magnetic resonance imaging. *J Am Coll Cardiol* 1994; **23**: 951–958.

69. Kon MW, Myerson SG, Moat NE *et al.* Quantification of regurgitant fraction in mitral regurgitation by cardiovascular magnetic resonance: Comparison of techniques. *J Heart Valve Dis* 2004; **13**: 600–607.

70. Wyttenbach R, Bremerich J, Saeed M *et al.* Integrated MR imaging approach to valvular heart disease. *Cardiol Clin* 1998; **16**: 227–294.

71. Eichenberger AC, Jenni R, von Schulthess GK. Aortic valve pressure gradients in patients with aortic valve stenosis: Quantification with velocity encoded cine MR imaging. *Am J Roentgenol* 1993; **160**: 971–977.

72. Caruthers SD, Lin SJ, Brown P *et al.* Practical value of cardiac magnetic resonance imaging for clinical quantification of aortic valve stenosis: Comparison with echocardiography. *Circulation* 2003; **108**: 2236–2243.

73. Heidenreich PA, Steffens J, Fujita N *et al.* Evaluation of mitral stenosis with velocity encoded cine-magnetic resonance imaging. *Am J Cardiol* 1995; **75**: 365–369.

74. Lin SJ, Brown PA, Watkins MP *et al.* Quantification of stenotic mitral valve area with magnetic resonance imaging and comparison with Doppler ultrasound. *J Am Coll Cardiol* 2004; **44**: 133–137.

75. Caputo GR, Kondo C, Masui T *et al.* Right and left lung perfusion: *In vitro* and *in vivo* validation with oblique-angle, velocity encoded cine MR imaging. *Radiology* 1991; **180**: 693–698.

76. Bellenger NG, Burgess M, Ray SG *et al.* Comparison of left ventricular ejection fraction and volumes in heart failure by two-dimensional echocardiography, radionuclide ventriculography and cardiovascular magnetic resonance: Are they interchangeable? *Eur Heart J* 2000; **21**: 1387–1396.

77. Van Rugge FP, van der Wall EE, Spanjersberg SJ *et al.* Magnetic resonance imaging during dobutamine stress for detection of coronary artery disease: Quantitative wall motion analysis using a modification of the centerline method. *Circulation* 1994; **90**: 127–138.

78. Haag UJ, Maier SE, Jakob M *et al.* Left ventricular wall thickness measurements by magnetic resonance: A validation study. *Int J Card Imaging* 1991; **7**: 31–41.

79. Baer FM, Smolarz K, Theissen P *et al.* Regional ^{99m}Tc-methoxyisobutyl-isonitrile uptake at rest in patients with myocardial infarcts: Comparison with morphological and functional parameters obtained from gradient-echo magnetic resonance imaging. *Eur Heart J* 1994; **15**: 97–107.

80. Azhari H, Sideman S, Weiss JL *et al.* Three-dimensional mapping of acute ischemic regions using MRI: Wall thickening versus motion analysis. *Am J Physiol* 1990; **259**: H1492–H1503.

81. Sheehan FH, Bolson EL, Dodge HT *et al.* Advantages and applications of the centerline method for characterizing regional ventricular function. *Circulation* 1986; **74**: 293–305.

82. Von Land CD, Rao SR, Reiber JHC. Development of an improved centerline wall motion model. *Comput Cardiol* 1990; **17**: 687–690.

83. Holman ER, Buller VGM, de Roos A *et al.* Detection and quantification of dysfunctional myocardium by magnetic resonance imaging: A new three-dimensional method for quantitative wall thickening analysis. *Circulation* 1997; **95**: 924–931.

84. McVeigh ER, Zerhouni EA. Non-invasive measurement of transmural gradients in myocardial strain with MR imaging. *Radiology* 1991; **180**: 677–683.

85. Gerber BL, Garot J, Bluemke DA *et al.* Accuracy of contrast enhanced resonance magnetic imaging in predicting improvement of regional myocardial function in patients after acute myocardial infarction. *Circulation* 2002; **106**: 1083–1089.

86. Paelinck BP, Lamb HJ, Bax JJ *et al.* Assessment of diastolic function by cardiovascular magnetic resonance. *Am Heart J* 2002; **144**: 198–205.

87. Van der Geest RJ, Reiber JH. Quantification in cardiac MRI. *J Magn Reson Imaging* 1999; **10**: 602–608.

88. Suzuki JI, Caputo GR, Masui T *et al.* Assessment of right ventricular diastolic and systolic function in patients with dilated cardiomyopathy using cinemagnetic resonance imaging . *Am Heart J* 1991; **122**: 1035–1040.

89. Fujita N, Hartiala J, O'Sullivan M *et al.* Assessment of left ventricular diastolic function in dilated cardiomyopathy with cine-magnetic resonance imaging: Effect of an angiotensin converting enzyme inhibitor, benazepril. *Am Heart J* 1993; **125**: 171–178.

90. Yamanari H, Kakishita M, Fujimoto Y *et al.* Regional myocardial perfusion abnormalities and regional myocardial early diastolic dysfunction in patients with hypertrophic cardiomyopathy. *Heart Vessels* 1997; **12**: 192–198.

91. Kudelka AM, Turner DA, Liebson PR *et al.* Comparison of cine-magnetic resonance imaging and Doppler echocardiography for evaluation of left ventricular diastolic function. *Am J Cardiol* 1997; **80**: 384–386.

92. Mohiaddin RH, Gatehouse PD, Henien M *et al.* Cine MR Fourier velocimetry of blood through cardiac valves: Comparison with Doppler echocardiography. *J Magn Reson Imaging* 1997; **7**: 657–663.

93. Hartiala JJ, Mostbeck GH, Foster E *et al.* Velocity encoded cine MRI in the evaluation of left ventricular diastolic function. Measurement of mitral valve and pulmonary vein flow velocities and flow volume across the mitral valve. *Am Heart J* 1993; **125**: 1054–1066.

94. Fyrenius A, Wigstrom L, Bolger AF *et al.* Pitfalls in Doppler evaluation of diastolic function: Insights from three-dimensional magnetic resonance imaging. *J Am Soc Echocardiogr* 1999; **12**: 817–826.

95. Hartiala JJ, Foster E, Fujita N *et al.* Evaluation of left atrial contribution to left ventricular filling in aortic stenosis by velocity encoded cine MRI. *Am Heart J* 1994; **127**: 593–600.

96. Karwatowski SP, Brecker SJD, Yang GZ *et al*. Mitral valve flow measured with cine MR velocity mapping in patients with ischemic heart disease: Comparison with Doppler echocardiography. *J Magn Reson Imaging* 1995; **5**: 89–92.

97. Buchalter MB, Weiss JL, Rogers WJ *et al*. Non-invasive quantification of left ventricular rotational deformation in normal humans using magnetic resonance imaging myocardial tagging. *Circulation* 1990; **81**: 1236–1244.

98. Nagel E, Stuber M, Lakatos M *et al*. Cardiac rotation and relaxation after anteroseptal myocardial infarction. *Coron Artery Dis* 2000; **10**: 261–267.

99. Kroeker CA, Tyberg JV, Beyar R. Effects of ischemia on left ventricular apex rotation. An experimental study in anesthetized dogs. *Circulation* 1995; **92**: 3539–3548.

100. Paetsch I, Foell D, Kaluza A *et al*. Magnetic resonance stress tagging in ischemic heart disease. *Am J Physiol Heart Circ Physiol* 2005; **288**: H2708-14.

101. Sensky PR, Jivan A, Hudson NM *et al*. Coronary artery disease: combined stress MR imaging protocol- one stop evaluation of myocardial perfusion and function. *Radiology* 2000; **215**: 608–614.

102. Plein S, Ridgway JP, Jones TR *et al*. Coronary artery disease: Assessment with a comprehensive MR imaging protocol—initial results. *Radiology* 2002; **225**: 300–307.

103. Chiu CW, So NM, Lam WW *et al*. Combined first-pass perfusion and viability study of MR imaging in patients with non-ST segment-elevation acute coronary syndromes: Feasibility study. *Radiology* 2003; **226**: 717–722.

104. Kwong RY, Schussheim AE, Rekhraj S *et al*. Detecting acute coronary syndrome in the emergency department with cardiac magnetic resonance imaging. *Circulation* 2003; **107**: 531–537.

105. Moon JC, de Arenaza DP, Elkington AG *et al*. The pathologic basis of Q-wave and non-Q-wave myocardial infarction: A cardiovascular magnetic resonance study. *J Am Coll Cardiol* 2004; **44**: 554–560.

106. Finn AV, Antman EM. Images in clinical medicine: Isolated right ventricular infarction. *N Engl J Med* 2003; **349**: 1636.

107. Wagner A, Mahrholdt H, Holly TA *et al*. Contrast enhanced MRI and routine single photon emission computed tomography (SPECT) perfusion imaging for detection of subendocardial myocardial infarcts: An imaging study. *Lancet* 2003; **361**: 374–379.

108. Choi KM, Kim RJ, Gubernikoff G *et al*. Transmural extent of acute myocardial infarction predicts long term improvement in contractile function. *Circulation* 2001; **104**: 1101–1107.

109. Mahrholdt H, Wagner A, Holly TA *et al*. Reproducibility of chronic infarct size measurement by contrast enhanced magnetic resonance imaging. *Circulation* 2002; **106**: 2322–2327.

110. Garcia-Dorado D, Oliveras J, Gili J *et al*. Analysis of myocardial edema by magnetic resonance imaging early after coronary artery occlusion with or without reperfusion. *Cardiovasc Res* 1993; **27**: 1462–1469.

111. Abdel-Aty H, Zagrosek A, Schulz-Menger J *et al*. Delayed enhancement and T2-weighted cardiovascular magnetic resonance imaging differentiate acute from chronic myocardial infarction. *Circulation* 2004; **109**: 2411–2416.

112. Bellenger NG, Rajappan K, Rahman SL *et al*. Effects of carvedilol on left ventricular remodeling in chronic stable heart failure: A cardiovascular magnetic resonance study. *Heart* 2004; **90**: 760–764.

113. Schulman SP, Weiss JL, Becker LC *et al*. Effect of early enalapril therapy on left ventricular function and structure in acute myocardial infarction. *Am J Cardiol* 1995; **76**: 764–70.

114. Foster RE, Johnson DB, Barilla F *et al*. Changes in left ventricular mass and volumes in patients receiving angiotensin-converting enzyme inhibitor therapy for left ventricular dysfunction after Q-wave myocardial infarction. *Am Heart J* 1998; **136**: 269–75.

115. Sakuma H, Koskenvuo JW, Niemi P *et al*. Assessment of coronary flow reserve using fast velocity encoded cine MR imaging: Validation study using positron emission tomography. *Am J Roentgenol* 2000; **165**: 1029–1033.

116. Clarke GD, Eckels R, Chaney C *et al*. Measurements of absolute epicardial coronary artery flow and flow reserve with breath-hold cine phase-contrast magnetic resonance imaging. *Circulation* 1995; **91**: 2627–2634.

117. Sakuma H, Saeed M, Takeda K *et al*. Quantification of coronary artery volume flow rate using fast velocity encoded cine MR imaging. *Am J Roentgenol* 1997; **168**: 1363–1367.

118. Nagel E, Thouet T, Klein C *et al*. Non-invasive determination of coronary blood flow velocity with cardiovascular magnetic resonance in patients after stent deployment. *Circulation* 2003; **107**: 1738–1743.

119. Al-Saadi N, Nagel E, Gross M *et al*. Non-invasive detection of myocardial ischemia from perfusion reserve based on cardiovascular magnetic resonance. *Circulation* 2000; **101**: 1379–1383.

120. Nagel E, Klein C, Paetsch I *et al*. Magnetic resonance perfusion measurements for the non-invasive detection of coronary artery disease. *Circulation* 2003; **108**: 432–437.

121. Al-Saadi N, Nagel E, Gross M *et al*. Improvement of myocardial perfusion reserve early after coronary intervention: Assessment with cardiac magnetic resonance imaging. *J Am Coll Cardiol* 2000; **36**: 1557–1564.

122. Lauerma K, Virtanen KS, Sipila L *et al*. Multislice MRI assessment of myocardial perfusion in patients with single-vessel proximal left anterior descending

coronary artery disease before and after revascularization. *Circulation* 1997; **96**: 2859–2867.

123. Rehwald WG, Fieno DS, Chen EL *et al.* Myocardial magnetic resonance imaging contrast agent concentrations after reversible and irreversible ischemic injury. *Circulation* 2002; **105**: 224–229.

124. Ingkanisorn WP, Rhoads KL, Aletras AH *et al.* Gadolinium delayed enhancement cardiovascular magnetic resonance correlates with clinical measures of myocardial infarction. *J Am Coll Cardiol* 2004; **43**: 2253–2259.

125. Steuer J, Bjerner T, Duvernoy O *et al.* Visualisation and quantification of perioperative myocardial infarction after coronary artery bypass surgery with contrast enhanced magnetic resonance imaging. *Eur Heart J* 2004; **25**: 1293–1299.

126. Ricciardi JM, Wu E, Davidson CJ *et al.* Visualization of discrete micro-infarction after percutaneous coronary intervention associated with mild creatine kinase-MB elevation. *Circulation* 2001; **103**: 2780–2783.

127. Gallegos RP, Swingen C, Xu XJ *et al.* Infarct extent by MRI correlates with peak serum troponin level in the canine model. *J Surg Res* 2004; **120**: 266–271.

128. Kim RJ, Wu E, Rafael A *et al.* The use of contrast enhanced magnetic resonance imaging to identify reversible myocardial dysfunction. *N Engl J Med* 2000; **343**: 1445–1453.

129. Weiss CR, Aletras AH, London JF *et al.* Stunned, infarcted, and normal myocardium in dogs: Simultaneous differentiation by using gadolinium enhanced cine MR imaging with magnetization transfer contrast. *Radiology* 2003; **226**: 723–730.

130. Wassmuth R, Erdbruegger U, Leritzsch S *et al.* Magnetic resonance imaging for monitoring cardiac function and tissue characterization in anthracyclines therapy. *Circulation* 2000; **102**: 809–810.

131. McCrohon JA, Moon JC, Prasad SK *et al.* Differentiation of heart failure related to dilated cardiomyopathy and coronary artery disease using gadolinium enhanced cardiovascular magnetic resonance. *Circulation* 2003; **108**: 54–59.

132. Manning WJ, Li W, Edelman RR. A preliminary report comparing magnetic resonance coronary angiography with conventional angiography. *N Engl J Med* 1993; **328**: 828–832.

133. Post JC, van Rossum AC, Hofman MB *et al.* Three-dimensional respiratory-gated MR angiography of coronary arteries: Comparison with conventional coronary angiography. *Am J Roentgenol* 1996; **166**: 1399–1404.

134. Van Geuns RJ, Wielopolski PA, de Bruin HG *et al.* MR coronary angiography with breath-hold targeted volumes: Preliminary clinical results. *Radiology* 2000; **217**: 270–277.

135. Huber A, Nikolaou K, Gonschior P *et al.* Navigator echo-based respiratory gating for three-dimensional MR coronary angiography: Results from healthy volunteers and patients with proximal coronary artery stenoses. *Am J Roentgenol* 1999; **173**: 95–101.

136. Kim WY, Danias PG, Stuber M *et al.* Coronary magnetic resonance angiography for the detection of coronary stenoses. *N Engl J Med* 2001; **345**: 1863–1869.

137. Langerak SE, Vliegen HW, de Roos A *et al.* Detection of vein graft disease using high resolution magnetic resonance angiography. *Circulation* 2002; **105**: 328–333.

138. Stuber M, Botnar RM, Kissinger KV *et al.* Free-breathing black blood coronary MR angiography: Initial results. *Radiology* 2001; **219**: 278–283.

139. Stuber M, Botnar RM, Spuentrup E *et al.* Three-dimensional high resolution fast spin-echo coronary magnetic resonance angiography. *Magn Reson Med* 2001; **45**: 206–211.

140. Fayad ZA, Fuster V, Fallon JT *et al.* Non-invasive *in vivo* human coronary artery lumen and wall imaging using black blood magnetic resonance imaging. *Circulation* 2000; **102**: 506–510.

141. Sodickson DK, Manning WJ. Simultaneous acquisition of spatial harmonics (SMASH)—fast imaging with radio-frequency coil arrays. *Magn Reson Med* 1997; **38**: 591–603.

142. Pruessmann KP, Weiger M, Scheidegger MB *et al.* SENSE: Sensitivity encoding for fast MRI. *Magn Reson Med* 1999; **42**: 952–962.

143. Stuber M, Botnar RM, Danias PG *et al.* Contrast agent-enhanced, free-breathing, three-dimensional coronary magnetic resonance angiography. *J Magn Reson Imag* 1999; **10**: 790–799.

144. Li D, Dolan B, Walovitch RC *et al.* Three-dimensional MR imaging of coronary arteries using an intravascular contrast agent. *Magn Reson Med* 1998; **39**: 1014–1018.

145. Stuber M, Botnar RM, Fischer SE *et al.* Preliminary report on *in vivo* coronary MRA at 3 Tesla in humans. *Magn Reson Med* 2002; **48**: 425–429.

146. Nayak KS, Cunningham CH, Santos JM *et al.* Real time cardiac MRI at 3 Tesla. *Magn Reson Med* 2004; **51**: 655–660.

147. Peters DC, Korosec FR, Grist TM *et al.* Undersampled projection reconstruction applied to MR angiography. *Magn Reson Med* 2000; **43**: 91–101.

148. Larson AC, Simonetti OP, Li D. Coronary MRA with 3D undersampled projection reconstruction TrueFISP. *Magn Reson Med* 2002; **48**: 594–601.

149. Bornert P, Stuber M, Botnar RM *et al.* Direct comparison of 3D spiral vs Cartesian gradient-echo coronary magnetic resonance angiography. *Magn Reson Med* 2001; **46**: 789–794.

150. Taylor AM, Keegan J, Jhooti P *et al.* A comparison between segmented k-space FLASH and interleaved

spiral MR coronary angiography sequences. *J Magn Reson Imaging* 2000; **11**: 394–400.

151. Taylor AM, Thorne SA, Rubens MB *et al*. Coronary artery imaging in grown up congenital heart disease: Complementary role of magnetic resonance and x-ray coronary angiography. *Circulation* 2000; **101**: 1670–1678.

152. McConnell MV, Ganz P, Selwyn AP *et al*. Identification of anomalous coronary arteries and their anatomic course by magnetic resonance coronary angiography. *Circulation* 1995; **92**: 3158–3162.

153. Post JC, van Rossum AC, Bronzwaer JG *et al*. Magnetic resonance angiography of anomalous coronary arteries: A new gold standard for delineating the proximal course? *Circulation* 1995; **92**: 3163–3171.

154. Drory Y, Turetz Y, Hiss Y *et al*. Sudden unexpected death in persons less than 40 years of age. *Am J Cardiol* 1991; **68**: 1388–1392.

155. Kasper EK, Agema WR, Hutchins GM *et al*. The causes of dilated cardiomyopathy: A clinicopathologic review of 673 consecutive patients. *J Am Coll Cardiol* 1994; **23**: 586–590.

156. Liu PP, Mason JW. Advances in the understanding of myocarditis. *Circulation* 2001; **104**: 1076–1082.

157. Laissy JP, Messin B, Varenne O *et al*. MRI of acute myocarditis: A comprehensive approach based on various imaging sequences. *Chest* 2002; **22**: 1638–1648.

158. Friedrich MG, Strohm O, Schulz-Menger J *et al*. Contrast media-enhanced magnetic resonance imaging visualizes myocardial changes in the course of viral myocarditis. *Circulation* 1998; **97**: 1802–1809.

159. Yasuda T, Palacios IF, Dec GW *et al*. Indium 111-monoclonal antimyosin antibody imaging in the diagnosis of acute myocarditis. *Circulation* 1987; **76**: 306–311.

160. Morguet AJ, Munz DL, Kreuzer H *et al*. Scintigraphic detection of inflammatory heart disease. *Eur J Nucl Med* 1994; **21**: 666–674.

161. Davis MJ, Ward DE. How can myocarditis be diagnosed and should it be treated? *Br Heart J* 1992; **68**: 346–347.

162. Mason JW, O'Connell JB, Herskowitz A *et al*. A clinical trial of immunosuppressive therapy for myocarditis: The Myocarditis Treatment Trial Investigators. *N Engl J Med* 1995; **333**: 269–275.

163. Alpert JS, Cheitlin M. Update in cardiology: myocarditis. *Ann Intern Med* 1996; **125**: 40–46.

164. Brown CA, O'Connell JB. Implications of the Myocarditis Treatment Trial for clinical practice. *Curr Opin Cardiol* 1996; **11**: 332–336.

165. Sasse-Klaassen S, Probst S, Gerull B *et al*. Novel gene locus for autosomal dominant left ventricular non-compaction maps to chromosome 11p15. *Circulation* 2004; **109**: 2720–2723.

166. Hermida-Prieto M, Monserrat L, Castro-Beiras A *et al*. Familial dilated cardiomyopathy and isolated left ventricular non-compaction associated with lamin A/C gene mutations. *Am J Cardiol* 2004; **94**: 50–54.

167. Ichida F, Tsubata S, Bowles KR *et al*. Novel gene mutations in patients with left ventricular non-compaction or Barth syndrome. *Circulation* 2001; **103**: 1256–1263.

168. Oechslin EN, Attenhofer Jost CH, Rojas JR *et al*. Long term follow-up of 34 adults with isolated left ventricular non-compaction: A distinct cardiomyopathy with poor prognosis. *J Am Coll Cardiol* 2000; **36**: 493–500.

169. Ritter M, Oechslin E, Sutsch G *et al*. Isolated non-compaction of the myocardium in adults. *Mayo Clin Proc* 1997; **72**: 26–31.

170. Pignatelli RH, McMahon CJ, Dreyer WJ *et al*. Clinical characterization of left ventricular non-compaction in children. A relatively common form of cardiomyopathy. *Circulation* 2003; **108**: 2672–678.

171. Agmon Y, Connolly HM, Olson LJ *et al*. Non-compaction of the ventricular myocardium. *J Am Soc Echocardiogr* 1999; **12**: 859–863.

172. Chin TK, Perloff JK, Williams RG *et al*. Isolated non-compaction of left ventricular myocardium. A study of eight cases. *Circulation* 1990; **82**: 507–513.

173. Stollberger C, Finsterer J. Left ventricular hypertrabeculation/non-compaction. *J Am Soc Echocardiogr* 2004; **17**: 91–100.

174. Tamborini G, Pepi M, Celeste F *et al*. Incidence and characteristics of left ventricular false tendons and trabeculations in the normal and pathologic heart by second harmonic echocardiography. *J Am Soc Echocardiogr* 2004; **17**: 367–374.

175. Chung T, Yiannikas J, Lee LC *et al*. Isolated non-compaction involving the left ventricular apex in adults. *Am J Cardiol* 2004; **94**: 1214–1216.

176. Hamamichi Y, Ichida F, Hashimoto I *et al*. Isolated non-compaction of the ventricular myocardium: Ultrafast computed tomography and magnetic resonance imaging. *Int J Cardiovasc Imaging* 2001; **17**: 305–314.

177. Korcyk D, Edwards CC, Armstrong G *et al*. Contrast enhanced cardiac magnetic resonance in a patient with familial isolated ventricular non-compaction. *J Cardiovasc Magn Reson* 2004; **6**: 569–576.

178. Soler R, Rodriguez E, Monserrat L *et al*. MRI of subendocardial perfusion deficits in isolated left ventricular non-compaction. *J Comput Assist Tomogr* 2002; **26**: 373–375.

179. McCrohon JA, Richmond DR, Pennell DJ *et al*. Isolated non-compaction of the myocardium. A rarity or missed diagnosis? *Circulation* 2002; **106**: e22–e23.

180. Maron BJ, Bonow RO, Cannon RO *et al*. Hypertrophic cardiomyopathy: Interrelations of clinical

manifestations, pathophysiology, and therapy. *N Engl J Med* 1987; **316**: 780–789, 844–852.

181. Wigle ED, Rakowski H, Kimball BP *et al.* Hypertrophic cardiomyopathy. Clinical spectrum and treatment. *Circulation* 1995; **92**: 1680–1692.

182. Spirito P, Seidman CE, McKenna WJ *et al.* The management of hypertrophic cardiomyopathy. *N Engl J Med* 1997; **336**: 775–785.

183. Varnava AM, Elliott PM, Mahon N *et al.* Relation between myocyte disarray and outcome in hypertrophic cardiomyopathy. *Am J Cardiol* 2001: **88**: 275–279.

184. Richard P, Charron P, Carrier L *et al.* Hypertrophic cardiomyopathy. Distribution of disease genes, spectrum of mutations, and implications for a molecular diagnosis strategy. *Circulation* 2003; **107**: 2227–2232.

185. Maron BJ, Shen WK, Link MS *et al.* Efficacy of implantable cardioverter-defibrillators for the prevention of sudden death in patients with hypertrophic cardiomyopathy. *N Engl J Med* 2000; **342**: 365–373.

186. Park JH, Kim YM, Chung JW *et al.* MR imaging of hypertrophic cardiomyopathy. *Radiology* 1992; **185**: 441–446.

187. Sardanelli F, Molinari G, Petillo A *et al.* MRI in hypertrophic cardiomyopathy: A morphofunctional study. *J comput Assist Tomogr* 1993; **17**: 862–872.

188. Arrive L, Assayag P, Russ G *et al.* MRI and cine MRI of asymmetric septal hypertrophic cardiomyopathy. *J Comput Assist Tomogr* 1994; **18**: 376–382.

189. Amano Y, Takayama M, Amano M *et al.* MRI of cardiac morphology and function after percutaneous transluminal septal myocardial ablation for hypertrophic obstructive cardiomyopathy. *Am J Roentgenol* 2004; **182**: 523–527.

190. Webb JG, Sasson Z, Rakowski H *et al.* Apical hypertrophic cardiomyopathy: Clinical follow-up and diagnostic correlates. *J Am Coll Cardiol* 1990; **15**: 83–90.

191. Suzuki J, Watanabe F, Takenaka K *et al.* New subtype of apical hypertrophic cardiomyopathy identified with nuclear magnetic resonance imaging as an underlying cause of markedly inverted T waves. *J Am Coll Cardiol* 1993; **22**: 1175–1181.

192. Young AA, Kramer CM, Ferrari VA *et al.* Three-dimensional left ventricular deformation in hypertrophic cardiomyopathy. *Circulation* 1994; **90**: 854–867.

193. Sipola P, Lauerma K, Husso-Saastamoien M *et al.* First-pass MR imaging in the assessment of perfusion impairment in patients with hypertrophic cardiomyopathy and the Asp 175 Asn mutation of the alpha-tropomyosin gene. *Radiology* 2003; **226**: 129–137.

194. Choudhury L, Mahrholdt H, Wagner A *et al.* Myocardial scarring in asymptomatic or mildly symptomatic patients with hypertrophic cardiomyopathy. *J Am Coll Cardiol* 2002; **40**: 2156–2164.

195. Basso C, Thiene G, Corrado D *et al.* Hypertrophic cardiomyopathy and sudden death in the young: Pathologic evidence of myocardial ischemia. *Hum Pathol* 2000; **8**: 988–998.

196. Teraoka K, Hirano M, Ookubo H *et al.* Delayed contrast enhancement of MRI in hypertrophic cardiomyopathy. *Magn Reson Imaging* 2004; **2**: 155–161.

197. Tiso N, Stephan DA, Nava A *et al.* Identification of mutations in the cardiac ryanodine receptor gene in families affected with arrhythmogenic right ventricular cardiomyopathy type 2 (ARVD2). *Hum Mol Genet* 2001; **10**: 189–194.

198. Rampazzo A, Nava A, Malacrida S *et al.* Mutation in human desmoplakin domain binding to plakoglobin causes a dominant form of arrhythmogenic right ventricular cardiomyopathy. *Am J Hum Genet* 2002; **71**: 1200–1206.

199. Thiene G, Nava A, Corrado D *et al.* Right ventricular cardiomyopathy and sudden death in young people. *N Engl J Med* 1988; **318**: 129–133.

200. Fontaine G, Fontaliran F, Frank R. Arrhythmogenic right ventricular cardiomyopathies: Clinical forms and main differential diagnoses. *Circulation* 1998; **97**: 1532–1535.

201. Richardson P, McKenna W, Bristow M *et al.* Report of the 1995 World Health Organization/International Society and Federation of Cardiology Task Force on the Definition and Classification of cardiomyopathies. *Circulation* 1996; **93**: 841–842.

202. Basso C, Thiene G, Corrado D *et al.* Arrhythmogenic right ventricular cardiomyopathy: Dysplasia, dystrophy, or myocarditis? *Circulation* 1996; **94**: 983–991.

203. Burke AP, Farb A, Tashko G *et al.* Arrhythmogenic right ventricular cardiomyopathy and fatty replacement of the right ventricular myocardium: Are they different diseases? *Circulation* 1998; **97**: 1571–1580.

204. Carlson MD, White RD, Trohman RG *et al.* Right ventricular outflow tract ventricular tachycardia: Detection of previously unrecognized anatomic abnormalities using cine-magnetic resonance imaging. *J Am Coll Cardiol* 1994; **24**: 720–727.

205. Proclemer A, Basadonna PT, Slavich GA *et al.* Cardiac magnetic resonance imaging findings in patients with right ventricular outflow tract premature contractions. *Eur Heart J* 1997; **18**: 2002–2010.

206. Castillo E, Tandri H, Rene Rodriguez ER *et al.* Arrhythmogenic right ventricular dysplasia: *ex vivo* and *in vivo* fat detection with black blood MR imaging. *Radiology* 2004; **232**: 38–48.

207. Auffermann W, Wichter T, Breithardt G *et al.* Arrhythmogenic right ventricular disease: MR imaging vs angiography. *Am J Roentgenol* 1993; **161**: 549–555.

208. Appleton CP, Hatle LK, Popp RL. Relation of transmitral flow velocity patterns to left ventricular diastolic function: New insights from a combined hemodynamic and Doppler echocardiographic study. *J Am Coll Cardiol* 1988; **12**: 426–440.

209. Kayser H, Schalij M, van der Wall E *et al.* Biventricular function in patients with non-ischemic right ventricular tachyarrhythmias assessed with MR imaging. *Am J Roentgenol* 1997; **159**: 995–999.

210. Talreja DR, Edwards WD, Danielson GK *et al.* Constrictive pericarditis in 26 patients with histologically normal pericardial thickness. *Circulation* 2003; **108**: 1852–1857.

211. Masui T, Finck S, Higgins CB. Constrictive pericarditis and restrictive cardiomyopathy: Evaluation with MR imaging. *Radiology* 1992; **182**: 369–373.

212. Fattori R, Rocchi G, Celletti F *et al.* Contribution of magnetic resonance imaging in the differential diagnosis of cardiac amyloidosis and symmetric hypertrophic cardiomyopathy. *Heart J* 1998; **136**: 824–830.

213. Mana J. Nuclear imaging: Gallium-67, 201 thallium, ^{18}F- labeled fluoro-2 deoxy-D glucose position emission tomography. *Clin Chest Med* 1997; **18**: 799–811.

214. Kinney E, Caldwell J. Do thallium myocardial perfusion scan abnormalities predict survival in sarcoid patients without cardiac symptoms? *Angiology* 1990: **41**: 573–576.

215. Uemura A, Morimoto S, Hiramitsu S *et al.* Histologic diagnostic rate of cardiac sarcoidosis: Evaluation of endocardial biopsies. *Am Heart J* 1999; **138**: 299–302.

216. Chandra M, Silverman ME, Oshinski J *et al.* Diagnosis of cardiac sarcoidosis aided by MRI. *Chest* 1996; **110**: 562–565.

217. Matsuki M, Matsuo M. MR findings of myocardial sarcoidosis. *Clin Radiol* 2000; **55**: 323–325.

218. Serra JJ, Monte GU, Mello ES *et al.* Cardiac sarcoidosis evaluated by delayed enhanced magnetic resonance imaging. *Circulation* 2003; **107**: e188–e189.

219. Nemeth MA, Muthupillai R, Wilson JM *et al.* Cardiac sarcoidosis detected by delayed hyperenhancement magnetic resonance imaging. *Tex Heart Inst J* 2004; **31**: 99–102.

220. Vignaux O, Dhote R, Duboc D *et al.* Clinical significance of myocardial magnetic resonance abnormalities in patients with sarcoidosis: A 1-year follow-up study. *Chest* 2002; **122**: 1895–1901.

221. Shimida J, Shimida K, Sakane T *et al.* Diagnosis of sarcoidosis and evaluation of the effects of steroid therapy by gadolinium-DTPA enhanced magnetic resonance imaging. *Am J Med* 2001; **110**: 525–527.

222. Paz H, McCormick D, Kutalek S *et al.* The automatic implantable defibrillator prophylaxis in cardiac sarcoidosis. *Chest* 1994; **106**: 1603–1607.

223. Smith SC Jr, Dove JT, Jacobs AK *et al.* ACC/AHA guidelines for percutaneous coronary intervention —executive summary: A report of the American College of Cardiology/American Heart Association task force on practice guidelines (committee to revise the 1993 guidelines for percutaneous transluminal angioplasty) endorsed by the Society for Cardiac Angiography and Interventions. *Circulation* 2001; **103**: 3019–3041.

224. Isjkander S, Iskandrian AE. Risk assessment using single-photon emission computed tomographic technetium-99m sestamibi imaging. *J Am Coll Cardiol* 1998; **32**: 57–62.

225. Ladenheim ML, Pollock BH, Rozanski A *et al.* Extent and severity of myocardial hypoperfusion as predictors of prognosis in patients with suspected coronary artery disease. *J Am Coll Cardiol* 1986; **7**: 464–471.

226. Hendel RC, Berman DS, Cullom SJ *et al.* Multicenter clinical trial to evaluate the efficacy of correction for photon attenuation and scatter in SPECT myocardial perfusion imaging. *Circulation* 1999; **99**: 2742–2749.

227. Taillefer R, De Duey EG, Udelson JE *et al.* Comparative diagnostic accuracy of Tl-201 and Tc-99m sestamibi SPECT imaging (perfusion and ECG-gated SPECT) in detecting coronary artery disease in women. *J Am Coll Cardiol* 1997; **29**: 69–77.

228. Gould KL, Kirkeeide RL, Buchi M. Coronary flow reserve as a physiological measure of stenosis severity. *J AM Coll Cardiol* 1990; **15**: 459–474.

229. Ellis S, Alderman EL, Cain K *et al.* Morphology of left anterior descending coronary territory lesions favoring acute occlusion and myocardial infarction: A quantitative angiographic study. *J Am Coll Cardiol* 1989; **13**: 1481–1491.

230. Ellis S, Alderman EL, Cain K *et al.* Prediction of risk of anterior myocardial infarction by lesion severity and measurement method of stenoses in the left anterior descending coronary distribution: A CASS registry study. *J Am Coll Cardiol* 1988; **11**: 908–916.

231. Kim RJ, Feino DS, Parish TB *et al.* Relationship of MRI delayed contrast enhancement to irreversible injury, infarct age, and contractile function. *Circulation* 1999; **100**: 1992–2002.

232. Werns SW, Walton JA, Hsia HH *et al.* Evidence of endothelial dysfunction in angiographically normal coronary arteries of patients with coronary artery disease. *Circulation* 1989; **79**: 287–291.

233. Uren NG, Melin JA, De Bruyne B *et al.* Relation between myocardial blood flow and the severity of coronary artery stenosis. *N Engl J Med* 1994; **330**: 1782–1788.

234. Sambuceti G, Parodi O, Marcassa C *et al.* Alterations in regulation of myocardial blood flow in one-vessel coronary artery disease determined by positron emission tomography. *Am J Cardiol* 1993; **72**: 538–543.

235. Di Carli M, Czernin J, Hoh CK *et al.* Relation among stenosis severity, myocardial blood flow, and flow reserve in patients with coronary disease. *Circulation* 1995; **91**: 1944–1951.

236. Noeske R, Seifert F, Rhein KH *et al.* Human cardiac imaging at 3 Tesla using phased array coils. *Magn. Reson. Med.* 2000; **44**: 978–982.

237. Schwitter J, Nanz D, Kneifel S *et al.* Assessment of myocardial perfusion in coronary artery disease by magnetic resonance: A comparison with positron emission tomography and coronary angiography. *Circulation* 2001; **103**: 2230–2235.

238. Walsh EG, Doyle M, Lawson MA *et al.* Multislice first-pass myocardial perfusion imaging on a conventional clinical scanner. *Magn Reson Med* 1995; **34**: 39–47.

239. Hartnell G, Cerel A, Kamalesh M *et al.* Detection of myocardial ischemia: Value of combined myocardial perfusion and cine-angiographic MR imaging. *Am J Roentgenol* 1994; **163**: 1061–1067.

240. Saeed M, Wendland MF, Sakuma H *et al.* Coronary artery stenosis: Detection with contrast enhanced MR imaging in dogs. *Radiology* 1995; **196**: 79–84.

241. Schwitter J, Saeed M, Wendland MF *et al.* Assessment of myocardial function and perfusion in a canine model of non-occlusive coronary artery stenosis using fast magnetic resonance imaging. *J Magn Reson Imaging* 1998; **9**: 101–110.

242. Keijer JT, van Rossum AC, van Eenige MJ *et al.* Magnetic resonance imaging of regional myocardial perfusion in patients with single vessel coronary disease: Quantitative comparison with 201 thallium-SPECT and coronary angiography. *Am Heart J* 1995; **130**: –93-901.

243. Panting JR, Gatehouse PD, Yang GZ *et al.* Abnormal subendocardial perfusion in cardiac syndrome X detected by cardiovascular magnetic resonance imaging. *N Engl J Med* 2002; **346**: 1948–1953.

244. Eichenberger AC, Schuiki E, Kochli VD *et al.* Ischemic heart disease: Assessment with gadolinium enhanced ultrafast MR imaging and dipyridamole stress. *J Magn Reson Imaging* 1994; **4**: 425–431.

245. Bertschinger KM, Nanz D, Buechi M *et al.* Magnetic resonance myocardial first-pass perfusion imaging: Parameter optimization for signal response and cardiac coverage. *J Magn Reson Imaging* 2001; **14**: 556–62.

246. Wilke N, Simm C, Zhang J *et al.* Contrast enhanced first-pass myocardial perfusion imaging: Correlation between myocardial blood flow in dogs at rest and during hyperemia. *Magn Reson Med* 1993; **29**: 485–497.

247. Lombardi M, Jones RA, Westby J *et al.* Use of the mean transit time of an intravascular contrast agent as an exchange-insensitive index of myocardial perfusion. *J Magn Reson Imaging* 1999; **9**: 402–408.

248. Klocke FJ, Simonetti OP, Judd RM *et al.* Limits of detection of regional differences in vasodilated flow in viable myocardium by first-pass magnetic resonance perfusion imaging. *Circulation* 2001; **104**: 2412–2416.

249. Holland AE, Goldfarb JW, Edelman RR. Diaphragmatic and cardiac motion during suspended breathing: Preliminary experience and implications for breath-hold MR imaging. *Radiology* 1998; **209**: 483–489.

250. McConnell MV, Khasgiwala VC, Savord BJ *et al.* Prospective adaptive navigator correction for breath-hold MR coronary angiography. *Magn Reson Med* 1997; **37**: 148–152.

251. Chuang ML, Chen MH, Khasgiwala VC *et al.* Adaptive correction of imaging plane position in segmented k-space cine cardiac MRI. *J Magn Reson Imaging* 1997; **7**: 811–814.

252. Manning WJ, Atkinson DJ, Grossman W *et al.* First-pass nuclear magnetic resonance imaging studies using gadolinium-DTPA in patients with coronary artery disease. *J Am Coll Cardiol* 1991; **18**: 959–965.

253. Matheijssen NA, Louwerenburg HW, van Rugge F *et al.* Comparison of ultrafast dipyridamole magnetic resonance imaging with dipyridamole sestamibi SPECT for detection of perfusion abnormalities in patients with one-vessel disease: Assessment by quantitative model fitting. *Magn Reson Med* 1996; **35**: 221–228.

254. Larsson HB, Fritz Hansen T, Rostrup E *et al.* Myocardial perfusion modeling using MRI. *Magn Reson Med* 1996; **35**: 716–726.

255. Muhling OM, Dickson ME, Zenovich A *et al.* Quantitative magnetic resonance first-pass perfusion analysis: Inter and intra-observer agreement. *J Cardiovasc Magn Reson* 2001; **3**: 247–256.

256. Wilke N, Jerosch HM, Wang Y *et al.* Myocardial perfusion reserve: Assessment with multisection, quantitative, first-pass MR imaging. *Radiology* 1997; **204**: 373–384.

257. Slavin GS, Wolff SD, Gupta SN *et al.* First-pass myocardial perfusion MR imaging with interleaved notched saturation: Feasibility study. *Radiology* 2001; **219**: 258–263.

258. Sakuma H, O'Sullivan M, Lucas J *et al.* Effect of magnetic susceptibility contrast medium on myocardial signal intensity with fast gradient-recalled echo and spin-echo MR imaging: Initial experience in humans. *Radiology* 1994; **190**: 161–166.

259. Panting JR, Taylor AM, Gatehouse PD *et al.* First-pass myocardial perfusion imaging and equilibrium signal changes using the intravascular contrast agent NC 100150 injection. *J Magn Reson Imaging* 1999; **10**: 404–410.

260. Ding S, Wolff SD, Epstein FH. Improved coverage in dynamic contrast enhanced cardiac MRI using interleaved gradient-echo EPI. *Magn Reson Med* 1998; **39**: 514–519.

261. Cullen JH, Horsfield MA, Reek CR *et al*. A myocardial perfusion reserve index in humans using first-pass contrast enhanced magnetic resonance imaging. *J Am Coll Cardiol* 1999; **33**: 1386–1394.

262. Weiger M, Pruessmann KP, Boesiger P. Cardiac real time imaging using SENSE. Sensitivity encoding scheme. *Magn Reson Med* 2000; **43**: 177–184.

263. Gheorghiade M, Bonow RO. Chronic heart failure in the United States: a manifestation of coronary artery disease. *Circulation* 1998; **97**: 282–9.

264. Hammermeister KE, DeRouen TA, Dodge HT. Variables predictive of survival in patients with coronary artery disease. Selection by univariate and multivariate analyses from the clinical, electrocardiographic, exercise, arteriographic, and quantitative angiographic evaluations. *Circulation* 1979; **59**: 421–30.

265. Harris PJ, Harell FE, Lee KL *et al*. Survival in medically treated coronary artery disease. *Circulation* 1979; **60**: 1259–1269.

266. Mock MB, Ringqvist I, Fisher LD *et al*. Survival of medically treated patients in the Coronary Artery Surgery Study (CASS) registry. *Circulation* 1982; **66**: 562–568.

267. Rees G, Bristow JD, Kremkau EL *et al*. Influence of aortocoronary bypass surgery on left ventricular performance. *N Engl J Med* 1971; **284**: 1116–1120.

268. Chatterjee K, Swan HJ, Parmley WW *et al*. Influence of direct myocardial revascularization on left ventricular asynergy and function in patients with coronary heart disease: With and without previous myocardial infarction. *Circulation* 1973; **47**: 276–286.

269. Horn HR, Teichholz LE, Cohn PF *et al*. Augmentation of left ventricular contraction pattern in coronary artery disease by an inotropic catecholamine: The epinephrine ventriculogram. *Circulation* 1974; **49**: 1063–1071.

270. Cohn PF, Gorlin R, Herman MV *et al*. Relation between contractile reserve and prognosis in patients with coronary artery disease and a depressed ejection fraction. *Circulation* 1975; **51**: 414–420.

271. Diamond GA, Forrester JS, de Luz PL *et al*. Postextrasystolic potentiation of ischemic myocardium by atrial stimulation. *Am Heart J* 1978; **95**: 204–209.

272. Rahimtoola SH. The hibernating myocardium. *Am Heart J* 1989; **117**: 211–221.

273. Heyndrickx GR, Millard RW, McRitchie RJ *et al*. Regional myocardial functional and electrophysiological alterations after brief coronary artery occlusion in conscious dogs. *J Clin Invest* 1975; **56**: 978–985.

274. Braunwald E, Kloner RA. The stunned myocardium: Prolonged, postischemic ventricular dysfunction. *Circulation* 1982; **66**: 1146–1149.

275. Kloner RA, Bolli R, Marban E *et al*. Medical and cellular implications of stunning, hibernation and preconditioning: An NHLBI workshop. *Circulation* 1998; **97**: 1848–1867.

276. Bolli R. Mechanism of myocardial stunning. *Physiol Rev* 1999; **79**: 609–634.

277. Kusuoka H, Marban E. Cellular mechanisms of myocardial stunning. *Annu Rev Physiol* 1992; **54**: 243–256.

278. Anselmi M, Golia G, Cicoira M *et al*. Prognostic value of detection of myocardial viability using low dose dobutamine echocardiography in infarcted patients. *Am J Cardiol* 1998; **81**: 21G–28G.

279. Picano E, Sicari R, Landi P *et al*. Prognostic value of myocardial viability in medically treated patients with global left ventricular dysfunction early after an uncomplicated myocardial infarction: A dobutamine stress echocardiography study. *Circulation* 1998; **98**: 1078–84.

280. Previtali M, Fetiveau R, Lanzarini L *et al*. Prognostic value of myocardial viability and ischemia detected by dobutamine stress echocardiography early after myocardial infarction treated with thrombolysis. *J Am Coll Cardiol* 1998; **32**: 380–386.

281. Allman KC, Shaw LJ, Hachamovitch R *et al*. Myocardial viability testing and impact of revascularization on prognosis in patients with coronary artery disease and left ventricular dysfunction: A meta-analysis. *J Am Coll Cardiol* 2002; **39**: 1151–1158.

282. Schwarz ER, Schaper J, von Dahl J *et al*. Myocyte degeneration and cell death in hibernating human myocardium. *J Am Coll Cardiol* 1996; **27**: 1577–1585.

283. Nagel E, Lehmkuhl HB, Bocksch W *et al*. Non-invasive diagnosis of ischemia-induced wall motion abnormalities with the use of high dose dobutamine stress MRI: Comparison with dobutamine stress echocardiography. *Circulation* 1999; **99**: 763–770.

284. Hoffman R, Lethen H, Marwick T *et al*. Analysis of interinstitutional observer agreement in interpretation of dobutamine stress echocardiograms. *J Am Coll Cardiol* 1996; **27**: 330–336.

285. Dubnow MH, Burchell HB, Titus JL. Postinfarction ventricular aneurysm. A clinicomorphologic and electrocardiographic study of 80 cases. *Am Heart J* 1965; **70**: 753–760.

286. Baer FM, Smolarz K, Jungehulsing M *et al*. Chronic myocardial infarction: Assessment of morphology, function, and perfusion by gradient echo magnetic resonance imaging and 99m Tc-methoxy-isobutyl-isonitrile SPECT. *Am heart J* 1992; **123**: 636–645.

287. Baer FM, Voth E, Schneider CA *et al*. Comparison of low-dose dobutamine-gradient-echo magnetic resonance imaging and positron emission tomography with [^{18}F] fluorodeoxyglucose in patients with chronic coronary artery disease. A functional and morphological approach to the detection of residual myocardial viability. *Circulation* 1995; **91**: 1006–1015.

288. Dendale P, Franken PR, Waldman GJ *et al.* Low dosage dobutamine magnetic resonance imaging as an alternative to echocardiography in the detection of viable myocardium after acute infarction. *Am Heart J* 1995; **130**: 134–140.

289. Sandstede JJ, Bertsch G, Beer M. Detection of myocardial viability by low dose dobutamine cine MR imaging. *Magn Reson Imaging* 1999; **17**: 1437–1443.

290. Dendale P, Franken PR, Block P *et al.* Contrast enhanced and functional magnetic resonance imaging for the detection of viable myocardium after infarction. *Am Heart J* 1998; **135**: 875–880.

291. Baer FM, Voth E, La Rosee K *et al.* Comparison of low dose dobutamine transesophageal echocardiography and dobutamine magnetic resonance imaging for detection of residual myocardial viability. *Am J Cardiol* 1996; **78**: 415–419.

292. Zoghbi WA, Barasch E. Dobutamine MRI: A serious contender in pharmacological stress imaging? *Circulation* 1999; **99**: 730–732.

293. Beller GA. Comparison of ²⁰¹Tl scintigraphy and low dose dobutamine echocardiography for the noninvasive assessment of myocardial viability. *Circulation* 1996; **94**: 2681–2684.

294. Bonow RO. Identification of viable myocardium. *Circulation* 1996; **94**: 2674–2680.

295. Perone-Filardi P, Pace L, Prastaro M *et al.* Assessment of myocardial viability in patients with chronic coronary artery disease. Rest-4-hour-24-hour 201 T₁ tomography versus dobutamine echocardiography. *Circulation* 1996; **94**: 2712–2719.

296. Ausma J, Schaart G, Thone F *et al.* Chronic ischemic viable myocardium in man: Aspects of dedifferentiation. *Cardiovasc Pathol* 1995; **4**: 29–37.

297. De Roos A, Doornbos J, van der Wall E *et al.* MR imaging of acute myocardial infarction: Value of Gd-DTPA. *Am J Roentgenol* 1998; **150**: –31-534.

298. De Roos A, van Rossum AC, van der Wall E *et al.* Reperfused and non-reperfused myocardial infarction: Diagnostic potential of Gd-DTPA enhanced MR imaging. *Radiology* 1989; **172**: 717–20.

299. Yokota C, Nonogi H, Miyazaki S *et al.* Gadolinium enhanced magnetic resonance imaging in acute myocardial infarction. *Am J Cardiol* 1995; **75**: 577–581.

300. Edelman RR, Wallner B, Singer A *et al.* Segmented turbo-FLASH: Method for breath-hold MR imaging of the liver with flexible contrast. *Radiology* 1990; **177**: 515–521.

301. Simonetti OP, Kim RJ, Fieno DS *et al.* An improved MR imaging technique for the visualization of myocardial infarction. *Radiology* 2001; **218**: 215–223.

302. Eichstaedt HW, Felix R, Danne O *et al.* Imaging of acute myocardial infarction by magnetic resonance tomography (MRT) using the paramagnetic relaxation substance gadolinium-DTPA. *Cardiovasc Drugs Ther* 1989; **3**: 779–788.

303. Lima JA, Judd RM, Bazille A *et al.* Regional heterogeneity of human myocardial infarcts demonstrated by contrast enhanced MRI. Potential mechanisms. *Circulation* 1995; **92**: 1117–1125.

304. Van Rossum AC, Visser FC, van Eenige MJ *et al.* Value of gadolinium-diethylene-triamine pentaacetic acid dynamics in magnetic resonance imaging of acute myocardial infarction with occluded and reperfused coronary arteries after thrombolysis. *Am J Cardiol* 1990; **65**: 845–851.

305. Wu E, Judd RM, Vargas JD *et al.* Visualization of presence, location, and transmural extent of healed Q-wave and non-Q wave myocardial infarction. *Lancet* 2001; **357**: 21–28.

306. Jennings RB, Schaper J, Hill ML *et al.* Effect of reperfusion late in the phase of reversible ischemic injury. Changes in cell volume, electrolytes, metabolites and ultrastructure. *Circ Res* 1985; **56**: 262–278.

307. Whalen DA, Hamilton DG, Ganote CE *et al.* Effect of a transient period of ischemia on myocardial cells. I. Effects on cell volume regulation. *Am J Pathol* 1974; **74**: 381–397.

308. Koenig SH, Spiller M, Brown RD 3ʳᵈ *et al.* Relaxation of water protons in the intra and extracellular regions of blood containing Gd (DTPA). *Magn Reson Med* 1986; **3**: 791–795.

309. Rochitte CE, Lima JA, Bluemke DA *et al.* Magnitude and time course of microvascular obstruction and tissue injury after acute myocardial infarction. *Circulation* 1998; **98**: 1000–1114.

310. Judd RM, Lugo-Olivieri CH, Arai M *et al.* Physiological basis of myocardial contrast enhancement in fast magnetic resonance images of two-day-old reperfused canine infarcts. *Circulation* 1995; **92**: 1902–1910.

311. Hillenbrand HB, Kim RJ, Parker MA *et al.* Early assessment of myocardial salvage by contrast enhanced magnetic resonance imaging. *Circulation* 2000; **102**: 1678–1683.

312. Lieberman AN, Weiss JL, Jugdutt BI *et al.* Two-dimensional echocardiogarphy and infarct size: Relationship of regional wall motion and thickening to the extent of myocardial infarction in the dog. *Circulation* 1981; **63**: 739–46.

313. Force T, Kemper A, Perkins L *et al.* Overestimation of infarct size by quantitative two-dimensional echocardiography: The role of tethering and of analytic procedures. *Circulation* 1986; **73**: 1360–1368.

314. Armstrong WF. "Hibernating" myocardium: Asleep or part dead? *J Am Coll Cardiol* 1996; **28**: 530–535.

315. Weiss JL, Bulkley BH, Hutchins GM *et al.* Two-dimensional echocardiographic recognition of myocardial injury in man: Comparison with postmortem studies. *Circulation* 1981; **63**: 401–408.

316. Mahrholdt H, Wagner A, Choi K *et al.* Contrast MRI detects subendocardial infarcts in regions of normal wall motion. *Circulation* 2001; **104** (Suppl 2): 341.

317. Kuikka J, Yang J, Kilainen H. Physical performance of Siemens E.Cam gamma camera. *Nucl Med Commun* 1998; **19**: 457–462.

318. Garvin AA, James J, Garcia EV. Myocardial perfusion imaging using single-photon emission computed tomography. *Am J Card Imaging* 1994; **8**: 189–198.

319. Kannel WB, Abbott RD. Incidence and prognosis of unrecognized myocardial infarction. An update on the Framingham study. *N Engl J Med* 1984; **311**: 1144–1147.

320. Sigurdsson E, Thorgeirsson, Sigvaldason H *et al.* Unrecognized myocardial infarction: Epidemiology, clinical characteristics, and the prognostic role of angina pectoris. The Reykjavik study. *Ann Intern Med* 1995; **122**: 96–102.

321. Nadelmann J, Frishman WH, Ooi WL. Prevalence, incidence and prognosis of recognized and unrecognized myocardial infarction in persons aged 75 years or older: The Bronx Aging Study. *Am J Cardiol* 1990; **66**: 533–537.

322. Kim H, Wu E, Meyers SN *et al.* Prognostic significance of unrecognized myocardial infarction detected by contrast enhanced MRI. *Circulation* 2002; **106**: 11–38.

323. Weiss RG, Bottomley PA, Hardy CJ *et al.* Regional myocardial metabolism of high energy phosphates during isometric exercise in patients with coronary artery disease. *N Engl J Med* 1990; **323**: 1593–1600.

324. Buchthal SD, den Hollander JA, Merz CN *et al.* Abnormal myocardial phosphorus-31 nuclear magnetic resonance spectroscopy in women with chest pain but normal coronary angiograms. *N Engl J Med* 2000; **23**: 829–835.

325. Johnson BD, Shaw CJ, Buchthal SD *et al.* National Institute of Health-National Heart, Lung, Blood Institute. Prognosis in women with myocardial ischemia in the absence of obstructive coronary disease: results from the National Institute of Health-National Heart, Lung, Blood Institute – sponsored Women's Ischemia Syndrome Evaluation (WISE). *Circulation* 2004; **109**: 2993–2999.

CHAPTER 8

MSCT coronary imaging

Koen Nieman

Introduction

Over recent years we have witnessed rapid technical advancement of multislice, or multidetector-row spiral computed tomography (MSCT), with current technology allowing practically motionless imaging of the heart and detailed visualization of the coronary arteries. It has been shown that MSCT can accurately detect lumenal narrowing in the coronary arteries, as well as bypass grafts, and it may develop into a clinically useful alternative to conventional angiography in selected patients. In addition, early reports indicate that MSCT may have a role in the detection and characterization of atherosclerotic material in the coronary wall.

Data acquisition and evaluation

Technology

Contrary to sequential computed tomography, which applies a step-and-shoot approach, spiral CT scanners acquire data continuously while the patient is moved through the scanner gantry. Among a number of advantages is the increased coverage speed, which has advanced the development of CT (coronary) angiography. While the first spiral CT scanners were equipped with only one row of detectors, current multislice spiral CT scanners are capable of acquiring up to 64 slices simultaneously. In addition to the expansion of the number of detector rows, the rotation time of the roentgen tube and detector system has decreased dramatically form one second down to 330 ms per rotation, which is of pivotal importance to the feasibility of cardiac CT. Finally the individual detector width has decreased to 0.5–0.625 mm to allow detailed visualization of the small coronary branches.

Acquisition protocol

The sequence of procedures in coronary MSCT is outlined in Fig. 8.1. Imaging of the coronary arteries requires contrast enhancement of the coronary vessel lumen, which is accomplished by an intravenous injection of an iodine-containing medium through a peripheral vein. Either a small test bolus is injected to determine the time interval between injection and contrast arrival at the ascending aorta, or bolus tracking is applied, in which case the entire contrast dose is injected and the scan is automatically initiated as soon as contrast enhancement is detected within the aortic root. The patient moves in a supine position through the scanner gantry while CT data is acquired continuously and the

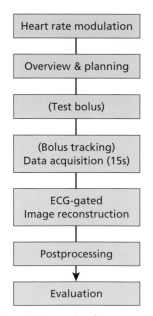

Fig. 8.1 Data acquisition protocol.

ECG is recorded. While the table advancement per rotation is more than the width of the detectors for non-gated acquisitions, the table increment is approximately a third of the total detector width in ECG-gated scans to assure availability of CT data for each position during multiple cardiac phases. The total acquisition time is 20 s or fewer for standard acquisition protocols, during which time the patient maintains an inspiratory breath-hold.

Image reconstruction

Contrary to ECG-triggered sequential scan protocols, spiral CT images are reconstructed after all data has been acquired. Isocardiophasic slices are created using CT data that was acquired during the same phase of each cardiac cycle based on the recorded ECG (Fig. 8.2). The minimal amount of data required for the reconstruction of a single image is collected during a 180 degree gantry rotation. If the rotation time is 400 ms, then the temporal resolution is 200 ms.

For motionless imaging of the coronary arteries 200 ms is still rather long, particularly in patients with a fast heart rate. Several methods can be used

to reduce the occurrence of motion related image artifacts. The most straightforward solution is acceleration of the gantry rotation speed. But since gantry acceleration is limited by mechanical constraints, additional measures are used to assure optimal image quality. When there is a fast heart rate, in relation to the table speed, each long axis, or z-position will be sampled by different detectors during two or more heart cycles. This creates the opportunity to combine isophasic data of these two cycles to reduce the effective temporal resolution. For certain favorable heart rates the acquired data during both cycles, equal to a 90 degree gantry rotation each, is entirely non-complementary, resulting in the most optimal temporal resolution (100 ms in this example). But when the duration of the heart cycle results in the same x-tube position (or exactly an opposite position) the data at each time point is complementary and no improvement of temporal resolution is possible. When the table advancement in relation to the heart rate is further reduced, three or more heart cycles can be combined with a potentially even better temporal resolution, at the price of a relatively high radiation exposure. Considering the unpredictable efficiency and the disadvantages of a high heart rate and/or higher radiation exposure, most CT users prefer using β-receptor blockers to improve the relative temporal resolution. Rather than shortening of the reconstruction window, the total cycle time is prolonged by administration of a short acting beta-receptor blocking substance.

In an attempt to reduce the radiation exposure of the examination, prospectively ECG-triggered x-tube modulation can be applied to lower the x-tube output during the systolic cardiac phase. The systolic phase is rarely used for high resolution image reconstruction of the coronary arteries in patients with a low and stable heart rate. Particularly in patients with a low heart rate, the total exposure can be reduced substantially without losing the possibility of varying the positioning of the reconstruction window within the diastolic cardiac phase [1].

The result of the reconstruction procedure is a large stack of two-dimensional (axial) images. These approximately 250–300 images with a slice thickness between 0.5–1.0 mm can overlap by 0.2–0.4 mm, which improves the (subjective) z-resolution. The three-dimensional resolution of this data set is approximately $0.5 \times 0.5 \times 0.5$ mm.

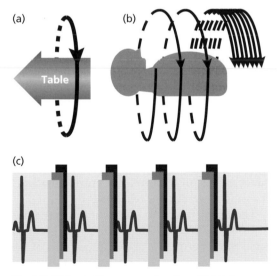

Fig. 8.2 ECG-gated image reconstruction: CT data is continuously acquired while the table is advanced through the gantry at a constant speed (a) and (b). CT data that has been acquired during the same ECG phase of each cycle is extracted to reconstruct isocardiophasic slices of the heart (c). Different phases can be reconstructed, indicated by the different shades of blue.

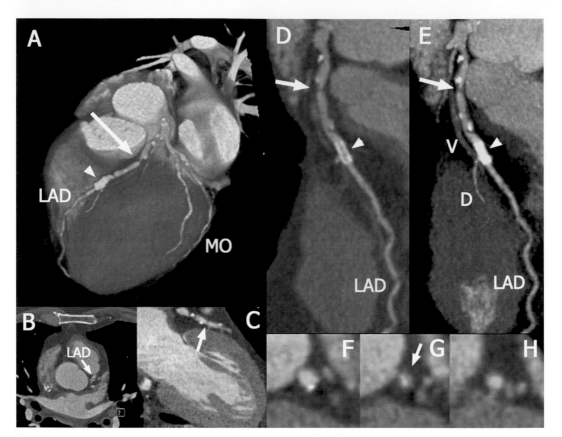

Fig. 8.3 Image postprocessing: Various postprocessing applications in a patient who underwent PCI of the left anterior descending coronary artery (LAD) in the past and now complains of recurrent angina. Multiple lesions, partially calcified, can be seen in the proximal LAD (D, E), as well as the stent in the mid-LAD. A complete 3D reconstruction of the heart (A) shows a significant lesion in the LAD (arrow) and the high-density stent (arrow head). Only a small section of the LAD can be visualized on a single axial slice (B), while multiplanar reformations can be created along the vessel and show extended sections (C). Curved multiplanar reformations (D) and maximum intensity projections (E) can be used to show the entire vessel in a single image. Panels F, G and H show cross-sections of the LAD at the proximal reference, the stenosis and the distal reference level, respectively. Marginal branch (MO), diagonal branch (D), cardiac vein (V).

Image processing and analysis

To facilitate the evaluation of the large amount of CT images various postprocessing tools have been developed (Fig. 8.3). Thin slab maximum intensity projections (MIP) are selective 2D displays of the highest densities, contrast medium, calcium or metal, within a positioned slab. It allows for quick assessment of the data set and the lumenal integrity, but is less effective in the presence of severe coronary calcification or stents. In these situations multiplanar reformation (MPR), which are 2D cross-sections at freely selectable positions or angles, are more suitable. The MPR images also provide more information regarding the vessel wall.

Three-dimensional reconstruction of the coronary arteries, from an external or internal (virtual endoscopy) perspective allows an overview of the coronary morphology, and its relation to the cardiac anatomy. Three-dimensional reconstructions are less suited for initial assessment of the coronary lumen, particularly in the presence of stents and calcified plaque tissue. Confirmation of a detected lesion on the original source images is therefore recommended.

Coronary lumenography

Detection of coronary stenosis

With ongoing technical innovation the diagnostic accuracy with respect to the detection and (semi) quantification of obstructive coronary artery disease is steadily improving. At the time of writing data from five studies that compared 16-MSCT with conventional angiography for the diagnosis of coronary stenosis were available (Table 8.1). In all studies β-receptor blockers were applied to reduce the heart rate during data acquisition and prevent motion artifacts. Two early studies used a 16-slice scanner with a rotation time of 420 ms, collimation 12 × 0.75 mm [2, 3]. Mollet *et al.*, and Hoffmann *et al.* used a similar scanner but could apply all detector rows: 16 × 0.75 mm [4, 5]. Martuscelli *et al.* used a different scanner type with a slower rotation

speed (500 ms), but a thinner detector collimation (16 × 0.625 mm) [6].

The results in these studies varied mainly as a result of population characteristics, scanner parameters and methods of analysis. We evaluated entire coronary vessels with a minimal diameter of 2.0 mm in a population (N = 58) with a high disease prevalence and very low (medically induced) heart rate (57 bpm). Without exclusion of less assessable vessels, this resulted in a high (overall) sensitivity (95%) for the detection of significantly narrowed vessels, and a slightly lower positive predictive value (80%) because of overestimation of particularly calcified vessels [2]. Ropers *et al.* examined 77 patients with a relatively lower disease prevalence and a slightly higher heart rate (52 bpm), and included vessels down to 1.5 mm diameter. After exclusion of non-assessable vessels (12%) sensitivity was 92%

Table 8.1 Diagnostic performance of 4- and 16-slice MSCT to detect coronary stenosis, with conventional coronary angiography as reference standard.

	Coll. (mm)	RT (ms)	N	β	Analysis	Excl. (%)	Sens. (%)	Spec. (%)	PPV (%)	NPV (%)	Sens.[a] (%)
4-MSCT											
Nieman [8]	4 × 1.0	500	31	–	S	27	81	97	81	97	68
Achenbach [9]	4 × 1.0	500	64	–	V	32	85	76	56	93	55
Knez [10]	4 × 1.0	500	43	–	S	6	78	98	84	96	51
Vogl [11]	4 × 1.0	500	64	–	S	28	75	99	92	98	–
Kopp[b] [12]	4 × 1.0	500	102	–	S	15	86	96	76	98	86
							93	97	81	99	93
Giesler[c] [13]	4 × 1.0	500	100	+/–	S	29	91	89	66	98	49
Nieman[c] [14]	4 × 1.0	500	78	–	S	32	84	95	67	98	63
Sato [15]	4 × 1.0	500	54	+	V	5	94	97	94	97	81
Kuettner [16]	4 × 1.0	500	66	–	S	43	66	98	83	95	37
8-MSCT				–							
Maruyama [7]	8 × 1.25	500	25	–	S	14	90	99	93	99	73
16-MSCT				–							
Nieman [2]	12 × .75	420	58	+	V	–	95	86	80	97	95
Ropers [3]	12 × .75	420	77	+	V	12	92	93	79	97	85
Mollet [4]	16 × .75	420	128	+	S	–	92	95	79	98	92
Martuscelli [6]	16 × .63	500	64	+	S	16	89	98	90	98	78
Hoffmann [5]	16 × .75	420	33	+	S	17	70	94	58	97	63

Collimation as the number of detector rows times the width of the individual detector rows (coll.); X-tube rotation time in ms (RT); study population size (N); use of β-receptor blocker (β); analysis of segments (S) or vessels (V); excluded segments/branches (Excl.); sensitivity (Sens.); specificity (Spec.); positive (PPV) and negative predictive value (NPV), all with respect to the assessable segments/branches.

[a] Sensitivity including missed lesions in non-assessable segments/branches.

[b] Results by two observers, without consensus reading.

[c] Studies include patients from earlier publications.

and specificity was 93%, but if lesions in non-assessable segments were included as false-negative results the overall sensitivity dropped to 73%. In patients with a heart rate below 60 bpm few vessels needed exclusion (4%) and the overall sensitivity improved (92%) [3]. Evaluating segments down to 1.5 mm diameter, Martuscelli *et al.* achieved similar results in a population with an intermediate disease prevalence: exclusion rate 16%, sensitivity 89%, specificity 98%, and overall sensitivity of 78% [6]. Mollet *et al.* evaluated >2.0 mm segments in a high prevalence population (N = 128) with a low (induced) heart rate (58 bpm) and detected significant obstruction with a high accuracy [4]. Finally, Hoffmann *et al.* evaluated all 17 coronary segments, as defined by the American Heart Association, regardless of the vessel diameter (N = 33), and found a lower overall sensitivity (70%), but high specificity (94%). The sensitivity was higher for the larger proximal segments (85%) [5]. In these studies the accuracy of classification of patients as to whether or not they had obstructive coronary artery disease varied between 78% and 90% [2–6].

Maruyama *et al.* used an eight-slice scanner (collimation 8 × 1.25 mm, rotation time 500 ms) to examine 25 patients with an intermediate disease prevalence. All 17 coronary segments, as defined by the American Heart Association, were evaluated. Using a 1.5 mm threshold 26% of the segments needed exclusion, while with a 2.0 mm threshold only 15% were considered non-evaluable. Sensitivity

and specificity for all assessable >1.5 mm segments was 90% and 99%, but including non-assessable segments the sensitivity dropped to 73%. This study confirmed earlier observations regarding the heart rate dependency of the diagnostic performance of MSCT [7].

The sensitivity and specificity of four-slice MSCT, after exclusion of 20–30% of the segments or vessels that were regarded as non-assessable, was reported as being between 75–90%, and between 85–90%, respectively [8–16]. The negative influence of a fast heart rate on the image interpretability and diagnostic accuracy of four-slice MSCT coronary angiography was confirmed in two studies, and encouraged use of beta-receptor blocking medication prior to the examination (Fig. 8.4) [13, 14]. Examples of MSCT coronary angiographys finding can be found in Fig. 8.5, Fig. 8.6, and Fig. 8.7.

Imaging of stents

The high roentgen attenuation of the metal in standard cardiovascular stents causes artifacts that complicate evaluation of the coronary lumen in the proximity of stent material. These artifacts are most impairing when the stent and (coronary) vessel are small and limitations of the spatial resolution of CT come into play [17]. Although no dedicated studies have been performed, the general impression is that complete occlusion can often be detected in the proximal coronary stents, but mild stenosis, particularly in smaller coronary branches, cannot be

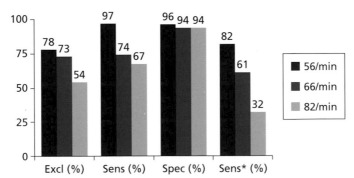

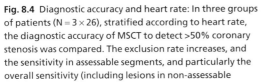

Fig. 8.4 Diagnostic accuracy and heart rate: In three groups of patients (N = 3 × 26), stratified according to heart rate, the diagnostic accuracy of MSCT to detect >50% coronary stenosis was compared. The exclusion rate increases, and the sensitivity in assessable segments, and particularly the overall sensitivity (including lesions in non-assessable segments as false-negative scores) decreases in patients with a higher heart rate. (Figure adapted from: Reference 14, Nieman K, Rensing BJ, van Geuns RJM *et al.* Non-invasive coronary angiography with multislice spiral computed tomography: Impact of heart rate. *Heart* 2002; **88**: 470–474.)

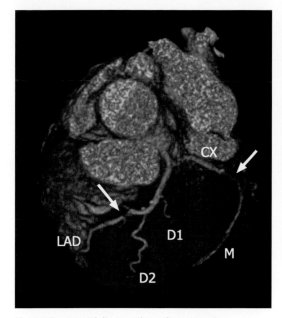

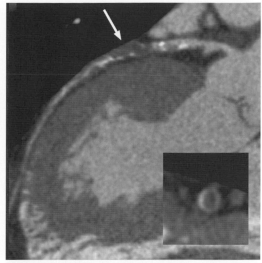

Fig. 8.6 Occluded left anterior descending coronary artery (arrow). Both calcified material as well as low density material, presumably thrombus material, can be visualized. Considering the length of the occlusion, the opacification of the distal vessel is probably due to collateral filling. The insert shows the cross-sectional view of the occluded vessel.

Fig. 8.5 Two-vessel disease: Three dimensional reconstruction of an MSCT coronary angiogram of a patient with a short stenosis in the left anterior descending coronary artery (LAD), and a long, more severe lesion in the left circumflex coronary artery (CX). Marginal branch (M), first and second marginal branch (D1 and D2).

reliably imaged. While the assessability of coronary stents has already improved with 16-MSCT compared to four-MSCT, even better stent imaging is expected by newer scanners with thinner detectors and usage of dedicated data processing that minimize stent artifacts (Fig. 8.8).

Graft imaging

Because of their large diameter, limited calcification and relative immobility bypass grafts, and particularly saphenous vein grafts, are well visualized by CT, although surgical material may cause artifacts (Fig. 8.9).

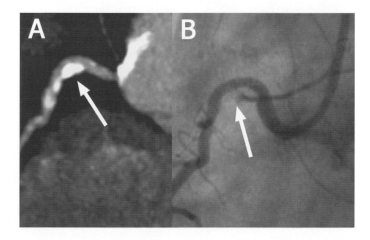

Fig. 8.7 Calcified proximal right coronary artery (arrow) by MSCT (A) and conventional coronary angiography (B).

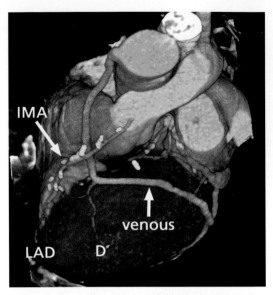

Fig. 8.8 Graft imaging: Three-dimensional reconstruction of a patient with a venous graft with a proximal anastomosis to the ascending aorta, an anastomosis to a diagonal branch (D) and continuing to the diaphragmatic surface of the heart, and a left internal mammary artery graft (IMA) connected to the middle segment of the left anterior descending coronary artery (LAD). While the grafts are well visualized, assessment of the native coronary arteries, particularly the LAD, is more complicated.

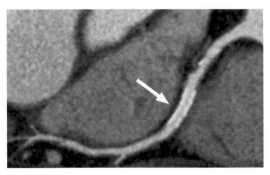

Fig. 8.9 MSCT stent imaging: Patent stent in the right coronary artery. (Figure reproduced courtesy of: Reference 4, Mollet NR, Cademartiri F, Nieman K *et al*. Multislice spiral computed tomography coronary angiography in patients with stable angina pectoris. *J Am Coll Cardiol* 2004; **43**: 2265–2270.)

Detection of graft patency was demonstrated with single-slice spiral CT as well as EBCT [18–25]. The diagnostic accuracy of detection of graft occlusion of current MSCT scanners comes close to 100%, without non-assessable exclusions [26–29]. MSCT

also allows detection of graft stenosis, without occlusion, as well as lesions in the distal segments of sequential grafts with a reasonable sensitivity (60–83%) and specificity (88–92%), although it should be noted that (venous) graft stenosis is relatively rare and the published studies contain only few cases (Table 8.2) [26, 28, 29].

Ischemic symptoms in patients after bypass surgery can be caused by obstruction of bypass grafts, or by progression of disease in the native coronary arteries. Therefore, evaluation cannot be limited to the bypass grafts but should include the coronary arteries as well, which proves to be more complicated because of the diffuse coronary degeneration and excessive presence of coronary calcification [28].

Clinical interpretations of the CT findings can be difficult as graft occlusion can occur without symptoms [30]. It may be hard, particularly in post-CABG patients with diffuse coronary artery disease to estimate the hemodynamic significance of a coronary or graft lesion without establishing the presence of (stress induced) myocardial ischemia, considering the likely existence of collateral vessels and microvascular disease in these patients. Therefore, functional information is crucial, and with the current state of technology, the clinical role of MSCT in patients who have undergone CABG may be limited.

Functional imaging

During the MSCT scan the heart is sampled throughout the cardiac cycle. In general, coronary evaluations are performed using diastolic data because the motion of the coronary arteries is limited during this phase. While the systolic reconstructions may be non-interpretable with respect to the coronary arteries, image quality is generally sufficient to evaluate larger structures and determine the left ventricular performance (Fig. 8.10). Multiple contraction phases can be reconstructed covering the entire cardiac cycle. From the end-diastolic and end-systolic phase images, the global ventricular function, i.e. stroke volume, ejection fraction, and cardiac output, can be calculated, and has shown promising results in comparison to established techniques [31–33]. Because the temporal resolution of MSCT (165–250 ms) is lower than echocardiography it is less suitable for demonstrating

Table 8.2 Diagnostic performance of spiral CT after bypass surgery.

Author	CT	N	Graft types		Total occlusion			Stenosis (50–99%)		
			Art. (n)	Ven. (n)	Excl. (%)	Sens. (%)	Spec. (%)	Excl. (%)	Sens. (%)	Spec. (%)
Ropers [26]	4	65	20	162	–	97	98	38	75	92
Yoo [27]	4	42	70	55	NR	98	100	–	–	–
Nieman* [28]	4	24	18 (26)	23 (60)	8	100	97	9	60	88
					16	95	94	5	83	90
Martuscelli [29]	64	96	96	189	13	100	100	13	90	100

Scanner type (CT); number of patients (N); arterial (Art.) and venous grafts (Ven.); exclusions (Excl.); sensitivity (Sens.); specificity (Spec.). Number of graft segments in sequential grafts between brackets. Not reported (NR).
* Analysis of graft segments by two observers. Only venous grafts evaluated for non-complete obstruction.

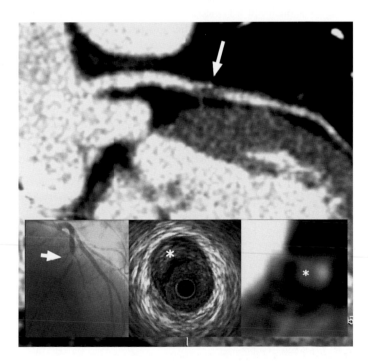

Fig. 8.10 Plaque imaging: Left anterior descending coronary artery with a significant stenosis (arrow), mostly consisting of non-calcified material. The inserts show the corresponding conventional coronary angiogram, the IVUS image with the plaque (*), and the MSCT cross-sectional view of the lesion, confirming the presence of the plaque(*).

dynamic wall motion abnormalities, but seems sufficient to depict abnormal ventricular wall thickening. Although evaluation of ventricular performance will rarely be the primary purpose of the CT examination, except perhaps in patients with contraindications to both ultrasound and MRI, functional information is available without the need for additional radiation exposure.

Areas with reduced myocardial perfusion have been demonstrated in animal studies [34] and retrospectively in non-gated and gated thoracic CT scans [35, 36]. Wada *et al.* have demonstrated how left ventricular recovery after percuataneous coronary intervention can be predicted based on the transmural contrast enhancement gradient [37]. As with the more established method of MR, late enhancement of the myocardium by CT 5–10 min after contrast injection has been demonstrated in animal studies and may represent a clinically relevant application [38].

Wall motion imaging as well as perfusion imaging would be more useful if resting and exercised conditions could be compared. Because repeated radiation exposure would be required, such protocols seem unattractive given the availability of alternatives such as nuclear imaging, stress echocardiography, PET and MRI.

Imaging of non-obstructive coronary atherosclerosis

Non-enhanced atherosclerosis imaging

Without the use of contrast media CT can be used for the detection and quantification of coronary calcium. While most clinical data have been gathered using electron beam CT, calcium scoring can be performed with MSCT using either prospectively ECG-triggered scanning or retrospectively ECG-gated image reconstruction [39–41].

Finding calcium proves that there is coronary atherosclerosis, but the opposite is not always true. This technique has a high sensitivity, but a low positive predictive value for the detection of significant coronary obstruction, which means it is of limited use for the detection of coronary stenosis [42, 43].

While it remains unclear to what extent the presence of calcium within a specific plaque determines the likelihood that it will rupture, there is an undeniable correlation between the amount of coronary calcium and the occurrence of acute coronary events [44–47]. Whether the added prognostic value of a calcium score, in addition to traditional risk factors, justifies widespread screening of asymptomatic individuals remains a matter of debate [48]. At present, calcium scoring seems most sensible in patients with an intermediate risk for coronary events, to determine whether they need intensive risk factor modification [49].

Contrast enhanced plaque imaging

In contrast enhanced coronary CT scans the diseased coronary artery wall can be imaged beyond the mere presence of calcium. Non-calcified plaque tissue appears as low density material, between the contrast enhanced coronary lumen and the lower density pericardial fat tissue (Fig. 8.11). Lipid-rich and fibrous plaques, a distinction with potential clinical consequences, have different but overlapping CT densities, and are therefore hard to differentiate in the small coronary arteries [50–52]. It is

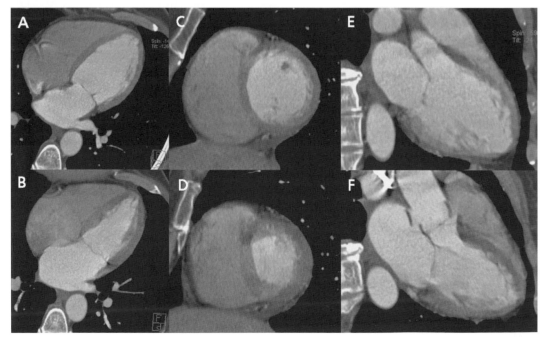

Fig. 8.11 Functional imaging: 4-chamber view (A and B), short axis view (C and D) and 2-chamber view (E and F) of the left ventricle during end-diastole (A, C and E) and end-systole (B, D, F).

conceivable that imaging of extensive non-enhanced material, in addition to calcified material, provides a better impression of the extent of the atherosclerotic plaque burden, although limited clinical data are available [53]. To what extent non-calcified plaque imaging may be useful for plaque characterization, risk stratification, disease progression or monitoring of treatment effect, will need to be evaluated further.

Limitations

Limitations of MSCT coronary angiography are related to scanner characteristics, ECG-gating, patient characteristics and safety issues (Table 8.3).

The temporal resolution of current MSCT scanners is less than 200 ms which is sufficient for motion-sparse imaging of the coronary arteries in patients at a low heart rate. In patients with a heart rate higher than 70–80 min image quality tends to be unpredictable, and the use of beta-blockers is advised in coronary imaging studies [3, 13, 14]. The maximum spatial resolution, which is approaching 0.5 mm in all directions, allows detailed appreci-

ation of the cardiac morphology and the proximal coronary arteries. Smaller coronary branches down to 1–2 mm are usually visible, but luminal assessment for the detection of significant stenosis becomes unreliable, particularly in the presence of extensive calcified disease [2–6].

Because the data for one CT angiogram are acquired during several heart cycles, the heart rhythm needs to be constant. For instance, in cases of arrhythmia, atrial fibrillation or single premature contractions, the end-diastolic filling state of the heart alternates, resulting in a disruption or displacement of the vessel between slices that were acquired during the consecutive heart cycles.

In obese patients image signal-to-noise is often insufficient for accurate coronary artery evaluation and cannot always be compensated with a higher roentgen tube output. Patients with impaired renal function, thyroid dysfunction or an allergy to iodine-containing contrast media are generally contraindicated for MSCT coronary angiography.

Apart from economic considerations, widespread use of cardiac CT has been stalled by concerns with regard to the radiation exposure. The radiation

Table 8.3 Limitations of MSCT coronary angiography.

Limitations		Potential solutions
Patient-related	obesity	increased radiation dose
	reduced kidney function	prehydration
		smaller contrast bolus
		shorter scan time
	calcified atherosclerosis	exclusion based calcium load on a non-enhanced scan
		improved spatial resolution
		software-based artifact reduction
Scanner-related	spatial resolution	thinner detector rings
	temporal resolution	beta-blocking
		faster gantry rotation
		faster x-tube rotation
		multisegmental reconstruction algorithms
	radiation exposure	(ECG-triggered) x-tube output modulation
Gating-related	arrhythmia	systolic gating or exclusion
	fast heart rate	beta-blocking
		improved temporal resolution
Interpretation-related	detection of ischemia	modality fusion (SPECT/PET)
	semiquantification	software applications
		improved spatial and temporal resolution

exposure of a standard 16-slice MSCT coronary angiogram is estimated at 8.1 mSv for males and 10.9 mSv for females. The radiation dose can be reduced to 4.3 mSv using ECG-triggered tube modulation [54]. Whether this exposure is justified depends on the indication and the availability, of diagnostic alternatives. While this disadvantage may outweigh the risks, discomfort and cost of invasive coronary angiography under certain conditions, few would support contrast enhanced screening of individuals without symptoms. Meanwhile, development efforts are being made to reduce the radiation exposure of MSCT without forfeiting the diagnostic accuracy.

Future development

The current state of the art MSCT technology is equipped with 32–64 detector rows with a detector width between 0.6–0.75 mm. The rotation time now approaches 300 ms, with a temporal resolution close to 150 ms. While more and thinner detector rows increase the performance of the scanner and make the examination more practical, the true challenge lies in the acceleration of the gantry, or the improvement of the temporal resolution by other means.

Quantification of stenosis severity is important. While the reliability of quantification tools will depend on the overall quality and the spatial resolution of the images, it is eagerly expected that quantification software will provide an objective and reproducible assessment of the stenosis severity.

Particularly in the absence of accurate stenosis quantification tools, functional information is essential to assess the hemodynamic significance of obstructive coronary artery disease. The feasibility of functional CT imaging, i.e. stress induced perfusion of wall motion imaging, is currently not regarded as a realistic option. CT findings can, however, be correlated to functional imaging results by other modalities, such as nuclear imaging, PET or MRI. Rather than collectively interpreting both results, scanner units that physically fuse CT with other modalities such as PET (hybrid PET/CT) have been introduced [55].

Conclusion

The achievements in the field of non-invasive coronary imaging are considerable. Today multislice spiral CT appears the most accurate and consistent modality for non-invasive angiographic identification of coronary stenosis. The exact role of this fast and relatively straightforward procedure within clinical cardiovascular practice remains to be determined.

References

1. Jakobs TF, Becker CR, Ohnesorge B *et al*. Multislice helical CT of the heart with retrospective ECG gating: Reduction of radiation exposure by ECG-controlled tube current modulation. *Eur Radiol* 2002; **12**: 1081–1086.
2. Nieman K, Cademartiri F, Lemos PA *et al*. Reliable non-invasive coronary angiography with fast submillimeter multislice spiral computed tomography. *Circulation* 2002; **106**: 2051–2054.
3. Ropers D, Baum U, Pohle K *et al*. Detection of coronary artery stenoses with thin-slice multidetector-row spiral computed tomography and multiplanar reconstruction. *Circulation* 2003; **107**: 664–666.
4. Mollet NR, Cademartiri F, Nieman K *et al*. Multislice spiral computed tomography coronary angiography in patients with stable angina pectoris. *J Am Coll Cardiol* 2004; **43**: 2265–2270.
5. Hoffmann U, Moselewski F, Cury RC *et al*. Predictive value of 16-slice multidetector spiral CT to detect significant obstructive coronary artery disease in patients at high risk for CAD: Patient vs segment-based analysis. *Circulation* 2004; **110**: 2638–2643.
6. Martuscelli E, Romagnoli A, D'Eliseo A *et al*. Accuracy of thin slice computed tomography in the detection of coronary stenoses. *Eur Heart J* 2004; **25**: 1043–1048.
7. Maruyama T, Yoshizumi T, Tamura R *et al*. Comparison of visibility and diagnostic capability of non-invasive coronary angiography by eight slice multidetector-row computed tomography versus conventional coronary angiography. *Am J Cardiol* 2004; **93**: 537–542.
8. Nieman K, Oudkerk M, Rensing BJ *et al*. Coronary angiography with multislice computed tomography. *Lancet* 2001; **357**: 599–603.
9. Achenbach S, Giesler T, Ropers D *et al*. Detection of coronary artery stenoses by contrast enhanced, retro-spectively electrocardiographically-gated, multislice spiral computed tomography. *Circulation* 2001; **103**: 2535–2538.
10. Knez A, Becker CR, Leber A *et al*. Usefulness of multislice spiral computed tomography angiography for determination of coronary artery stenoses. *Am J Cardiol* 2001; **88**: 1191–1194.
11. Vogl TJ, Abolmaali ND, Diebold T *et al*. Techniques for the detection of coronary atherosclerosis: multidetector-row CT coronary angiography. *Radiology* 2002; **223**: 212–220.

12. Kopp AF, Schröder S, Kuettner A *et al.* Non-invasive coronary angiography with high resolution multidetector-row computed tomography: Results in 102 patients. *Eur Heart J* 2002; **23**: 1714–1725.

13. Giesler T, Baum U, Ropers D *et al.* Non-invasive visualization of coronary arteries using contrast enhanced multidetector CT: Influence of heart rate on image quality and stenosis detection. *Am J Roentgenol* 2002; **179**: 911–916.

14. Nieman K, Rensing BJ, van Geuns RJM *et al.* Non-invasive coronary angiography with multislice spiral computed tomography: Impact of heart rate. *Heart* 2002; **88**: 470–474.

15. Sato Y, Matsumoto N, Kato M *et al.* Non-invasive assessment of coronary artery disease by multislice spiral computed tomography using a new retrospectively ECG-gated image reconstruction technique. *Circ J* 2003; **67**: 401–405.

16. Kuettner A, Kopp AF, Schroeder S *et al.* Diagnostic accuracy of multidetector computed tomography coronary angiography in patients with angiographically proven coronary artery disease. *J Am Coll Cardiol* 2004; **43**: 831–839.

17. Nieman K, Cademartiri F, Raaijmakers R *et al.* Non-invasive angiographic evaluation of coronary stents with multislice spiral computed tomography. *Herz* 2003; **28**: 136–142.

18. Bateman TM, Gray RJ, Whiting JS *et al.* Cine computed tomographic evaluation of aortocoronary bypass graft patency. *J Am Coll Cardiol* 1986; **8**: 693–698.

19. Bateman TM, Gray RJ, Whiting JS *et al.* Prospective evaluation of ultrafast cardiac computed tomography for determination of coronary bypass graft patency. *Circulation* 1987; **75**: 1018–1024.

20. Stanford W, Brundage BH, MacMillan R *et al.* Sensitivity and specificity of assessing coronary bypass graft patency with ultrafast computed tomography: Results of a multicenter study. *J Am Coll Cardiol* 1988; **12**: 1–7.

21. Achenbach S, Moshage W, Ropers D *et al.* Non-invasive, three-dimensional visualization of coronary artery bypass grafts by electron beam tomography. *Am J Cardiol* 1997; **79**: 856–61.

22. Ha JW, Cho SY, Shim WH *et al.* Non-invasive evaluation of coronary artery bypass graft patency using three-dimensional angiography obtained with contrast enhanced electron beam CT. *Am J Roentgenol* 1999; **172**: 1055–1059.

23. Lu B, Dai RP, Jing BL *et al.* Evaluation of coronary artery bypass graft patency using three-dimensional reconstruction and flow study on electron beam tomography. *J Comput Assist Tomogr* 2000; **24**: 663–670.

24. Engelmann MG, von Smekal A, Knez A *et al.* Accuracy of spiral computed tomography for identifying arterial and venous coronary graft patency. *Am J Cardiol* 1997; **80**: 569–574.

25. Tello R, Costello P, Ecker C *et al.* Spiral CT evaluation of coronary artery bypass graft patency. *J Comput Assist Tomogr* 1993; **17**: 253–259.

26. Ropers D, Ulzheimer S, Wenkel E *et al.* Investigation of aortocoronary artery bypass grafts by multislice computed tomography with electrocardiographic-gated image reconstruction. *Am J Card* 2001; **88**: 792–795.

27. Yoo KJ, Choi D, Choi BW *et al.* The comparison of the graft patency after coronary artery bypass grafting using coronary angiography and multislice computed tomography. *Eur J Cardiothor Surg* 2003; **24**: 86–91.

28. Nieman K, Pattynama PMT, Rensing BJ *et al.* CT angiographic evaluation of postCABG patients: Assessment of grafts and coronary arteries. *Radiology* 2003; **229**: 749–756.

29. Martuscelli E, Romagnoli A, D'Eliseo A *et al.* Evaluation of venous and arterial conduit patency by 16-slice spiral computed tomography. *Circulation* 2004; **110**: 3234–3238.

30. Bryan AJ, Angelini GD. The biology of saphenous vein occlusion: Etiology and strategies for prevention. *Curr Opin Cardiol* 1994; **9**: 614–619.

31. Dirksen MS, Bax JJ, de Roos A *et al.* Usefulness of dynamic multislice computed tomography and left ventricular function in unstable angina pectoris and comparison with echocardiography. *Am J Cardiol* 2002; **90**: 1157–1160.

32. Juergens KU, Grude M, Maintz D *et al.* Multidetector-row CT of left ventricular function with dedicated analysis software versus MR imaging: initial experience. *Radiology* 2004; **230**: 403–10.

33. Mahnken AH, Spuentrup E, Niethammer M *et al.* Quantitative and qualitative assessment of left ventricular volume with ECG-gated multislice spiral CT: Value of different image reconstruction algorithms in comparison to MRI. *Acta Radiol* 2003; **44**: 604–11.

34. Hoffmann U, Millea R, Enzweiler C *et al.* Acute myocardial infarction: Contrast enhanced multidetector-row CT in a porcine model. *Radiology* 2004; **231**: 697–701.

35. Nikolaou K, Knez A, Sagmeister S *et al.* Assessment of myocardial infarctions using multidetector-row computed tomography. *J Comput Assist Tomogr* 2004; **28**: 286–92.

36. Gosalia A, Haramati LB, Sheth MP *et al.* CT detection of acute myocardial infarction. *AJR Am J Roentgenol* 2004; **182**: 1563–6.

37. Wada H, Kobayashi Y, Yasu T *et al.* Multidetector computed tomography for imaging of subendocardial infarction: Prediction of wall motion recovery after reperfused anterior myocardial infarction. *Circ J* 2004; **68**: 512–514.

38. Park JM, Choe YH, Chang S *et al.* Usefulness of multidetector-row CT in the evaluation of reperfused myocardial infarction in a rabbit model. *Korean J Radiol* 2004; **5**: 19–24.

39. Becker CR, Kleffel T, Crispin A *et al.* Coronary artery calcium measurement: Agreement of multirow detector

and electron beam CT. *AJR Am J Roentgenol* 2001; **176**: 1295–1298.

40. Horiguchi J, Nakanishi T, Ito K. Quantification of coronary artery calcium using multidetector CT and a retrospective ECG-gating reconstruction algorithm. *AJR Am J Roentgenol* 2001; **177**: 1429–1435.

41. Carr JJ, Crouse JR 3rd, Goff DC Jr *et al.* Evaluation of subsecond gated helical CT for quantification of coronary artery calcium and comparison with electron beam CT. *AJR Am J Roentgenol* 2000; **174**: 915–921.

42. Budoff MJ, Georgiou D, Brody A *et al.* Ultrafast computed tomography as a diagnostic modality in the detection of coronary artery disease: A multicenter study. *Circulation* 1996; **93**: 898–904.

43. Haberl R, Becker A, Leber A *et al.* Correlation of coronary calcification and angiographically documented stenoses in patients with suspected coronary artery disease: Results of 1,764 patients. *J Am Coll Cardiol* 2001; **37**: 451–457.

44. Raggi P, Callister TQ, Cooil B *et al.* Identification of patients at increased risk of first unheralded acute myocardial infarction by electron beam computed tomography. *Circulation* 2000; **101**: 850–855.

45. Detrano RC, Wong ND, Doherty TM *et al.* Coronary calcium does not accurately predict near term future coronary events in high risk adults. *Circulation* 1999; **99**: 2633–2638.

46. Arad Y, Spadaro LA, Goodman K *et al.* Prediction of coronary events with electron beam computed tomography. *J Am Coll Cardiol* 2000; **36**: 1253–1260.

47. Raggi P, Cooil B, Callister TQ. Use of electron beam tomography data to develop models for prediction of hard coronary events. *Am Heart J* 2001; **141**: 375–382.

48. O'Rourke RA, Brundage BH, Froelicher VF *et al.* American College of Cardiology/American Heart Association expert consensus document on electron beam computed tomography for the diagnosis and prognosis of coronary artery disease. *Circulation* 2001; **102**: 126–1140.

49. Greenland P, Smith SC Jr, Grundy SM. Improving coronary heart disease risk assessment in asymptomatic people: Role of traditional risk factors and non-invasive cardiovascular tests. *Circulation* 2001; **104**: 1863–1867.

50. Schroeder S, Kopp AF, Baumbach A *et al.* Non-invasive detection and evaluation of atherosclerotic coronary plaques with multislice computed tomography. *J Am Coll Cardiol* 2001; **37**: 1430–1435.

51. Leber AW, Knez A, Becker A *et al.* Accuracy of multidetector spiral computed tomography in identifying and differentiating the composition of coronary atherosclerotic plaques: A comparative study with intracoronary ultrasound. *J Am Coll Cardiol* 2004; **43**: 1241–1247.

52. Becker CR, Nikolaou K, Muders M *et al.* Ex vivo coronary atherosclerotic plaque characterization with multidetector-row CT. *Eur Radiol* 2003; **13**: 2094–2098.

53. Achenbach S, Moselewski F, Ropers D *et al.* Detection of calcified and non-calcified coronary atherosclerotic plaque by contrast enhanced, submillimeter multidetector spiral computed tomography: A segment based comparison with intravascular ultrasound. *Circulation* 2004; **109**: 14–17.

54. Trabold T, Buchgeister M, Kuttner A *et al.* Estimation of radiation exposure in 16-detector row computed tomography of the heart with retrospective ECG-gating. *Rofo* 2003; **175**: 1051–1055.

55. Koepfli P, Hany TF, Wyss CA *et al.* CT attenuation correction for myocardial perfusion quantification using a PET/CT hybrid scanner. *J Nucl Med* 2004; **45**: 537–542.

CHAPTER 9

Cardiac computed tomography: Evaluation of myocardial function, perfusion and viability

Subha V. Raman & Patrick M. Colletti

With recent advances in multidetector row technology, computed tomography (CT) has emerged as a viable alternative to invasive angiography for visualization of coronary arteries, bypass grafts, and other vascular anatomy. Care of the patient with cardiovascular disease, however, requires understanding of both anatomic as well as physiological considerations. For example, in patients with ischemic cardiomyopathy, the clinician is faced with two fundamental questions: (1) are there targets for revascularization and (2) if revascularized, will left ventricular function improve? This chapter reviews current and future capability for myocardial assessment with CT that provides physiological information complementary to anatomic visualization. Techniques described here assume the use of contrast enhanced 16-slice or 64-slice CT (multidetector or MDCT) [1] or electron beam CT (EBCT) [2].

Technical considerations

Timing and delivery of contrast agent
Iodinated CT contrast agents for cardiovascular imaging distribute [3] primarily to the blood pool and myocardial extracellular space. Non-ionic, low osmolality contrast agents are preferable, especially for patients with cardiovascular conditions. The amount of iodinated contrast agent required for satisfactory cardiac CT depends on patient mass, with 0.5 gm of iodine per kg body mass as the usual dose [4]. Using standard low osmolality contrast agents with concentrations of 300–400 mg iodine/ml, typically 50–100 ml of contrast agent is administered at 4–5 ml/s

via a programmable injector system. This is followed by a bolus flush of 50 ml of normal saline [5].

Timing the CT image acquisition to the contrast agent bolus arrival for left ventricular anatomic and functional analysis is identical to timing used for coronary artery CT examinations [6]. There may be considerable variability in circulation time from patient to patient. The time between peripheral contrast injection and appearance of contrast in the aorta can be determined using a small volume test contrast agent bolus of 20 ml and rapid, repeated imaging of a single transaortic plane [7]. Alternatively, a Hounsfield Unit (HU) threshold may be set such that the volume acquisition is triggered to begin once a certain HU value is detected in the ascending aorta. This is referred to as bolus tracking.

The uniform programmed injection delivery of intravenous contrast agent requires 40–75 s. During this time, intravascular concentration rises, peaks, and declines. It has been demonstrated that tailored injection protocols with exponentially decelerated profiles yield a consistently more uniform intravascular contrast agent level [8].

Cardiac triggering
Cardiac CT must be acquired during suspended respiration with cardiac gating. Two approaches to cardiac gating may be applied: Prospective ECG triggering and retrospective ECG gating [1]. Prospective ECG triggering uses the ECG signal to modulate scanning, so that x-rays are generated and projection data are acquired only during selected portions of the cardiac cycle, i.e. diastole. There are

important limitations to prospective triggering techniques [1]:

- Sensitive to heart rate variations and arrhythmias
- Limited spatial z-axis resolution in order to cover the entire heart in a single breath-hold (this is less of a problem with 64-slice techniques)
- Effective only for lower heart rates
- Perform poorly with arrhythmias, such as in atrial fibrillation

To overcome these limitations, retrospective ECG gating is commonly used. With retrospective techniques, partially overlapping MDCT projections are continuously acquired, and the ECG signal is simultaneously recorded. Algorithms are then applied to sort the data from different phases of the cardiac cycle by progressively shifting the temporal window of acquired helical projection data relative to the R wave. Every position of the heart must be covered by a detector row at every point during the cardiac cycle. This means that the scanner table must not advance more than the total width of the active detectors for each heartbeat. Helical pitch can be varied proportionally to the heart rate to achieve continuous volume coverage, at the expense of a higher radiation dose.

Retrospective gating techniques allow [1]:

- Faster continuous cardiac volume coverage
- Improved z-axis resolution
- Imaging of the entire cardiac cycle for functional analysis.

Radiation exposure

The cardiac CT techniques described here depend upon the ability for rapid, repetitive scanning. With this, considerations of patient radiation exposure become important. Cardiac CT radiation exposure is highly dependent on the protocol utilized. EBCT generally delivers considerably less radiation to the patient when compared to MDCT [9–11] (Table 9.1). Doses in the 1–2 mSv (millisievert) range are typically reported for the prospective gating of only a portion of the cardiac cycle generally used for CT calcium scoring. For contrast enhanced coronary stenosis assessment, with retrospective gating and imaging throughout the cardiac cycle, much higher doses in the range of 8–12 mSv are reported [12–19]. For comparison, the radiation dose of an uncomplicated coronary angiography is 4–6 mSv [12, 18]. Efforts to reduce the high dose accumulated in retrospective gating, termed dose modula-

Table 9.1 *Radiation doses with cardiac CT (in millisieverts) refs. 8–20.*

Method Exam	Catheter angiography	EBCT	MDCT
Calcium score		1–1.3	1–2
Coronary arteries ventriculography	2.1–2.5	1.5–2	8–12
Perfusion		1–8	8–12
Delayed (viability)		1–2	4–10

Compared to males, females may receive up to 40% greater absorbed radiation dose during CT of the chest.

tion, are directed at reducing the tube current during parts of the cardiac cycle, particularly systole, where poorer image quality can be tolerated because assessment of the coronary arteries is generally more important near diastole. Dose modulation allows a 30–50% dose reduction [19, 20]. Although CT ventriculography does not have the resolution requirements of coronary CT, it is important to consider the effect of electrocardiographic (ECG) dose modulation when generating multiphase data. If radiation dose is excessively restricted to end-diastole, as is the case on most systems with ECG dose modulation, reduced signal-to-noise ratio (SNR) in the reformatted systolic images may render delineation of endocardial borders in these phases problematic. Satisfactory volumetric analysis may require relatively less dose modulation. A repeat exposure, perhaps with reduced dosage, is needed if delayed contrast enhanced myocardial viability CT is to be performed. Strategies for reduced exposure would be required for rapid sequential imaging of myocardial perfusion.

Myocardial function

Ventricular function

Cardiac gated CT acquired for the evaluation of possible pulmonary emboli, aortic dissection, or coronary artery disease may be reformatted into standard two, three, and four chamber and short axis views (Fig. 9.1). With these standard cardiac views, regional left and right ventricular wall motion and thickening [21, 22] may be evaluated. Cine cardiac CT may be viewed in two or three dimensions (Fig. 9.2). Hypokinesia, akinesia, dyskinesia, and asynergy are reported in a manner similar to

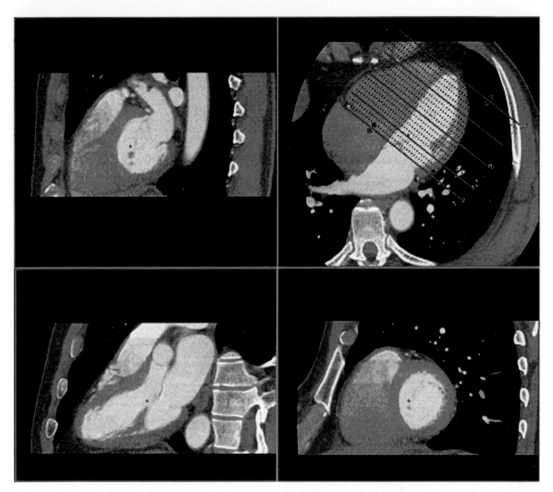

Fig. 9.1 Depiction of short axis image generation from multiphase data (CardIQ Function©, GE Healthcare). Standard cardiac views are reconstructed from the 3D axial image data set. The short axis views, lower right are formatted from the four-chamber view, upper right.

echocardiography and cardiac MR. An example of segmental wall motion abnormality in a patient with anterior wall akinesis is shown in Fig. 9.3. As in other tomographic and volumetric imaging techniques, CT regional LV wall motion results may be displayed as a color coded functional image (Fig. 9.4). At the same time as the myocardial wall motion is reviewed, heart valves and the aortic root may also be inspected for morphological and functional abnormalities.

Left ventricular ejection fraction (LVEF) is by far the most widely used global measurement of ventricular systolic function [23–25]. While the evaluation of regional and global left ventricular function is unlikely to be the sole reason for referral for a volume CT examination, multiphase reformatting of volume CT data can provide quantifica-

tion of ventricular volumes and function. This is particularly likely when conflicting data exists from other modalities and there is a concomitant need to define the coronary arteries or other complex cardiovascular anatomy.

Left ventricular systolic function: Methodologically, measurement of end-diastolic volume, end-systolic volume, stroke volume, and LVEF by CT is straightforward with appropriately timed contrast enhanced acquisition that results in adequate contrast between LV cavity and myocardium for postprocessing [24–26].

Multiphase acquisition can be accomplished on EBCT as well as MDCT systems, though the technique varies among platforms. To accurately quantify ventricular function, sufficient phases covering

(a)

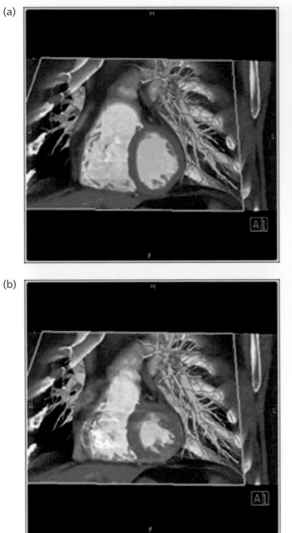

(b)

(a)

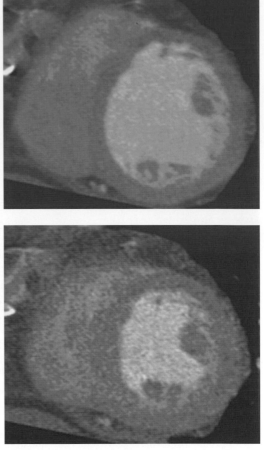

(b)

Fig. 9.3 Example of segmental contraction motion abnormality demonstrated by comparing end-diastolic (a) to end-systolic (b) frames in a representative short axis slice of the left ventricle in a patient with anterior wall akinesis.

Fig. 9.2 4D cardiac CT (64 slices) image reconstructed through the cardiac cycle. These "sub-MIP" (sub-maximum intensity projections) are reconstructed at end-diastole (a) and end-systole (b). (Figure reproduced with permission from: Reference 22, Lawler LP, Ney D, Pannu HK *et al.* Four-dimensional imaging of the heart based on near-isotropic MDCT data sets. *AJR and AJR Online* 2005; **184**: 774–776, **http://www.ajronline.org/**)

the cardiac cycle are required. Particular attention should be paid to temporal resolution such that end-systole and end-diastole are captured in two of these phases. Based on the nuclear cardiology literature, eight-frame acquisition is sufficient for clinically useful measures of EF. However, eight-frame nuclear medicine techniques may underestimate

EF and left ventricular volumes and are generally insufficient for estimates of diastolic function [27, 28]. Using the 5% window temporal reconstruction advocated by many coronary CT investigators, 20 cardiac phases may be reconstructed. This typically allows for the generation of volumetric curves and more accurate CT evaluation of ventricular volumes and EF. Diastolic function may then be estimated from a calculated peak filling rate and time to peak filling rate.

Different vendors have varying techniques to generate multiphase data; one approach is to generate the entire axial data set at multiple phases, then generate multislice short axis images from this large image set (several thousand images for the average

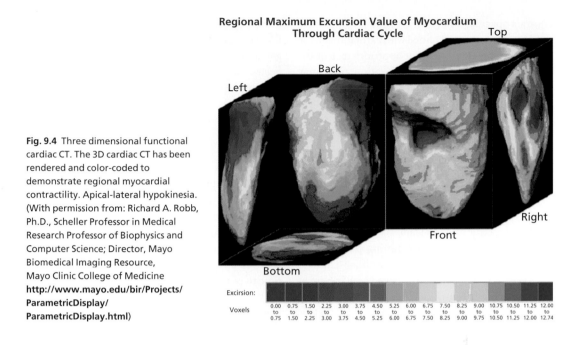

Fig. 9.4 Three dimensional functional cardiac CT. The 3D cardiac CT has been rendered and color-coded to demonstrate regional myocardial contractility. Apical-lateral hypokinesia. (With permission from: Richard A. Robb, Ph.D., Scheller Professor in Medical Research Professor of Biophysics and Computer Science; Director, Mayo Biomedical Imaging Resource, Mayo Clinic College of Medicine **http://www.mayo.edu/bir/Projects/ ParametricDisplay/ ParametricDisplay.html)**

volume coverage). Alternatively, multiphase short axis images are generated directly from the raw data. The advantage of the former approach is that the multiphase axial image set can be stored and retrieved for subsequent analysis in various planes. The latter approach generates only the short axis images (several hundred images) resulting in reduced storage requirements. Subsequent reformatting in, for example the long axis planes, requires special attention to the processing and possible storage of the raw data on current platforms. In both approaches, an iterative process requiring minimal user input to identify the short axis relative to the interventricular septum rapidly generates multi-slice, multiphase images in contiguous short axis planes (Fig. 9.1).

Postprocessing of the short axis image set is very similar to techniques used in cardiac magnetic resonance, and can be done using a variety of software platforms. Essentially this involves application of Simpson's rule, which states that the volume of the LV cavity is the sum of individual slice volumes computed as areas enclosed by the LV endocardial contour in a given slice multiplied by slice thickness. Thus, end-diastolic volume and end-systolic volume are measured. Stroke volume and ejection fraction are then calculated [21, 29–48]. LV epicardial outlines are then detected and outlined, and the LV myocardial mass is measured as the sum of volumes of the space between epicardial and endocardial outlines totaled for all short axis slices at end-diastole [49].

Left ventricular wall thickening: While virtually all publications to date regarding ventricular function with cardiac CT have focussed on global measures of ventricular volumes and ejection fraction, most postprocessing software platforms currently available also provide methods to compute regional wall thickening [50]. This requires some use input to identify, for example the inferior RV-LV junction from which the short axis is divided evenly into multiple sectors. Displacement of the endocardial contour relative to the epicardial contour in each sector can be quantified, providing regional wall thickening and therefore a measure of regional systolic function [51].

Right ventricular systolic function: RV systolic function has important prognostic and therapeutic implications, particularly in patients with conditions such as valvular heart disease, pulmonary hypertension, and various forms of congenital heart disease [52]. Cardiac CT allows accurate quantification of right ventricular ejection fraction if acquisition timing is modified to optimize contrast opacification of the RV, and is comparable to RV measurement obtained with cardiac magnetic resonance [53–55]. Without appropriate acquisition timing for right heart visualization, there may be insufficient contrast for RV endocardial border delineation. Optimal RV timing usually differs from that used for routine coronary CTA. Given the usual relationship of the great vessels and ventricular concordance, RV opacification is optimized by triggering acquisition once the contrast agent reaches the main pulmonary artery. RV delineation in transposition or other abnormal great vessel-ventricular relationships requires a prior knowledge of the anatomy and relevant surgical history to select the correct region for timing prescription. As an alternative, prolonged optimal contrast enhancement levels may be achieved with the use of tailored injection protocols with exponentially decelerated profiles [8].

One advantage CMR holds over cardiac CT for myocardial function is the ability to obtain excellent contrast for both RV and LV quantification in the same examination. Further investigations will determine how to reliably achieve sufficient contrast in both ventricles with CT. This has important implications in the growing population of adult congenital heart disease patients, where CT holds the promise of providing comprehensive non-invasive assessment of right heart structures along with the ageing coronary arteries.

Suspected pulmonary thromboembolism (PE) represents a common clinical scenario requiring CT examination where RV function holds prognostic importance. Even the simple transverse plane RV to LV diameter ratio is useful to predict outcomes with pulmonary emboli [56]. The positive predictive value for PE related mortality with an RV/LV ratio greater than 1.0 was 10.1% (95% confidence interval [CI]: 2.9%, 17.4%). The negative predictive value for an uneventful outcome with an RV/LV ratio of 1.0 or less was 100% (95% CI: 94.3%, 100%). There was an 11.2-fold increased risk of dying of PE for patients with an obstruction index (% of pulmonary artery cross-section obliterated by embolus) of 40% or higher (95% CI: 1.3, 93.6) [56–59].

Coche *et al.* studied 10 patients suspected of having PE, four with actual PE, by CT angiography, with both 16-slice gated CT and equilibrium radionuclide imaging, calculating RV and LV ejection fractions with both techniques [59]. In this hemo-dynamically stable group, CT tended to overestimate RV systolic function compared to radionuclide gated blood pool studies. Further studies, as have been done with echocardiography, are warranted to demonstrate the clinical utility of RVEF by CT in the acute evaluation of patients with pulmonary thromboembolic disease.

Left and right ventricular diastolic function: Diastolic function is an important phenomenon with significant clinical applications. Time-volume curves can be generated with any modality producing multiphase contiguous short-axis images, including cardiac CT. Temporal resolution of 5% of each cardiac cycle can be used to derive accurate early and late ventricular filling curves and peak filling rates and time to peak filling measurements.

Non-ischemic cardiomyopathies: Late postgadolinium imaging with CMR, also termed delayed myocardial enhancement (DME), has emerged as an excellent technique to distinguish ischemic from non-ischemic cardiomyopathy [60]. However, patients with cardiomyopathy increasingly have implantable cardiac devices, particularly in the era of resynchronization therapy, which preclude examination with magnetic resonance. Simultaneous ability to evaluate ventricular function and coronary artery anatomy with cardiac CT may be useful in such instances.

Several authors have documented cases of arrythmogenic right ventricular dysplasia with cardiac CT using both electron beam and multidetector scanners [61–63]. The characteristic findings of scalloping of the anterior wall of the RV, fatty infiltration of the RV myocardium, and regional RV wall motion abnormalities all appear readily on thin-slice gated cardiac CT imaging (Fig. 9.5). Occasionally, unusual causes of cardiomyopathy such as ventricular non-compaction may be detected by careful examination of myocardial morphology on reformatted CT images (Fig. 9.6).

Atrial evaluation: Right and left atrial anatomy and volumes may be evaluated with contrast enhanced CT [64]. Pulmonary vein anatomy is useful for planning electrophysiology ablation procedures [65, 66]. Occasionally, atrial thrombus may be detected. Atrial tumors and anomalous pulmonary veins are uncommon, but important findings, that are routinely searched for on routine cardiac CT studies.

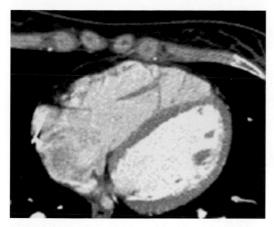

Fig. 9.5 Arrhythmogenic right ventricular cardiomyopathy by cardiac CT with dilatation and increased RV trabeculations. Note the presence of a pacemaker lead precluding CMR examination in this case.

Perfusion and viability

Epicardial coronary artery disease is significant only to the extent that it impairs delivery of blood to viable cardiac myocytes. Myocardial perfusion can be visualized with invasive coronary angiography [67], contrast echocardiography, nuclear scintigraphy, or magnetic resonance imaging. Resting perfusion abnormalities may be helpful in evaluating patients presenting with acute chest pain or anginal equivalent and no known history of CAD; however, detection of myocardial ischemia requires comparison

of perfusion at rest to perfusion with exercise or pharmacological stress. Particularly in patients with obstructive CAD with left ventricular systolic dysfunction, measurement of myocardial viability with well validated techniques such as rest-redistribution thallium imaging or DME-CMR can predict the likelihood of recovery of function with revascularization [68, 69]. While limited studies have shown promise for myocardial perfusion [70, 71] and viability assessment with CT, much work remains to be done to demonstrate the validity, accuracy, and predictive value of CT-based myocardial perfusion assessment.

Experimentally produced acute ischemia in dogs is readily detected *in vivo* by dynamic CT imaging as absent or markedly reduced myocardial contrast enhancement [72–74]. Because CT attenuation is directly proportional to iodine concentration, dynamic contrast enhanced CT has the potential for quantitation [75]. Based on 169 regional measurements in five dogs at rest and during hyperperfusion induced by chromonar, EBCT and microsphere-determined flows correlated moderately ($r = 0.68$) over a range of 0.4–8 mL/min/g [76]. However, when the data were divided into resting and hyperperfusion, (i.e. 20–30 min after the injection of the chromonar) states, a significant (P less than .001) increase in regional flow was determined from the EBCT measurements. The authors concluded that EBCT can distinguish between low and high

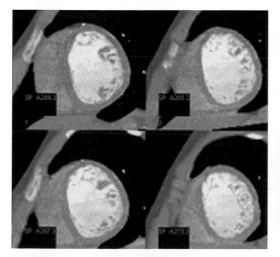

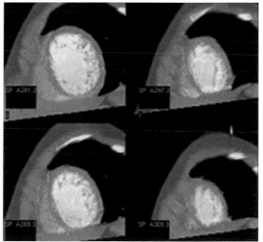

Fig. 9.6 A case of non-compaction of the LV myocardium diagnosed in a 14-year-old male undergoing CTA to exclude obstructive coronary artery disease as the etiology for new onset left ventricular dysfunction. Note in this set of short axis frames the characteristic spongy appearance of the LV endocardial surface.

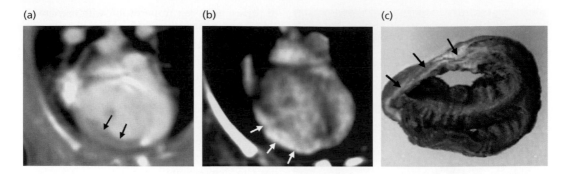

(a)   (b)   (c)

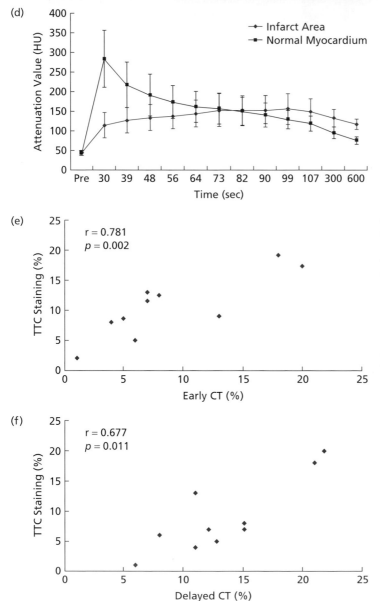

(d)

Fig. 9.7 Rabbit model coronary artery ligated-reperfused myocardial infarction, with sequential contrast enhanced CT. Infarct demonstrates early decreased enhancement and late increased enhancement. Early phase CT obtained at 27 s following administration of contrast material (a) showed hypoenhancement (arrows) and 10-min-delayed image (b) showed hyperenhancement (arrows) in the anterior wall compared with normal myocardium. 2'3'5-triphenyl tetrazolium chloride-stained specimen obtained at four weeks after coronary artery occlusion and reperfusion (c) shows damaged myocardium (arrows) as a TCC-unstained area with wall thinning. (d) is a data plot of CT attenuation value (HU) vs delay time (seconds) for normal myocardium and experimentally infarcted-reperfused myocardium. Plots of TCC% stain vs CT% abnormality for early (e) and late (f) imaging demonstrate histological correlation. (Figure reproduced with permission from: Reference 83, Park JM, Choe YH, Chang S *et al.* Usefulness of multidetector-row CT in the evaluation of reperfused myocardial infarction in a rabbit model. *Korean J Radiol* 2004; **5**: 19–24.)

myocardial flow states in dogs, with considerable potential for evaluating coronary flow reserve [76]. Initial animal data in a coronary ligation model [77, 78] with CT imaging and tissue analysis [79] was controversial [80, 81], leaving CT myocardial perfusion imaging less well defined when compared to the careful *ex vivo* correlative studies that have provided histopathological validity for delayed myocardial enhancement CMR [82] techniques. Detailed investigations have been done with radioisotopes and gadolinium chelates, quantifying their first pass and redistribution effects. Recently, Park *et al.* [83] have investigated the pharmacokinetics of CT contrast agents in a coronary artery ligation-reperfusion rabbit model with 2′3′5-triphenyl tetrazolium chloride (TTC) staining (Fig. 9.7a–d). They demonstrated correlation coefficients of $r = 0.781$ for early and $r = 0.677$ for late contrast enhanced reperfused infarction (Fig. 9.7e and Fig. 9.7f). Several small studies, which included other *in vivo* methods, suggest potential utility of perfusion abnormalities identified with CT. One study of 12 patients with anterior myocardial infarction compared perfusion defects by EBCT to Tc-sestamibi scintigraphy, and found that the two modalities correlated well over a range of infarct sizes [84], though EBCT may underestimate infarct size [85, 86]. More recently, 30 subjects who had undergone 16-detector CT as well as CMR including both DME and stress perfusion acquisitions were studied retrospectively [87]. CT performed well in delineating infarcts (Fig. 9.8), again underestimating infarct size, with an overall sensitivity of 91%, specificity of 79%, and accuracy of 83%. As expected, resting defects alone on CT performed poorly compared to adenosine stress CMR in identifying ischemia (sensitivity 50%).

Mahnken *et al.* have described a dual-phase technique where the late postcontrast cardiac CT acquisition is performed with additional but lower radiation dose compared to the initial full-dose angiogram; no additional contrast was administered beyond the 120 cc for the full-dose angiogram [88]. They tested this technique in 28 patients with reperfused myocardial infarction, all with their first infarct treated successfully with single vessel percutaneous revascularization. Fifteen-minute postgadolinium standard DME CMR images were compared to 15 min postcontrast CT examination using 16-slice MSCT, at 80 kVp, with an effective tube

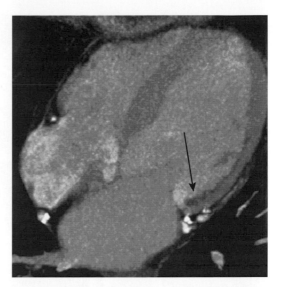

Fig. 9.8 Subendocardial perfusion defect involving the basal anterolateral wall of the left ventricle (arrow).

current-time product of 500 effective millampere-seconds (mAs_{eff}). CT axial images were reconstructed with a medium smooth convolution kernel (B30f), effective slice thickness of 1.0 mm, and an increment of 0.6 mm at 60% of the RR interval. Comparable to short axis DME images, 8-mm short axis multiplanar reformats were generated from the axial data set (Fig. 9.9). The results with first-pass perfusion defect on initial contrast CT acquisition showed poor agreement with DME CMR (kappa = 0.64), but late enhancement CT correlated well with DME CMR (kappa = 0.88). Paul *et al.* performed a comparison between 5 min postcontrast CT imaging with SPECT imaging and reported sensitivity, specificity, and overall accuracy in detecting residual defects in 34 patients with reperfused MI of 93%, 100%, and 94% [89].

The techniques described to identify perfusion abnormalities with cardiac CT vary, though the most clinically applicable technique simply uses data acquired during standard coronary CT examination reformatted to various LV long axis and short axis planes [89]. There is limited clinical data with respect to the optimal timing of contrast administration to maximize accuracy of CT-based detection of LV myocardial perfusion abnormalities. This will be helpful, given evidence from several studies suggesting underestimation of infarct size by CT. One group in Japan has described early defects (ED),

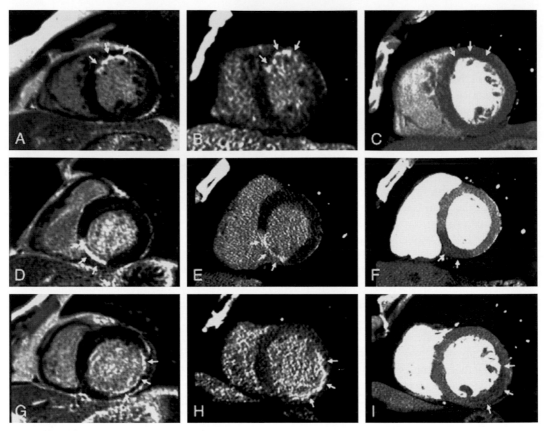

Fig. 9.9 DME-CMR infarct imaging (A, D, G) compared to late enhancement CT imaging (B, E, H) and initial CT imaging of perfusion abnormalities (C, F, I). (Figure re-printed from: Reference 88, Mahnken AH, Koos R, Katoh M *et al.* Assessment of myocardial viability in reperfused acute myocardial infarction using 16-slice computed tomography in comparison to magnetic resonance imaging. *J Am Coll Cardiol* 2005; **45**: 2042–2047. Reprinted with permission from the American College of Cardiology Foundation, 2005.)

residual defects (RD), and late enhancement (LE) by dual-phase imaging acquired at 45 s as well as 7 min after initial acquisitions with additional contrast infusion (Fig. 9.10) [51, 90]. Of 58 patients with acute myocardial infarction studied acutely and one-year postrevascularization, absence of any defect predicted best systolic function at follow-up. Presence of residual defects portended the worst LVEF, while wall thickness decreased more significantly for patients with early defects compared to those without ED. Concerns about double radiation dose may limit greater use of this dual-imaging CT technique, particularly with availability of other well validated viability assessment modalities such as PET and DME-CMR.

The reported good test performance to detect myocardial scar among 5 min, 7 min, and 15 min postcontrast CT acquisition protocols is intriguing, particularly given the careful inversion time selection required for DME-CMR imaging based on dynamic T1 properties of infarcted versus normal myocardium. None the less, the optimal timing for "late" postcontrast CT imaging for myocardial infarct detection has yet to be determined.

In summary, the volumetric nature of image acquisition with cardiac CT allows accurate measurement of ventricular size and function, particularly as this information complements the coronary anatomy not available non-invasively with any other imaging modality. Preliminary data suggest that cardiac CT images reformatted in the left ventricular long axis and short axis planes may be useful in identifying regions of myocardial infarction and non-viability. Further studies are needed to demon-

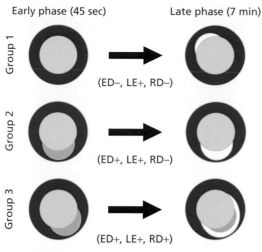

Early phase (45 sec)   **Late phase (7 min)**

Group 1 — (ED–, LE+, RD–)

Group 2 — (ED+, LE+, RD–)

Group 3 — (ED+, LE+, RD+)

Fig. 9.10 Early versus late phase CT imaging demonstrates perfusion defects and scar, respectively, in patients with myocardial infarction. ED = early defect; LE = late enhancement; RD = residual defect. Group 1 (ED–, LE+, RD–) – reperfused infarct; Group 2 (ED+, LE+, RD–) = reperfused infarct with resting perfusion defect; Group 3 (ED–, LE+, RD–) = reperfused infarct with microvascular occlusion. (Figure reproduced with permission from: Reference 51, Koyama Y, Matsuoka H, Mochizuki T *et al.* Assessment of reperfused acute myocardial infarction with two-phase contrast-enhanced helical CT: Prediction of left ventricular function and wall thickness. *Radiology* 2005; **235**: 804–811.)

strate validity compared to histopathological and clinical analysis as well as to provide multicenter data regarding prognostic value and reproducibility.

References

1. Desjardins B, Kazerooni. EA ECG-gated cardiac CT. *Am J Roentgenol* 2004; **182**: 993–1010.
2. Boyd DB. Computerized transmission tomography of the heart using scanning electron beams. In: Higgins CH, ed. *Computed Tomography of the Heart and Great Vessels*. Futura Publishing Company, Mount Kisco, New York, 1983: 45–55.
3. Newhouse JH. Fluid compartment distribution of intravenous iothalamate in the dog. *Invest Radiol* 1977; **12**: 364–367.
4. Newhouse JH, Murphy RX. Tissue distribution of soluble contrast: Effect of dose variation and changes with time. *Am J Roentgenol* 1981; **136**: 463–467.
5. Cademartiri F, Mollet N, van der Lugt A *et al.* Non-invasive 16-row multislice CT coronary angiography: Usefulness of saline chaser. *Eur Radiol* 2004; **14**: 178–183.
6. Awai K, Hiraishi K, Hori S. Effect of contrast material injection duration and rate on aortic peak time and peak enhancement at dynamic ct involving injection protocol with dose tailored to patient weight. *Radiology* 2004; **230**: 142–150.
7. Cademartiri F, Nieman K, van der Lugt A *et al.* Intravenous contrast material administration at 16-detector row helical CT coronary angiography: Test bolus versus bolus-tracking technique. *Radiology* 2004; **233**: 817–823.
8. Bae KT, Tran HQ, Heiken JP. Uniform vascular contrast enhancement and reduced contrast medium volume achieved by using exponentially decelerated contrast material injection method. *Radiology* 2004; **231**: 732–736.
9. Cohnen M, Poll LW, Püttmann C *et al.* Radiation exposure in multislice CT of the heart. *RöFo Fortschr Röntgenstr* 2001; **173**: 295–299.
10. Gerber TC, Kuzo RS, Morin RL. Techniques and parameters for estimating radiation exposure and dose in cardiac computed tomography. *Int J Cardiovasc Imaging* 2005; **21**: 165–176.
11. Hunold P, Vogt FM, Schmermund A *et al.* Radiation exposure during cardiac CT: Effective doses at multi-detector row CT and electron-beam CT. *Radiology* 2003; **226**: 145–152.
12. Becker CR, Schätzl M, Feist H *et al.* Estimation of the effective dose applied by routine investigation of the chest, heart and abdomen with conventional CT, electron-beam tomography and coronary angiography. *RöFo Fortschr Röntgenstr* 1999; **170**: 99–104 (in German).
13. Wisser G, Lehmann KJ, Scheck R *et al.* Dose and image quality of electron-beam CT compared with spiral CT. *Invest Radiol* 1999; **34**: 415–420.
14. Trabold T, Buchgeister M, Kuttner A *et al.* Estimation of radiation exposure in 16-detector row computed tomography of the heart with retrospective ECG-gating. *Rofo* 2003; **175**:1051–1055.
15. Jung B, Mahnken AH, Stargardt A *et al.* Individually weight-adapted examination protocol in retrospectively ECG-gated MSCT of the heart. *Eur Radiol* 2003; **13**: 2560–2566.
16. Morin RL, Gerber TC, McCollough CH. Radiation dose in computed tomography of the heart. *Circulation* 2003; **107**: 917–922.
17. Morin RL, Gerber TC, McCollough CH. Physics and dosimetry in computed tomography. *Cardiol Clin* 2003; **21**: 515–520.
18. Mochizuki T, Higashino H, Koyama Y *et al.* Clinical usefulness of the cardiac multi-detector-row CT. *Comput Med Imaging Graph* 2003; **27**: 35–42.
19. Jakobs TF, Becker CR, Ohnesorge B *et al.* Multislice helical CT of the heart with retrospective ECG gating: Reduction of radiation exposure by ECG-controlled tube current modulation. *Eur Radiol* 2002; **12**: 1081–1086.

20. Poll LW, Cohnen M, Brachten S *et al*. Dose reduction in multislice CT of the heart by use of ECG-controlled tube current modulation ("ECG pulsing"): Phantom measurements. *Rofo Fortschr Geb Rontgenstr Neuen Bildgeb Verfahr* 2002; **174**: 1500–1505.

21. Mahnken AH, Katoh M, Bruners P *et al*. Acute myocardial infarction: assessment of left ventricular function with 16-detector row spiral CT versus MR imaging—study in pigs. *Radiology* 2005; **236**: 112–117.

22. Lawler LP, Ney D, Pannu HK *et al*. Four-dimensional imaging of the heart based on near-isotropic MDCT data sets. *AJR and AJR Online* 2005; **184**: 774–776, **http://www.ajronline.org/**

23. Pfeffer MA, Braunwald E. Ventricular remodeling after myocardial infarction. Experimental observations and clinical implications. *Circulation* 1990; **81**: 1161–1172.

24. White HD, Norris RM, Brown MA *et al*. Left ventricular end-systolic volume as the major determinant of survival after recovery from myocardial infarction. *Circulation* 1987; **76**: 44–51.

25. Moss AJ, Hall WJ, Cannom DS *et al*. Improved survival with an implanted defibrillator in patients with coronary disease at high risk for ventricular arrhythmia. Multicenter Automatic Defibrillator Implantation Trial investigators. *N Engl J Med* 1996; **335**: 1933–1940.

26. Schuijf JD, Bax JJ, Jukema JW *et al*. Non-invasive angiography and assessment of left ventricular function using multislice computed tomography in patients with type 2 diabetes. *Diabetes Care* 2004; **27**: 2905–2910.

27. Germano GG, Berman DS, eds. *Quantitative Gated Perfusion SPECT*. Futura Publishing Company, Inc., Armonk, NY, 1999.

28. Green MV, Bacharach SL. Functional imaging of the heart: methods, limitations and examples from gated blood pool scintigraphy. *Prog Cardiovasc Dis* 1986; **28**: 319–348.

29. Raman SV, Shah M, McCarthy B *et al*. AK. Multidetector row cardiac CT accurately quantifies right and left ventricular size and function compared to cardiac magnetic resonance. *Am Heart J* 2005, in press.

30. Böhm T, Alkadhi H, Roffi M *et al*. Time-effectiveness, observer-dependence, and accuracy of measurements of left ventricular ejection fraction using 4-channel MDCT. *RöFo Fortschr Röntgenstr* 2004; **176**: 529–537.

31. Dirksen MS, Bax JJ, de Roos A *et al*. Usefulness of dynamic multislice computed tomography of left ventricular function in unstable angina pectoris and comparison to echocardiography. *Am J Cardiol* 2002; **90**: 1157–1160.

32. Ehrhard K, Oberholzer K, Gast K *et al*. Multislice CT (MSCT) in cardiac function imaging: Threshold-value-supported 3D volume reconstructions to determine the left ventricular ejection fraction in comparison to MRI. *RöFo Fortschr Röntgenstr* 2002; **174**: 1566–1569.

33. Grude M, Juergens KU, Wichter T *et al*. Evaluation of global left ventricular myocardial function with electrocardiogram-gated multidetector computed tomography: comparison with magnetic resonance imaging. *Invest Radiol* 2003; **38**: 653–661.

34. Heuschmid M, Küttner A, Schröder S *et al*. Left ventricular functional parameters using ECG-gated multidetector spiral CT in comparison with invasive ventriculography. *RöFo Fortschr Röntgenstr* 2003; **175**: 1349–1354.

35. Hundt W, Siebert K, Wintersperger BJ *et al*. Assessment of global left ventricular function: Comparison of cardiac multidetector-row computed tomography with angiocardiography. *J Comput Assist Tomogr* 2005; **29**: 373–381.

36. Juergens KU, Grude M, Fallenberg EM *et al*. Using ECG-gated multidetector CT to evaluate global left ventricular myocardial function in patients with coronary artery disease. *AJR* 2002; **179**: 1545–1550.

37. Juergens KU, Grude M, Maintz D *et al*. Multidetector row CT of left ventricular function with dedicated analysis software versus MR imaging: Initial experience. *Radiology* 2004; **230**: 403–410.

38. Juergens KU, Maintz D, Grude M *et al*. Multidetector row computed tomography of the heart: Does a multisegment reconstruction algorithm improve left ventricular volume measurements? *Eur Radiol* 2005; **15**: 111–117.

39. Koch K, Oellig F, Kunz P *et al*. Assessment of global and regional left ventricular function with a 16-slice spiral-CT using two different software tools for quantitative functional analysis and qualitative evaluation of wall motion changes in comparison with magnetic resonance imaging. *RöFo Fortschr Röntgenstr* 2004; **176**: 1786–1793 (in German).

40. Mahnken AH, Henzler D, Klotz E *et al*. Determination of cardiac output with multislice spiral computed tomography: A validation study. *Invest Radiol* 2004; **39**: 451–454.

41. Mahnken AH, Koos R, Katoh M *et al*. Sixteen-slice spiral CT versus MR imaging for the assessment of left ventricular function in acute myocardial infarction. *Eur Radiol* 2005; **15**: 714–720.

42. Mahnken AH, Spüntrup E, Wildberger JE *et al*. Quantification of cardiac function with multislice spiral CT using retrospective ECG-gating: comparison with MRI. *RöFo Fortschr Röntgenstr* 2003; **175**: 83–88 (in German).

43. Schlosser T, Pagonidis K, Herborn CU *et al*. Assessment of left ventricular parameters using 16-MDCT and new software for endocardial and epicardial border delineation. *AJR* 2005; **184**: 765–773.

44. Schuijf JD, Bax JJ, Salm LP *et al*. Non-invasive coronary imaging and assessment of left ventricular function using 16-slice computed tomography. *Am J Cardiol* 2005; **95**: 571–574.

45. Halliburton S, Petersilka M, Schvartzman PR *et al.* Evaluation of left ventricular dysfunction using multiphasic reconstructions of coronary multislice computed tomography data in patients with chronic ischemic heart disease: Validation against cine magnetic resonance imaging. *Int J Cardiovasc Imaging* 2003; **19**: 73–83.

46. Pujadas S, Reddy GP, Weber O *et al.* MR imaging assessment of cardiac function. *J Magn Reson Imaging* 2004; **19**: 789–799.

47. Kim TH, Hur J, Kim SJ *et al.* Two-phase reconstruction for the assessment of left ventricular volume and function using retrospective ECG-Gated MDCT: Comparison with echocardiography. *Am J Roentgenol* 2005; **185**: 319–325.

48. Reiter SJ, Rumberger JA, Stanford W *et al.* Quantitative determination of aortic regurgitant volumes in dogs by ultrafast computed tomography. *Circulation* 1987; **76**: 728–735.

49. Feiring AJ, Rumberger JA, Skorton SM *et al.* Determination of left ventricular mass in the dog with rapid acquisition cardiac CT scanning. *Circulation* 1985; **72**: 1355–1364.

50. Feiring AJ, Rumberger JA. Ultrafast computed tomography analysis of regional radius-to-wall thickness ratios in normal and volume overloaded human left ventricle. *Circulation* 1992; **85**: 1423–1432.

51. Koyama Y, Matsuoka H, Mochizuki T *et al.* Assessment of reperfused acute myocardial infarction with two-phase contrast-enhanced helical CT: Prediction of left ventricular function and wall thickness. *Radiology* 2005; **235**: 804–811.

52. Raman S, Cook S, McCarthy M *et al.* Usefulness of multidetector row computed tomography to quantify right ventricular size and function in adults with either tetralogy of Fallot or transposition of the great arteries. *Am J Cardiol* 2005; **95**: 683–686.

53. Helbing W, Rebergen S, Maliepaard C *et al.* Quantification of right ventricular function with magnetic resonance imaging in children with normal hearts and with congenital heart disease. *Am Heart J* 1995; **30**: 828–837.

54. Elgeti T, Lembcke A, Enzweiler CN *et al.* Comparison of electron beam computed tomography with magnetic resonance imaging in assessment of right ventricular volumes and function. *J Comput Assist Tomogr* 2004; **28**: 679–685.

55. Koch K, Oellig F, Oberholzer K *et al.* Assessment of right ventricular function by 16-detector-row CT: comparison with magnetic resonance imaging. *Eur Radiol* 2005; **15**: 312–318.

56. Van der Meer RW, Pattynama PMT, van Strijen MJL *et al.* Right ventricular dysfunction and pulmonary obstruction index at helical CT: Prediction of clinical outcome during 3-month follow-up in patients with acute pulmonary embolism. *Radiology* 2005; **235**: 798–803.

57. Mansencal N, Joseph T, Vieillard-Baron A *et al.* Diagnosis of right ventricular dysfunction in acute pulmonary embolism using helical computed tomography. *Am J Cardiol* 2005; **95**: 1260–1263.

58. Quiroz R, Kucher N, Schoepf UJ *et al.* Right ventricular enlargement on chest computed tomography: Prognostic role in acute pulmonary embolism. *Circulation* 2004; **109**: 2401–2404.

59. Coche E, Vlassenbroek A, Roelants V *et al.* Evaluation of biventricular ejection fraction with ECG-gated 16-slice CT: Preliminary findings in acute pulmonary embolism in comparison with radionuclide ventriculography. *Eur Radiol* 2005; **15**: 1432–1440.

60. McCrohon JA, Moon JCC, Prasad SK *et al.* Differentiation of heart failure related to dilated cardiomyopathy and coronary artery disease using gadolinium-enhanced cardiovascular magnetic resonance. *Circulation* 2003; **108**: 54–59.

61. Tada H, Shimizu W, Ohe T *et al.* Usefulness of electron-beam computed tomography in arrhythmogenic right ventricular dysplasia. Relationship to electrophysiological abnormalities and left ventricular involvement. *Circulation* 1996; **94**: 437–444.

62. Tandri H, Bomma C, Calkins H *et al.* Magnetic resonance and computed tomography imaging of arrhythmogenic right ventricular dysplasia. *J Magn Reson Imaging* 2004; **19**: 848–858.

63. Robles P, Olmedilla P, Jimenez JJ. Sixteen row cardiac computed tomography in the diagnosis of arrhythmogenic right ventricular cardiomyopathy. *Heart* 2005; **91**: 718.

64. Lawler LP, Fishman EK. Multidetector row CT of thoracic disease with emphasis on 3D volume rendering and CT angiography. *RadioGraphics* 2001; **21**: 1257–1273.

65. Schwartzman D, Lacomis J, Wigginton W. Characterization of left atrium and distal pulmonary vein morphology using multidimensional computed tomography. *J Am Coll Cardiol* 2003; **41**: 1349–1357.

66. Lacomis JM, Wigginton W, Fuhrman C *et al.* Multidetector row CT of the left atrium and pulmonary veins before radio frequency catheter ablation for atrial fibrillation. *RadioGraphics* 2003; **23**: 35–48.

67. Gibson CM, Cannon CP, Murphy SA *et al.* Relationship of TIMI myocardial perfusion grade to mortality after administration of thrombolytic drugs. *Circulation* 2000; **101**: 125–30.

68. Kim RJ, Wu E, Rafael A *et al.* The use of contrast enhanced magnetic resonance imaging to identify reversible myocardial dysfunction. *N Engl J Med.* 2000; **343**: 1445–1453.

69. Chareonthaitawee P, Gersh BJ, Araoz PA *et al.* Revascularization in severe left ventricular dysfunction: The role of viability testing. *J Am Coll Cardiol* 2005; **46**: 567–574.

70. Hessel SJ, Adams DF, Judy PF *et al.* Detection of myocardial ischemia *in vitro* by computed tomography. *Radiology* 1978; **127**: 413–418.

71. Bell MR, Lerman LO, Rumberger JA. Validation of minimally invasive measurement of myocardial perfusion using electron beam computed tomography and application in human volunteers. *Heart* 1999; **81**: 628–635.

72. Cipriano PR, Nassi M, Ricci MT *et al.* Acute myocardial ischemia detected *in vivo* by computed tomography. *Radiology* 1981; **140**: 727–731.

73. Rumberger JA, Feiring AJ, Lipton MJ *et al.* Use of ultrafast computed tomography to quantitate regional myocardial perfusion: A preliminary report. *J Am Coll Cardiol* 1987; **9**: 59–69.

74. Wolfkiel CJ, Ferguson JL, Chomka EV *et al.* Measurement of myocardial blood flow by ultrafast computed tomography. *Circulation* 1987; **76**: 1262–1273.

75. Weiss RM, Otoadese EA, Noel MP *et al.* Quantitation of absolute regional perfusion using cine computed tomography. *J Am Coll Cardiol* 1994; **23**: 1186–1193.

76. Gould RG, Lipton MJ, McNamara MT *et al.* Measurement of regional myocardial blood flow in dogs by ultrafast CT. *Invest Radiol* 1987; **23**: 348–353.

77. Gray WR Jr, Parkey RW, Buja LM *et al.* Computed tomography: *In vitro* evaluation of myocardial infarction. *Radiology* 1977; **122**: 511–513.

78. Higgins CB, Siemers PT, Schmidt W *et al.* Evaluation of myocardial ischemic damage of various ages by computerized transmission tomography. Time-dependent effects of contrast material. *Circulation* 1979; **60**: 284–291.

79. Fishbein MC, Meerbaum S, Rit J *et al.* Early phase acute myocardial infarct size quantification: Validation of the triphenyl tetrazolium chloride tissue enzyme staining technique. *Am Heart J* 1981; **101**: 593–600.

80. Slutsky RA, Peck WW, Mancini GB *et al.* Myocardial infarct size determined by computed transmission tomography in canine infarcts of various ages and in the presence of coronary reperfusion. *J Am Coll Cardiol* 1984; **3**: 138–142.

81. Retraction of two additional papers by Robert A Slutsky, M.D. *J Am Coll Cardiol* 1987; **9**: 973.

82. Kim RJ, Fieno DS, Parrish TB *et al.* Relationship of MRI delayed contrast enhancement to irreversible injury, infarct age, and contractile function. *Circulation* 1999; **100**: 1992–2002.

83. Park JM, Choe YH, Chang S *et al.* Usefulness of multidetector-row CT in the evaluation of reperfused myocardial infarction in a rabbit model. *Korean J Radiol* 2004; **5**: 19–24.

84. Schmermund A, Gerber T, Behrenbeck T *et al.* Measurement of myocardial infarct size by electron beam computed tomography: A comparison with ^{99m}Tc sestamibi. *Invest Radiol* 1998; **33**: 313–321.

85. Hilfiker PR, Weishaupt D, Marincek B. Multislice spiral computed tomography of subacute myocardial infarction. *Circulation* 2001; **104**: 1083.

86. Mochizuki T, Murase K, Higashino H *et al.* Demonstration of acute myocardial infarction by subsecond spiral computed tomography: Early defect and delayed enhancement. *Circulation* 1999; **99**: 2058–2059.

87. Nikolaou K, Sanz J, Poon M *et al.* Assessment of myocardial perfusion and viability from routine contrast enhanced 16-detector-row computed tomography of the heart: preliminary results. *Eur Radiol* 2005; **15**: 864–871.

88. Mahnken AH, Koos R, Katoh M *et al.* Assessment of myocardial viability in reperfused acute myocardial infarction using 16-slice computed tomography in comparison to magnetic resonance imaging. *J Am Coll Cardiol* 2005; **45**: 2042–2047.

89. Paul J-F, Wartski M, Caussin C *et al.* Late defect on delayed contrast enhanced multidetector row CT scans in the prediction of SPECT infarct size after reperfused acute myocardial infarction: Initial experience. *Radiology* 2005; **236**: 485–489.

90. Koyama Y, Mochizuki T, Higaki J. Computed tomography assessment of myocardial perfusion, viability, and function. *J Magn Reson Imaging* 2004; **19**: 800–815.

PART III

Concurrent noninvasive assessment of coronary anatomy, physiology, and myocellular integrity

CHAPTER 10

PET and MRI in cardiac imaging

Stephan G. Nekolla

Introduction

Magnetic resonance imaging (MRI) and positron emission tomography (PET) were developed around the same time. Since their development, however, they have taken very different paths with respect to their transition from research systems to commercial success. Without any doubt, the clinical use of computerised tomography (CT) and MRI surpasses PET by far. However, the introduction of combined PET/CT devices in 1998 [1, 2], together with a change in the reimbursement policy in the USA, resulted in an increased interest in PET. Within three years, PET/CT scanner sales rose from 0% to 85% of all sales [3], showing the demand for a system which provides high sensitivity for biological processes combined with the assessment of morphological structures.

Although this development was primarily driven by oncological applications, one could speculate that cardiac imaging with MRI and PET combined would also profit from a similar approach. Each of these modalities provides a powerful means for cardiovascular applications in research and clinical routine, a fact that is obvious and well documented [4, 5] and which will not be repeated here in detail.

But the technical issues arising from combining PET and CT into one system are minor compared to those from combining PET and MRI, because of the current detector modules' inability to operate in magnetic fields larger than 10 mT. There is, however, enough evidence in the literature to indicate the attractiveness of a combined MRI and PET cardiac imaging approach to support the development of such a system. In the following, an overview of combined PET/MRI imaging is presented in four steps. It starts with validation studies, where essen-

tially one modality uses the other as a reference (and indicating that there is the eventual potential to replace it). Then, projects are presented where the focus is on synergetic use of MRI and PET. In two methodological sections, software based co-registration solutions and their limitations are discussed. Finally, the current status of hardware-based solutions is summarized.

Use of PET and MRI in validation studies

By far the greatest number of validation studies conducted focus on the use of MRI and PET in the same patients, which is the most widespread use of MRI and PET. Three large fields of applications can be identified. The first area is the myocardial perfusion scan, which provides vital information regarding cardiac pathophysiology and is performed clinically in very large numbers. There is great interest in the possibility of such scans being performed with MRI. Accordingly, there are several papers validating MRI-derived perfusion using first-pass extraction techniques and comparing the relative or absolute flow values with PET. A second group of studies utilize PET as the gold standard in viability imaging, in order to identify hibernating or stunned myocardium treatable with revascularization procedures. Here, MRI delayed enhancement scans are performed, identifying scar tissue. These results are evaluated against results from a PET assessment with fluorodeoxyglucose (FDG) as marker of maintained cell integrity. Because of its efficient collection and assessment with no additional examination time required, the assessment of global and regional function with gated PET acquisitions makes up the third significant area of research. In this area, MRI provides a precise reference with excellent spatial and temporal resolution. Very similar studies were also performed using single photon emission tomography (SPECT) techniques, which enabled the assessment of wall motion and provided a means of avoiding or at least limiting attenuation artifacts.

Perfusion studies

The non-invasive, regional, quantitative assessment of myocardial blood flow in the left ventricle was the exclusive domain of PET [6–8] until the early 90s, when MRI challenged this position. First-pass perfusion studies using contrast agent enhanced, dynamic MR imaging with gadolinium diethylene-triamine pentaacetic acid (Gd-DTPA) were employed, demonstrating its technical feasibility in animal studies with microspheres [9, 10]. In humans, several comparative validation studies of this approach and PET were reported. However, a key problem in MR perfusion studies was the input function (describing the arterial delivery of tracer to the myocardial tissue), which was frequently distorted. The assumption of a linear relationship between signal intensity and tracer concentration holds true only for low concentrations; in nearly all imaging protocols, the actual concentration of contrast agents during the first bolus passage through the cardiac chambers is relatively high and, thus, produces unreliable results. Consequently, the aforementioned validation studies relied mostly on semi-quantitative measurements and calculated indices for the delineation of myocardial blood flow and flow reserve. Currently, technical solutions for this problem are under development; in clinical practice, however, a visual analysis of the dynamic sequences is mostly used.

As an alternative to the invasive assessment of coronary flow reserve (CFR) with intracoronary Doppler guidewires (which was validated against regional PET flow measurements in 1996 [11]), Hofman *et al.* suggested measuring intracoronary flow without the use of contrast agent, using phase contrast velocity imaging [12]. Similarly, Sakuma and colleagues [13] suggested using a breath-hold velocity encoded cine sequence as an alternative. Both methods were validated later against PET flow measurements. Phase contrast MRI in the coronary sinus was applied in sixteen healthy volunteers and

nine patients with orthotopic heart transplants and compared against ^{13}N-ammonia PET [14]. A high correlation was found between regional myocardial blood flows in the left ventricle obtained by PET and the MR derived absolute flow in the coronary sinus.

In a later study, Sakuma and colleagues measured the blood flow velocity in the proximal portion of the left anterior descending artery under resting and stress conditions and calculated flow reserve. In ten normal volunteers, results were compared to data from O-15 water PET studies and a significant correlation was observed [15]. However, neither of these two implementations were applied in clinical practice, despite their ability to assess absolute myocardial blood flow under rest and stress conditions. Instead, techniques focusing on the measurement of truly regional flow reserve indices were favoured. Manning and colleagues demonstrated in the early 1990s that dynamic MR imaging during first-pass extraction of paramagnetic contrast agents was capable of detecting coronary artery disease (CAD) in patients [10]. Since then, several validation studies using a variety of imaging techniques have been published and are discussed in previous chapters of this book. To date, only a few publications have correlated the MRI derived flow values against quantitative PET data. One study compared ^{13}N-ammonia PET and MRI, using a pixel wise upslope parameter as flow index of the signal intensity curve during contrast media passage. This study, performed on 18 healthy subjects and 48 patients, revealed a good correlation between the number of pathological segments per patient (PET CFR threshold: 1.65, MR threshold: derived from mean normal upslope values in rest and stress studies individually) and high accuracy when implementing PET as reference in a receiver operating characteristic (ROC) analysis (sensitivity 91%, specificity 94%). In a subsequent study, which added a direct comparison of flow reserve values, it was found that the coronary flow reserve as assessed by first-pass extraction MRI is significantly underestimated (Fig. 10.1) [16]. Because of the reduced extraction of Gd-DTPA during high myocardial blood flows, there is a substantial "roll off" as is known from SPECT radiopharmaceuticals [17, 18]. This resulted in a relatively low MRI threshold of 1.3 for the CFR as compared to a PET

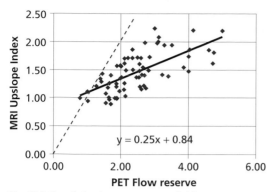

Fig. 10.1 Correlation between myocardial flow reserve as assessed with dynamic ^{13}N-ammonia versus semiquantitative flow reserve index from dynamic MRI imaging with Gd-DTPA bolus injection (upslope stress divided by upslope rest study). Although one appreciates that the correlation is good, the significant underestimation of the flow reserve is demonstrated as well. (Figure modified with permission from: Reference 16, Ibrahim T, Nekolla SG, Schreiber K. Assessment of coronary flow reserve: Comparison between contrast enhanced magnetic resonance imaging and positron emission tomography *J Am Coll Cardiol* 2002; **39**: 864–70.)

threshold of 2.5. A somewhat surprising finding is that, although MRI perfusion imaging offers excellent in plane spatial resolution (which gives access to subendocardial perfusion defects), the overall spatial coverage of the left ventricle, as well as the actual slice thickness, is limited. The time constraints of acquiring all slices within one heart-

beat in order to sample the signal intensity curve adequately are a limiting factor. Although the clinical relevance of this undersampling remains undetermined, the absolute quantitative measurement of myocardial blood flow is still a major advantage of PET.

Viability imaging and tissue characterization

The finding of limited effective spatial resolution does not hold true in the case of "delayed enhancement" imaging, utilized in viability and tissue characterization examinations. Lauerma *et al.* published an early study, performed on a limited patient group of ten subjects, in connection with this finding [19]. This paper combined MR first-pass perfusion, dobutamine stress cine, and "delayed enhancement" imaging, and compared the results to FDG PET. The authors concluded that the combination of MRI techniques clearly increased sensitivity and specificity, but indicated that the number of concordantly imaged slices of the three techniques needed to be increased for clinical usefulness. In addition, they found a need for more automated data analysis techniques to handle the substantial amount of multiparametric information. Klein and colleagues, from our research group, demonstrated in 31 patients with ischemic heart failure that the spatial location and extent of scar as delineated by delayed enhancement correlated very well with segments from PET [20] (Fig. 10.2). Somewhat

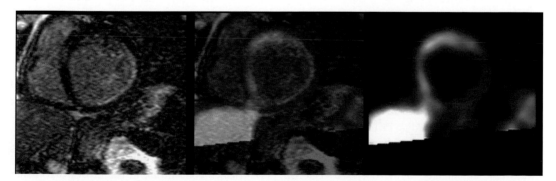

Fig. 10.2 Co-visualization of an MRI late enhancement image with ^{13}N-ammonia PET flow data. The subendocardial enhancement pattern in the MRI is matched with a reduced ^{13}N-ammonia uptake because of partial volume effects as well as reduced myocardial blood flow. Because of the limited spatial resolution of PET,

however, these effects cannot be separated. (Figure modified with permission from: Reference 20, Klein C, Nekolla SG, Bengel FM *et al.* Assessment of myocardial viability with contrast enhanced magnetic resonance imaging: Comparison with positron emission tomography. *Circulation* 2002; **105**: 162–167.)

contrary to the study carried out by Lauerma, the amount of scar in Klein *et al.*'s study was defined as the visually assessed extent from a single MRI "delayed enhancement" acquisition. This measurement was then correlated with the PET scar definition, which was derived from compound criteria related to flow (^{13}N-ammonia) and metabolism (FDG) PET data. The main source of fluctuation between the data sets was determined as the non-transmural enhancement patterns in MRI, which were not detected by PET due to the limited spatial resolution. In a similar patient group (n = 26), Kühl and colleagues, made similar findings. However, in their protocol, myocardial flow was assessed with tetrofosmin SPECT imaging [21]. Unfortunately, none of the previously mentioned studies had follow-up data available after treatment (e.g. revascularization). One can conclude from these studies that the definition of scar tissue can be performed with MRI in a very similar manner to PET, but with improved spatial resolution.

Assessment of regional and global function

In contrast to the two previous subsections, PET imaging of regional and global function utilizes MRI as the reference technique. Because of their limited spatial resolution, nuclear medicine techniques are not ideal for this task. However, as data can be acquired in a gated mode without any extra acquisition time, these techniques offer an attractive option of improving the diagnostic usefulness of the examinations. In addition, the presence of excellent tissue contrast, due to tracer uptake primarily from myocardial tissue, allows the use of fully automated analysis packages, avoiding the time consuming step of manual or computer assisted definition of endo- and epicardial contours.

The basic mechanism in gated PET makes use of the partial volume effect. As the effective spatial resolution in clinical cardiac PET scans is approximately 6–10 mm FWHM (full width at half maximum), the effect of regional wall thickening is measurable as changes in the observed regional count rates occur. Using assumptions, such as homogeneous tracer distribution over the myocardial wall, geometrical models can be adjusted to the count profiles over the myocardial wall and estimates of endo- and epicardial borders can be made.

This approach was extensively implemented and validated in SPECT imaging, where the spatial resolution is notably less [22, 23]. However, because of the substantial use of myocardial perfusion scintigraphy in clinical routine, these algorithms were soon available on a commercial basis, providing a high degree of reproducibility and offering nearly automatic data analysis.

Porenta and colleagues used a geometrical model containing three regional activity values of FDG (blood pool, regional myocardial activity, outside activity) and integrated this into the measured data [24]. In their study on 11 normal volunteers, seven subjects also received a gated MRI study. The authors found good correlation between their geometrical model and the actual wall thickness and motion parameters. The goal of this study was the accurate estimation of regional recovery coefficients, which is a crucial parameter in quantitative PET imaging. From the PET data alone, Buvat and co-authors derived a combined index of count increase and geometrical information. As opposed to the previously discussed study, they attempted to improve the classification of normal versus abnormal wall thickening patterns in PET [25]. For this purpose, simulated data from gated MRI studies were used and their results were compared in five patients. Following the line of this paper, several publications demonstrated gated FDG PET's ability to delineate global and regional function. A pilot study compared regional wall motion abnormalities, using visual analysis with a three-point scale in PET and MRI [26]. This was performed in four short axis slices in nine men. Another pilot study used ^{15}CO, which binds to the red blood cells and enables effective blood pool imaging in PET. In nine patients, the results of global function and volumes for both ventricles using a threshold technique were compared to gated MRI [27]. The results were promising, as the authors found reasonable to good correlations. However, almost all other research focusses on extracting regional and global myocardial function from tracers such as FDG, which concentrate in the myocardial tissue instead of the blood pool. Extending the work of Porenta, Khorsand *et al.* improved the geometrical model approach and demonstrated its feasibility even in the presence of large uptake defects [28]. The authors compared global function and volumes in twenty patients with MRI, enabling the almost simultaneous assessment of FDG metabolism and function. They showed good correlation although a clear trend to underestimate both volumes and ejection fraction is observed. Using a commercial, automated analysis package designed for SPECT studies [23], Schaefer *et al.* found a good to excellent agreement between MRI and gated FDG PET in thirty patients with severe CAD [29]. Although the assessment of end-systolic and end-diastolic volumes showed only non-significant trends for underestimation, the ejection fraction exhibits a significant underestimation for larger ejection fraction values. The authors attribute this difference to the reduced temporal resolution in PET (eight gates) as compared to MRI (twenty phases). The same group extended this work and evaluated two different automated analysis packages against MRI [30]. In 44 patients, the analysis results from two commercial programs (designed for gated SPECT) were correlated to cine MRI. As with their first study, the SPECT and MRI volumes correlated very well, but MRI ejection fraction was again slightly underestimated. It is interesting to note, however, that the reproducibility of the automated analysis of PET data was excellent.

The studies mentioned concentrated on global function only. Unfortunately, data on regional wall motion is limited. Slart and colleagues reproduced the findings for global function from Schaefer, using the same analysis program, but also correlated regional wall motion with a visual three score scheme in nine segments [31]. In 38 patients with chronic CAD, the correlation of the summed wall motion score was excellent and did not exceed a single grade difference in cases of disagreement. Finally, Freiberg and colleagues approached regional wall motion in PET with a geometrical model, incorporating a Gaussian distribution over the myocardial wall in short axis slices [32]. Using a heart model, as well as data from twelve normal volunteers, their model showed a considerable spread of absolute wall motion and wall thickness values, as compared to MRI. In this study, the limitations of both spatial and temporal resolution of gated PET became obvious.

In summary, the evaluation of global function and the delineation of indices of regional wall motion can be assessed by gated FDG as a part of the standard assessment of myocardial glucose metabolism. Myocardial glucose metabolism can be still considered the "gold standard" measurement of myocardial viability, although MRI delayed enhancement imaging continues increasingly to challenge this status.

Synergetic use of PET and MRI

The success of combined PET/CT devices in research, as well as routine applications, clearly demonstrates the advantage of combined assessment, producing high resolution morphological images and specific functional data. Precise localization of tumors dominates this field; the corresponding application in cardiac imaging would be the delineation of the coronaries, wall thickness and wall motion.

The success of gated SPECT myocardial perfusion studies over the last few years clearly shows the value that can be added by the assessment of global and regional function in large studies [33–35]. Nevertheless, as indicated above, the accuracy of the assessment of global and regional function in SPECT or PET studies is limited. MRI, however, offers excellent spatial and temporal resolution with short acquisition times. Recently, the hardware based PET/CT systems have become capable of producing high spatial and medium temporal resolution in combination with molecular imaging capabilities, but at the price of increased exposure to radiation even with sophisticated pulsing schemes over the cardiac cycle [36]. In the past, dual scanner acquisitions were used. However, additional coordination efforts were often required because of the logistical problem of scheduling measurement time on two systems. Furthermore, in most research institutions MRI and PET tomographs belong to different departments, resulting in non-technical considerations that increase the complexity of multimodal research. Despite these challenges, several studies have demonstrated the synergetic use of MRI and PET in cardiac imaging studies.

Viability imaging

The prospective identification of myocardial tissue, which would benefit from revascularization, is a highly relevant task in cardiac imaging. PET in conjunction with a combination of flow and metabolism tracer is still considered a reference method. However, as discussed previously, pure MRI techniques challenge this status. Although there is little data available on combined functional PET and morphological imaging with MRI, the combination could offer significant advantages.

Early examples of this strategy were published by Perrone-Filardi et al. [37, 38]. In patients with chronic CAD, myocardial uptake of FDG was assessed in parallel with regional wall motion and wall thickness. Taking all this information into consideration, an improved characterization of irreversible damaged myocardium, as well as hibernating myocardium, was achieved. This would not have been possible with the individual modalities alone. Baer et al. followed a similar approach, but included the response to low dose dobutamine stress in the MRI examination [39]. Although designed using FDG as a reference technique, the study showed (especially in its scatter plots between FDG uptake and MRI derived functional parameters) the complex situation of regional myocardial tissue. In a recent study carried out Schmidt et al., the functional recovery of akinetic but viable myocardium in 40 patients using a similar protocol was investigated [40]. The study concluded that dobutamine MRI and FDG are both well suited for evaluating viability. Interestingly, the article closes with the request for further comparative studies including studies on MRI and PET. The research group at my institution also believes that the pathophysiological base of viability in chronic heart disease is very complex and that patient specific variability is high. Thus, serial, multimodal imaging approaches could contribute extensively to this field.

Taking MR imaging into account, Knuesel further researched this strategy of improving tissue classification with respect to functional recovery after revascularization in nineteen patients [41]. The authors found that viable segments with a thick viable rim on ceMR recover function after revascularization, whereas all other classes showed low recovery rates of function. Despite the small patient number, this approach showed that the simple black/white pattern of a given imaging approach (such as MR) does not capture the great biological complexity and variability. Additionally, more specific techniques might have a significant impact

on clinical decision making, regardless of their reduced spatial resolution.

The failing heart

An interesting study on idiopathic dilated cardiomyopathy utilizes ^{11}C-acetate as PET tracer [42]. This tracer allows the quantitative assessment of the regional myocardial oxidative metabolism. Unfortunately, because of the tracer kinetics, the assessment of myocardial function with FDG, as described above, is impractical. Thus, the authors performed an additional gated MRI study in eleven normal patients to avoid unnecessary radiation. In ten patients, radionuclide ventriculography was performed. Thus, it was possible to assess myocardial efficiency non-invasively. The quantitative aspect of this approach, although not utilized in this particular study, makes this approach a potential candidate for assessing heart function during medical therapy.

Cardiac innervation

One of the most obvious fields in cardiac imaging where synergetic advantages will arise is the autonomic nervous system. This system contributes substantially to the control mechanisms of perfusion, metabolism and mechanical function and, thus, would be a highly attractive target for imaging. An in depth discussion is available in Chapter 5 of this book. As the concentrations of potential tracers fall in the subpicomolar range, nuclear imaging offers the only reasonable path to reliable imaging procedures. PET tracers, such as the catecholamine analogue ^{11}C-hydroxyphedrine, would offer an especially convenient means of absolute quantification of these dynamically acquired studies, as compared to its counterpart, the SPECT tracer ^{123}I-metaiodobenzylguanidin. Unfortunately, although both PET and SPECT tracers are technically available, these alternative imaging approaches are hardly used in clinical practice. Nevertheless, relevant research applications exist and profit from co-acquired morphological imaging.

Bengel and co-authors used either MRI or radionuclide ventriculography to assess global and regional myocardial function. These results were correlated to the results of ^{11}C-acetate studies (measuring oxidative metabolism) and HED in order to delineate regional innervation [43]. This protocol

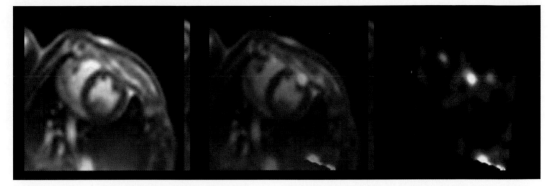

Fig. 10.3 Co-registration and fusion display in PET "hot spot" imaging using Iodine-124 2'-Fluoro-2'-deoxy-5-iodo-1-β-D-arabinofuranosyluracil (^{124}I-FIAU) as marker of gene expression in a pig model. Without anatomical reference, the tracer uptake is impossible to locate. For this display, a PET flow tracer study was aligned to the MRI and the co-registration matrix was subsequently applied to the FIAU data. (Figure reproduced with permission from: Reference 48, Bengel FM, Anton M, Richter T *et al.* Non-invasive imaging of transgene expression by use of positron emission tomography in a pig model of myocardial gene transfer. *Circulation* 2003; **108**: 2127–2133.)

was applied in normals, patients with severe dilated cardiomyopathy and finally, patients after symptom-free heart transplantation. This multimodal, multi-technique study makes it possible to take a detailed look at the control mechanisms of transplanted heart function.

Imaging of the vessel wall and vulnerable plaque and hot spot imaging in general

Although there are reports on plaque inflammation from PET/CT studies [44] and promising studies from the MRI field [45–47] there is no material available regarding the advantageous high spatial resolution in MRI in combination with the capabilities of molecular imaging from PET. From the perspective of PET, such an imaging strategy will very likely be by "hot spot imaging". This kind of imaging does not provide anatomical reference by nuclear imaging techniques. An example is the imaging of reporter gene expression with Iodine-124 2'-Fluoro-2-deoxy-5-iodo-1-β-D-arabinofuranosyluracil (^{124}I-FIAU) after regional intramyocardial injection of control adenovirus or adenovirus carrying the herpesviral thymidine kinase reporter gene (HSV1-tk) [48] (Fig. 10.3). The elevated FIAU retention during the first 30 minutes after injection could be co-visualized with the earlier acquired ^{13}N-ammonia flow studies as well. However, merging with the MRI data led to a clearly improved visualization and association with the location of virus injection.

Thus, the combination of PET and MRI, which avoids the substantial, additional radiation exposure and the limited temporal resolution from PET/CT systems, would be one of the most attractive imaging solutions. Whether or not the complex technical instrumentation and the expected high costs will offset the advantages of a combined PET and MRI remains to be seen.

MRI and PET in oncology of cardiac masses

The number of publications combining MRI and PET in oncology is virtually uncountable. In the cardiologic setting, the opposite is the case. In one case study, FDG-PET imaging was performed in a patient with metastatic breast carcinoma to delineate a mass visualized on a transthoracic echocardiogram and in gated cardiac MRI. Intense FDG uptake was found in the tumor, thus characterizing it as exhibiting high metabolic activity. A transjugular biopsy confirmed this mass as a sarcomatous-type tumor [49].

Software approaches for cardiac MRI and PET co-registration and fusion

In order to combine MRI and PET, the resulting image data from the two independent modalities must be combined in a single computer environment, aligned in the spatial domain, and analyzed. There has been substantial success in the implementation of a standardized image format (DICOM) and communication mechanisms in recent years. The first step towards technically combining MRI and PET image data has been greatly facilitated by the elimination of the previously experienced problems caused by various data formats and computer platforms, and limited computing resources. Despite this achievement, cardiac studies typically provide two additional challenges. Firstly, routine gated acquisitions performed in MRI are also possible in PET. Thus, the three spatial dimensions must be supplemented with a time dimension (this yields 4D data). Secondly, the highly varying acquisition times between PET and MRI are problematic. MRI scans are typically performed in a few seconds during breath-holds and PET scans have a minimum scan duration of five minutes. In addition, despite heart phased resolved data acquisition in PET, the effect of breathing motion is essentially ignored in all scanner systems and results in motional blurring. This creates the challenge of data co-registration of only one particular breathing state (MRI) with a mean breathing motion position (PET).

Practical co-registration

The methodological complexity described above is rarely, if at all, accounted for in validation studies or in studies incorporating both modalities. In most cases, mapping of the regional properties, such as wall motion or contrast media uptake in the left ventricle, is performed according to a standard model suggested by the American Heart Association [50]. This seventeen-segment model is typically filled out with the qualitative or quantitative information from both studies on a visual basis and subsequently statistically compared. Slice to slice comparisons are also used, but suffer from a limitation in MRI data acquisition. In contrast to CT and PET, where the complete data volume is sampled isotropically, MRI is in most cases slice based. In other words, arbitrary multiplanar reformatted images can be derived from the isotropic data volume. The foundation for this approach is similar voxel sizes in all spatial dimensions; this does not hold true for many MRI acquisitions, where the in plane resolution is much higher than the slice thickness. Thus, in order to create matching slices,

the CT or PET volume must be reformatted to the parameters at which the MR image was acquired. As this is a demanding and time consuming step, the pixel by pixel comparison is rarely found in publications.

Approaches to cardiac data co-registration

Two major groups of registration algorithms are known today. Feature based techniques identify common structures in both data sets and use, thereafter, an optimization routine to minimize the distance between the common structures as defined by these surfaces can be implemented . Thus, errors in the delineation of the surfaces limit the applicability of this approach. Those errors might stem from mistakes in the manual definition of common morphological elements. Or, if automatic feature extraction methods are used, the two imaging methods delineate inherently non-matching borders. This can be demonstrated by infarcted myocardial tissue, which shows excellent signal intensity in MRI delayed enhancement imaging, whereas normal tissue is blacked. PET perfusion imaging presents the exact opposite situation, in which normal perfused tissue shows significant tracer uptake and infarcted tissue shows little or even no uptake. In cardiac imaging, this poses an especially large problem, because of the limited number of accurate anatomical landmarks in the heart. For example, the rotational symmetry along the heart's long axis is much higher than the conditions found in the brain, making co-registration much more difficult.

The second class of registration algorithms focus on information from the data volumes, thus limiting the need for image segmentation steps. One of the early publications on the subject of MRI and PET co-registration appeared in 1993 [51]. Woods *et al.* used the standard deviation of signal intensity histograms in the brain from both modalities and calculated an optimal co-registration matrix to match MRI and PET. Other statistical properties, such as joint entropy [52] or mutual information [53−55] were investigated as well. The latter technique built the foundation for several commercial co-registration packages. The alignment precision, as found in thoracic image registration, is not available from MRI/PET studies, but might be estimated from PET/CT studies. Here, this value was found to be in the order of 2 mm in brain studies [56] and less than 10 mm in oncological studies of the thorax [57, 58].

So far, the discussed approaches have used linear registration. This allows translation in all three directions and rotation around three axes. As the heart is located in the thorax, non-linear techniques might apply as well, as substantial deformation occurs over both the breathing and cardiac cycles. Unfortunately, there is only limited data on this subject, even from PET/CT studies. One reason for the sparse number of publications may be the problems inherent in validation studies. Even sophisticated phantom studies fail to describe the complex motion and deformation patterns found in patients [59]. Thus, the practical consequences continue to be unclear, which also holds true for any dual modality acquisitions when not performed simultaneously [60, 61]. Interestingly, the displacement found in this hardware approach was in the order of the linear software fusion (< 10 mm) as mentioned above. However, this was considered to be modest from a clinical point of view, at least in oncology.

The previously mentioned co-registration of four-dimensional data sets (volume over time or volume over cardiac cycle) remains a challenging issue. Unfortunately, there is very limited data available to demonstrate its feasibility [62]. In this study, we utilized the cardiac analysis framework, "MunichHeart", developed at our institution for a model based approach to this issue. Data from PET acquisitions were analyzed using volumetric data analysis, which is facilitated by the fact that PET, as well as SPECT, data is acquired with near isotropic voxels [63, 64]. From static and gated MR studies, endo- and epicardial contours of the left ventricle were defined manually. Combined with the volume contours of the tracer distribution in static, dynamic or gated studies, this approach allowed the co-registration of the bimodal data sets (Fig. 10.4) in a two-step implementation. First, the two sets of contours describing the left ventricle in MRI and PET were matched as closely as possible, based on geometrical constraints. However, as already mentioned, the fundamental difference in imaging physics and physiology requires the assistance of a second step: a final, manual adjustment of the two modalities.

Klein and colleagues implemented a non-uniform, elastic model, described by 12 parameters, and adjusted the PET data within this model. Although this is not a multimodal application in the strictest sense, it shows great promise for this field [65, 66]. Another model-based technique was published recently [67], which also integrated the right ventricle and used external markers to integrate data from a third modality, magnetocardiography.

Aladl and colleagues [68, 69] recently described an approach to 4D SPECT-MRI co-registration and fusion, in which the MRI study was segmented, based on regional pixel value changes due to motion, essentially removing any static tissue; they subsequently applied mutual information measures to co-register the data sets. These results were compared to a co-registration performed manually by an expert. The translational differences were found to be in the order of 1 mm with MRI segmentation and 4 mm without it. For the rotational offset, 4° and 10° respectively were found. Technically, this technique can be applied to PET data as well and offers a high degree of automation.

All methods described so far require a substantial amount of user interaction or computing time. A scalable system, implementing algorithms based on voxel similarity, was developed by Shekhar *et al.* [70, 71]. Although focussing on gated 3D ultrasound heart data, their system has shown substantial potential, as it makes possible computationally very demanding procedures, which in turn allow for correction of misalignment between, for example pre- and poststress gated 3D echo data.

Image and parametric data integration

The high complexity of cardiac data acquisition co-registration would ideally require a multimodal integration of both image and parametric information, such as myocardial blood flow, which itself is derived from a series of temporal images. These parametric mapping techniques are common in functional imaging of the brain and were also used in MRI for perfusion and delayed enhancement studies [16]. However, very limited data is available on this issue, which goes beyond the visualization of so called 4D bimodal data sets (three dimension of space and one comprising the time, e.g. the offsets from the R wave). The work of Mäkela has already been mentioned above [67]. As the authors also

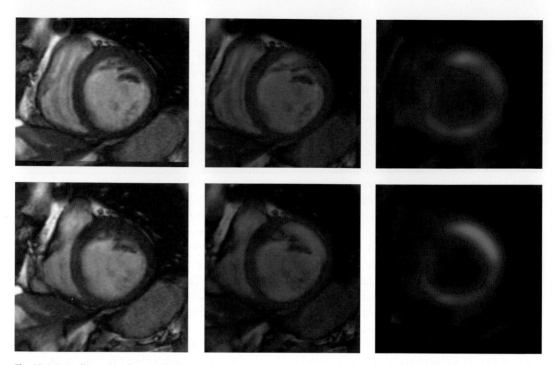

Fig. 10.4 Four-dimensional co-registration and fusion of a gated MRI and a gated FDG study in a patient with severe myocardial dysfunction. Only the end-systolic and the end-diastolic frame are displayed. The partial volume dependent FDG uptake is visible in the anterior wall because of the increasing proximity of myocardial wall and papillary muscle during systole.

added magnetocardiography to their study parameters, the amount of qualitative and quantitative data was even larger, as expected, and an efficient means of data visualization for the interpretation of the data was required. Although significant advances have been made in academic centres, complex cardiac data integration is still an ambitious project and commercial solutions have not yet come onto the market.

Limitations of spatial co-registration

Unfortunately, there is little data on the possible accuracy of aligning multimodal data in the chest from MRI and PET studies because of: a) gross patient motion, b) thoracic motion, and c) cardiac motion. The first two types of motion are very challenging, as they happen completely randomly and can produce irregular patterns. However, the availability of PET/CT systems has enabled studies to be conducted in the thorax. Although these limited

publications focus on oncological issues, they are briefly summarized here, as they provide a good estimate of the potential limitations.

Osman and co-authors evaluated the incidence of inaccurate lesion detection in 300 patients and found incorrect localizations in the liver/lung border zone in only six [72]. Other studies on respiratory induced motion, which focused more specifically on developing an optimal breathing protocol for the CT portion of the examination, reported displacements between PET and CT ranging between 5 and 20 mm [60, 73]. One conclusion of these papers was that co-registration can be achieved in the order of the spatial resolution of the PET system, which is between 6 and 10 mm. The study by Boucher and colleagues measured a mean $\pm$ SD motion in axial direction of the apex of the heart of 6.7 ± 3.0 mm (maximal displacement: 11.9 mm) for breathing triggered PET acquisition. This group used a temperature sensitive respiratory gating device installed in a breathing mask [74]. The derived apical motion was calculated from the reconstructed images. One should note that the transmission scan applied was ungated.

These numbers give some idea of the potential motion found in thorax imaging. Although animal models exist, which could serve as a validation platform [75], most research concentrates on retrospective alignment of complete patients. In their excellent review, Mäkela *et al.* summarized the registration accuracy for intra- and intermodal applications [76]. For MRI intramodal alignment, 1.5–3.0 mm accuracies were reported. With PET-PET co-registration, 1.0–2.5 mm was found and finally, PET-MRI showed 1.95 ± 1.6 mm [77] through the implementation of a rigid heart surface based approach for gated MRI and gated PET and 80 landmarks. A second reference calculated 2.8 ± 0.5 mm using an indirect measure for cardiac data (actually using thorax and lung surfaces for validation) [78].

In summary, patient, thorax and cardiac motion make co-registration of any imaging sequences not acquired simultaneously a major obstacle in inter- and intramodal data acquisition. Significant advances have been made in cardiac software co-registration, yielding accuracies in the range between 1–3 m. However, essentially none of the publications discussed in the validation and synergetic applications sections used these advanced software algorithms. Thus, major efforts are necessary to link the cardiological users with the image post-processing specialists in order to create user friendly applications, which will extract maximal information from multimodal studies.

Combined imaging in hardware

All previous results and discussions were based on separate examinations in the two modalities, MRI and PET. From a logistical and patient comfort point of view, this procedure is clearly suboptimal. The success of combined PET/CT devices is proof that more efficient methods can be obtained; certainly they are required. Even if the measurements cannot be performed simultaneously but only sequentially (as in PET/CT), the improvement in the solving of logistical problems and the gains in comfort for the patient will be significant. However, the absolute hardware costs, as well as cost efficiency, must be considered.

Technical challenges

The basic aim of PET is the detection of high energy photons resulting from an annihilation event during the decay of a positron emitting isotope. This isotope is typically bound to a pharmaceutical with the advantage that the concentration of these substances can be in the pico to femto molar range. The high energy photon (minimum 511 keV) is typically stopped by, and detected in, a detector crystal, where it is absorbed. After a short time, the particular atom emits a lower energy photon. This photon is detected by a photomultiplier tube, which is available in almost all PET scanners. In the photomultiplier, the photon releases an electron, which, in turn, is amplified at a high voltage cascade. Unfortunately, free electrons in the vacuum of the tube are displaced by even the smallest magnetic fields (approximately 1–10 mT), rendering the usual technique of photon detection and amplification in MR systems completely useless. For this reason, even the sequential approach of combining hardware in close proximity, as found in PET/CT systems is technically not feasible in PET/MRI.

Use of large magnetic fields to increase spatial resolution

Before discussing possible solutions, an interesting strategy, (which was discussed in the nineties) based on theoretical considerations and simulations, should be mentioned here. As described above, a positron is emitted during the decay of a radioisotope bound to the radiopharmaceutical. Depending on the actual isotope, the positron is emitted with substantial energy (examples of isotopes with special relevance in cardiac imaging: F-18 Emax = 0.64 MeV; C-11 Emax = 0.97 MeV; N-13 Emax = 1.2 MeV; O-15 Emax = 1.74 MeV, and Rb-82 Emax = 3.15 MeV). This energy allows it to travel several millimeters through water or biological substances before it forms the so called positronium with an electron, and before it finally annihilates with the emission of two 511 keV photons. This means that the spatial location of the emitting radioisotope does not coincide with the detected location of the annihilation. A large magnetic field, however, could force the positron on a circular path perpendicular to the magnetic field because of the Lorenz force, effectively improving the spatial resolution of a PET scanner. Following up on simulation studies by Iida *et al.* [79], Hammer and colleagues implemented an experimental set up, where four meter long optical light guides transported the photons to an area without disrupting magnetic fields [80–82]. Using Ge-68 (Emax = 1.90 MeV), they showed a clear improvement of spatial resolution at five Tesla (T) field strength and the full width at half maximum (FWHM) decreased by a factor of 1.42. They also concluded that the effect of using lower energy positron-emitters, such as Na-22 (Emax = 0.55 MeV) should have little or no effect. At least for the widely used Rb-82 in a hypothetical 3 T system, a certain gain in spatial resolution can be anticipated.

CMR spectroscopy and PET

Two years later, the next step from improvements of the spatial resolution of PET experiments in high magnetic fields towards the combination of the two modalities was performed at Guy's hospital in London, UK. A "minimal" PET scanner, consisting of a pair of electronically coupled sodium-iodine (NaI) detectors, was integrated within a 9.4 T wide bore spectroscopy system [83]. Again, long light guides were used to transfer the postannihilation photons to detectors outside of the main magnetic fields. This kind of PET system is not capable of acquiring image data, but is used at several PET centers to study the pharmacokinetics of various radiotracers in isolated rat or mouse heart models. This approach allowed the first simultaneous measurements of time resolved 31^P and 13^C spectra during FDG metabolic studies of isolated rat hearts. The temporal resolution was 15 s in both modalities.

Through a collaborative effort between the London group and the UCLA School of Medicine, the two coupled scintillation detectors were replaced by a miniature PET scanner [84]. Based on the UCLA group's micro-PET system [85], a single ring lutetium oxyorthosilicate (LSO) system with 72 crystals ($2 \times 2 \times 25$ mm) was built and inserted in a 7.3 cm bore, 9.4 T MR device. Once again, 4 m long optical fibres were used to transfer the scintillation photons to an external detection system. The disadvantage of long fibres, which attenuate the light

output from the scintillators, was partly offset by the use of LSO, which shows a significantly higher light yield compared to other PET detectors' materials. With this system, which is essentially a one-slice PET tomograph, a spatial PET resolution of 2 mm FWHM with an axial field-of-view of 25 mm was achieved inside and outside the magnetic field. Using an isolated rat heart model, simultaneous PET FDG images and 31^P spectra were acquired, thus demonstrating the feasibility of dual modality data acquisition. The operation of the PET subsystem within the CMR led to a 30% degradation of the 31^P line, which could not be improved with the shim coils. However, the authors concluded that such a degradation would not cause significant problems in biological CMR experiments.

In a subsequent study by Garlick *et al.* ^{31}P spectroscopy and PET FDG imaging was combined [86]. The authors were able to demonstrate that there is a differential effect of the uptake of the two glucose analogues, F-18 2-fluoro-2-deoxyglucose (as a standard PET tracer) and 2-deoxyglucose (DG), in a model of regional ischemia. Thus, the two modalities were able to trace two different glucose analogues, which are mutually exclusive to PET or MR in the very same physiological model. Very recently, the same group reported further findings, using ^{19}F spectroscopy [87], and was able to highlight the complex nature of FDG metabolism and the potential consequences in PET imaging. Although this was a pure CMR spectroscopy study, it clearly showed the potential for synergetic effects in basic research with hypothetical consequences for clinical routine examinations.

Simultaneous MRI and PET imaging

The next step was the generation of MR images, not only to accompany PET data, but acquired at the same time as the PET data was measured. A modified PET system, based on the device described above consisted of 48 $2 \times 2 \times 10$ mm^3 LSO crystals forming a 38 mm diameter ring. This modular scanner was inserted in 0.2 T vertical field open MRI system [88]. The coupling to the photo multiplier tubes was again achieved with 4 meter long optical fibres. Using a 2D FLASH sequence, a cylindrical phantom with seven 1 mm holes and a 5 mm separation, filled with a FDG and NiCl2 solution was acquired without visible artifacts.

In 1999, Slates and colleagues [89] utilized the setup as presented above in a series of imaging experiments in different MR scanners (0.2, 1.5, 4.7 and 9.4 T) and with a variety of MR image sequences, using a dedicated phantom and biological material (an orange). Susceptibility artifacts from the LSO scintillators and the optical fibres in the MR images were not observed. Other limitations, such as interactions with the scanners' magnetic field or electromagnetic interference with the PET acquisition, were not detected using various sequences (T_1 as well as T_2 spin echo, turbo spin echo and gradient echo). Although these results proved the feasibility of this concept, several limitations were observed [89]. Because of the one-ring concept and the optical fibre readout, the PET scanner showed an overall limited performance, as well as a very small field of view, when compared to dedicated small animal PET systems. In a review article, published in 2002, Paul Marsden and colleagues outlined the concept of a successor imaging device [90]. However, no further studies have been released so far. Although the concept of an optical readout is intriguing, the sensitivity of such an approach will always be limited because of substantial photon attenuation over long fiber optics. Whether concepts of integrated detectors utilizing avalanche photodiodes offer a possible solution for a complete, multi-ring PET scanner within an MR system is yet unknown although promising work has been published [91–93]. It is obvious, however, that detectors which can operate within the magnetic field, would simplify the construction of such a combined device.

Conclusion

This overview has discussed the wide range of applications in which MRI and PET acquisitions have been used in the same patients. Unfortunately, but understandably, validation studies represented the majority of the examples. Within the validation studies, one modality attempted to replace another in situations where there were potential clinical applications. This strategy is a result of cost pressures, clinical logistics and overall efficiency. However, it was also demonstrated that while the two modalities each had unique strengths, they were also able to complement each other extremely well.

There have been major achievements in software-based co-registration in the past. However, the migration of these techniques and tools to a wider application has not yet occurred. But the potential benefits of this kind of research and development are most definitely worth great effort.

Finally, a clinical success story for a combined MRI/PET device, as seen with PET/CT, will require much greater intellectual and financial investment.

Acknowledgments

The editorial assistance of Denise Lee is greatly appreciated. I thank Axel Martinez Möller and Frank Bengel for critically reading the manuscript.

References

1. Beyer T, Townsend DW, Brun T *et al*. A combined PET/CT scanner for clinical oncology. *J Nucl Med* 2000; **41**: 1369–1379.

2. Townsend DW. A combined PET/CT scanner: the choices. *J Nucl Med* 2001; **3**: 533–534.

3. Phelps ME. Comments and perspectives. *J Nucl Med* 2004; **45**: 1601–1603.

4. Schwaiger M, Melin J. Cardiological applications of nuclear medicine. *Lancet* 1999; **354**: 661–666.

5. Pohost GM, Hung L, Doyle M. Clinical use of cardiovascular magnetic resonance. *Circulation* 2003; **108**: 647–653.

6. Muzik O, Beanlands RS, Hutchins GD *et al*. Validation of nitrogen 13 ammonia tracer kinetic model for quantification of myocardial blood flow using PET. *J Nucl Med* 1993; **34**: 83–91.

7. Sawada S, Muzik O, Beanlands RS, Wolfe E, Hutchins GD, Schwaiger M. Interobserver and interstudy variability of myocardial blood flow and flow-reserve measurements with nitrogen 13 ammonia-labeled positron emission tomography. *J Nucl Cardiol* 1995; **2**: 413–422.

8. Kaufmann PA, Gnecchi-Ruscone T, Yap JT *et al*. Assessment of the reproducibility of baseline and hyperemic myocardial blood flow measurements with ^{15}O-labeled water and PET. *J Nucl Med* 1999; **40**: 1848–1856.

9. Weinmann HJ, Ebert W, Misselwitz B *et al*. Tissue-specific MR contrast agents. *Eur J Radiol* 2003; **46**: 33–44.

10. Manning WJ, Atkinson DJ, Grossman W *et al*. First-pass nuclear magnetic resonance imaging studies using gadolinium-DTPA in patients with coronary artery disease. *J Am Coll Cardiol* 1991; **18**: 959–965.

11. Miller DD, Donohue TJ, Wolford TL *et al*. Assessment of blood flow distal to coronary artery stenoses. Correlations between myocardial positron emission tomography

and poststenotic intracoronary Doppler flow reserve. *Circulation* 1996 ; **94**: 2447–2454.

12. Hofman MB, van Rossum AC, Sprenger M *et al.* Assessment of flow in the right human coronary artery by magnetic resonance phase contrast velocity measurement: Effects of cardiac and respiratory motion. *Magn Reson Med* 1996; **35**: 521–531.

13. Sakuma H, Blake LM, Amidon TM *et al.* Higgins CB. Coronary flow reserve: Non-invasive measurement in humans with breath-hold velocity encoded cine MR imaging. *Radiology* 1996; **198**: 745–750.

14. Schwitter J, De Marco T, Kneifel S, *et al.* Magnetic resonance based assessment of global coronary flow and flow reserve and its relation to left ventricular functional parameters: A comparison with positron emission tomography. *Circulation* 2000; **101**: 2696–2702.

15. Sakuma H, Koskenvuo JW, Niemi P *et al.* Assessment of coronary flow reserve using fast velocity encoded cine MR imaging: validation study using positron emission tomography. *Am J Roentgenol* 2000; **175**: 1029–1033.

16. Ibrahim T, Nekolla SG, Schreiber K. Assessment of coronary flow reserve: Comparison between contrast enhanced magnetic resonance imaging and positron emission tomography *J Am Coll Cardiol* 2002; **39**: 864–70.

17. Melon PG, Beanlands RS, De Grado TR *et al.* Schwaiger M. Comparison of technetium-99m sestamibi and thallium-201 retention characteristics in canine myocardium. *J Am Coll Cardiol* 1992; **20**: 1277–1283.

18. Ayalew A, Marie PY, Menu P *et al.* A comparison of the overall first-pass kinetics of thallium-201 and technetium-99m MIBI in normoxic and low-flow ischemic myocardium. *Eur J Nucl Med* 2000; **27**: 1632–1640.

19. Lauerma K, Niemi P, Hanninen H *et al.* Multimodality MR imaging assessment of myocardial viability: Combination of first-pass and late contrast enhancement to wall motion dynamics and comparison with FDG PET —initial experience. *Radiology* 2000; **217**: 729–736.

20. Klein C, Nekolla SG, Bengel FM *et al.* Assessment of myocardial viability with contrast enhanced magnetic resonance imaging: Comparison with positron emission tomography. *Circulation* 2002; **105**: 162–167.

21. Kühl HP, Beek AM, van der Weerdt AP *et al.* Myocardial viability in chronic ischemic heart disease: comparison of contrast enhanced magnetic resonance imaging with (18)F-fluorodeoxyglucose positron emission tomography. *J Am Coll Cardiol* 2003; **41**: 1341–1348.

22. Germano G, Kavanagh PB, Su HT *et al.* Automatic reorientation of three-dimensional, transaxial myocardial perfusion SPECT images. *J Nucl Med* 1995; **36**: 1107–1114.

23. Germano G, Kiat H, Kavanagh PB *et al.* Automatic quantification of ejection fraction from gated myocardial perfusion SPECT. *J Nucl Med* 1995; **36**: 2138–2147.

24. Porenta G, Kuhle W, Sinha S *et al.* Parameter estimation of cardiac geometry by ECG-gated PET imaging: Validation using magnetic resonance imaging and echocardiography. *J Nucl Med* 1995; **36**: 1123–1129.

25. Buvat I, Bartlett ML, Kitsiou AN *et al.* A "hybrid" method for measuring myocardial wall thickening from gated PET/SPECT images. *J Nucl Med* 1997; **38**: 324–329.

26. Waiter GD, Al-Mohammad A, Norton MY *et al.* Regional myocardial wall thickening assessed at rest by ECG gated (18)F-FDG positron emission tomography and by magnetic resonance imaging. *Heart* 2000; **84**: 332–333.

27. Rajappan K, Livieratos L, Camici PG *et al.* Measurement of ventricular volumes and function: A comparison of gated PET and cardiovascular magnetic resonance. *J Nucl Med* 2002; **43**: 806–810.

28. Khorsand A, Graf S, Frank H *et al.* Model-based analysis of electrocardiography-gated cardiac (18)F-FDG PET images to assess left ventricular geometry and contractile function. *J Nucl Med* 2003; **44**: 1741–1746.

29. Schaefer WM, Lipke CS, Nowak B *et al.* Validation of an evaluation routine for left ventricular volumes, ejection fraction and wall motion from gated cardiac FDG PET: A comparison with cardiac magnetic resonance imaging. *Eur J Nucl Med Mol Imaging* 2003; **30**: 545–553.

30. Schaefer WM, Lipke CS, Nowak B *et al.* Validation of QGS and 4D-MSPECT for quantification of left ventricular volumes and ejection fraction from gated 18F-FDG PET: Comparison with cardiac MRI. *J Nucl Med* 2004; **45**: 74–79.

31. Slart RH, Bax JJ, de Jong RM *et al.* Comparison of gated PET with MRI for evaluation of left ventricular function in patients with coronary artery disease. *J Nucl Med* 2004; **45**: 176–182.

32. Freiberg J, Hove JD, Kofoed KF *et al.* Absolute quantitation of left ventricular wall and cavity parameters using ECG-gated PET. *J Nucl Cardiol* 2004; **11**: 38–46.

33. Sharir T, Germano G, Kavanagh PB *et al.* Incremental prognostic value of poststress left ventricular ejection fraction and volume by gated myocardial perfusion single photon emission computed tomography. *Circulation* 1999; **100**: 1035–1034.

34. Sharir T, Berman DS, Lewin HC *et al.* Incremental prognostic value of rest-redistribution (201)Tl single-photon emission computed tomography. *Circulation* 1999; **100**: 1964–1970.

35. Meine TJ, Hanson MW, Borges-Neto S. The additive value of combined assessment of myocardial perfusion and ventricular function studies. *J Nucl Med* 2004; **45**: 1721–1724.

36. Trabold T, Buchgeister M, Kuttner A *et al.* Estimation of radiation exposure in 16-detector row computed tomography of the heart with retrospective ECG-gating. *Röfo* 2003; **175**: 1051–1055.

37. Perrone-Filardi P, Bacharach SL, Dilsizian V *et al.* Metabolic evidence of viable myocardium in regions with reduced wall thickness and absent wall thickening in patients with chronic ischemic left ventricular dysfunction. *J Am Coll Cardiol* 1992; **20**: 161–168.

38. Perrone-Filardi P, Bacharach SL, Dilsizian V *et al.* Regional left ventricular wall thickening. Relation to regional uptake of 18fluorodeoxyglucose and 201Tl in patients with chronic coronary artery disease and left ventricular dysfunction. *Circulation* 1992; **86**: 1125–1137.

39. Baer FM, Voth E, Schneider CA *et al.* Comparison of low-dose dobutamine-gradient-echo magnetic resonance imaging and positron emission tomography with [18F]fluorodeoxyglucose in patients with chronic coronary artery disease. A functional and morphological approach to the detection of residual myocardial viability. *Circulation* 1995; **91**: 1006–15 .

40. Schmidt M, Voth E, Schneider CA *et al.* F-18-FDG uptake is a reliable predictor of functional recovery of akinetic but viable infarct regions as defined by magnetic resonance imaging before and after revascularization. *Magn Reson Imaging* 2004; **22**: 229–236.

41. Knuesel PR, Nanz D, Wyss C *et al.* Characterization of dysfunctional myocardium by positron emission tomography and magnetic resonance: Relation to functional outcome after revascularization. *Circulation* 2003; **108**: 1095–1100.

42. Bengel FM, Permanetter B, Ungerer M *et al.* Non-invasive estimation of myocardial efficiency using positron emission tomography and carbon-11 acetate-comparison between the normal and failing human heart. *Eur J Nucl Med* 2000; **27**: 319–326.

43. Bengel FM, Ueberfuhr P, Schiepel N *et al.* Myocardial efficiency and sympathetic reinnervation after orthotopic heart transplantation: A non-invasive study with positron emission tomography. *Circulation* 2001; **103**: 1881–1886.

44. Rudd JH, Warburton EA, Fryer TD *et al.* Imaging atherosclerotic plaque inflammation with [18F]-fluorodeoxyglucose positron emission tomography. *Circulation* 2002; **105**: 2708–2711.

45. Yuan C, Miller ZE, Cai J *et al.* Carotid atherosclerotic wall imaging by MRI. *Neuroimaging Clin North Am* 2002; **12**: 391–401.

46. Botnar RM, Buecker A, Wiethoff AJ *et al. In vivo* magnetic resonance imaging of coronary thrombosis using a fibrin-binding molecular magnetic resonance contrast agent. *Circulation* 2004; **110**: 1463–1466.

47. Yuan C, Mitsumori LM, Ferguson MS *et al. In vivo* accuracy of multispectral magnetic resonance imaging for identifying lipid-rich necrotic cores and intraplaque hemorrhage in advanced human carotid plaques. *Circulation* 2001; **104**: 2051–2056.

48. Bengel FM, Anton M, Richter T *et al.* Non-invasive imaging of transgene expression by use of positron emission tomography in a pig model of myocardial gene transfer. *Circulation* 2003; **108**: 2127–2133.

49. Plutchok JJ, Boxt LM, Weinberger J *et al.* Differentiation of cardiac tumor from thrombus by combined MRI and F-18 FDG PET imaging. *Clin Nucl Med* 1998; **23**: 324–325.

50. Cerqueira MD, Weissman NJ, Dilsizian V *et al.* American Heart Association writing group on myocardial segmentation and registration for cardiac imaging. Standardized myocardial segmentation and nomenclature for tomographic imaging of the heart. *Circulation* 2002; **105**: 539–542.

51. Woods RP, Mazziotta JC, Cherry SR. MRI-PET registration with automated algorithm. *J Comput Assist Tomogr* 1993; **17**: 536–534.

52. Hill DL, Hawkes DJ, Gleeson MJ *et al.* Accurate frameless registration of MR and CT images of the head: Applications in planning surgery and radiation therapy. *Radiology* 1994; **191**: 447–454.

53. Wells WM, Viola P, Atsumi H *et al.* Multimodal volume registration by maximization of mutual information. *Med Image Anal* 1996; **1**: 35–51.

54. Maes F, Collignon A, Vandermeulen D *et al.* Multimodality image registration by maximization of mutual information. *IEEE Trans Med Imaging* 1997; **16**: 187–198.

55. Pluim JP, Maintz JB, Viergever MA. Mutual-information-based registration of medical images: A survey. *IEEE Trans Med Imaging* 2003; **22**: 986–1004.

56. West J, Fitzpatrick JM, Wang MY *et al.* Comparison and evaluation of retrospective intermodality brain image registration techniques. *J Comput Assist Tomogr* 1997; **21**: 554–566.

57. Skalski J, Wahl RL, Meyer CR. Comparison of mutual information-based warping accuracy for fusing body CT and PET by two methods: CT mapped onto PET emission scan versus CT mapped onto PET transmission scan. *J Nucl Med* 2002; **43**: 1184–1187.

58. Slomka PJ, Dey D, Przetak C *et al.* Automated 3-dimensional registration of stand-alone 18F-FDG whole-body PET with CT. *J Nucl Med* 2003; **44**: 1156–1167.

59. Visser JJ, Sokole EB, Verberne HJ *et al.* A realistic 3-D gated cardiac phantom for quality control of gated myocardial perfusion SPET: The Amsterdam gated (AGATE) cardiac phantom. *J Nucl Med Mol Imaging* 2004; **31**: 222–228.

60. Goerres GW, Kamel E, Heidelberg TH *et al.* PET-CT image co-registration in the thorax: Influence of respiration. *Eur J Nucl Med* 2002; **29**: 351–360.

61. Nakamoto Y, Tatsumi M, Cohade C *et al.* Accuracy of image fusion of normal upper abdominal organs visualized with PET/CT. *Eur J Nucl Med Mol Imaging* 2003; **30**: 597–602.

62. Nekolla SG, Ibrahim T, Balbach T *et al.* Co-registration and fusion of cardiac MRI and PET studies. In: Marzullo P, ed. *Understanding Cardiac Imaging Techniques: From Basic Pathology to Image Fusion.* IOS Press, Series 1: Life and Behavioural Sciences, vol 332, Amsterdam, 2001.

63. Nekolla S, Miethaner C, Nguyen N *et al.* Reproducibility of polar map generation, defect severity and extent assessment in tomographic myocardial PET perfusion imaging. *Eur J Nucl Med* 1998; **25**: 1313–1321.

64. Hattori N, Bengel FM, Mehilli J *et al.* Global and regional functional measurements with gated FDG PET in comparison with left ventriculography. *Euro J Nucl Med* 2001; **28**: 221–229.

65. Klein GJ, Huesman RH. Four-dimensional processing of deformable cardiac PET data. *Med Image Anal* 2002; **6**: 29–46.

66. Klein GJ, Reutter BW, Huesman RH. Four-dimensional affine registration models for respiratory-gated PET. *IEEE Trans Med Imaging* 2002; **48**: 756–760.

67. Mäkela T, Pham QC, Clarysse P *et al.* A 3-D model-based registration approach for the PET, MR and MCG cardiac data fusion. *Med Image Anal* 2003; **7**: 377–389.

68. Aladl UE, Dey D, Slomka PJ. Four-dimensional multi-modality image registration applied to gated SPECT and gated MRI. In: Hanson K, ed. *Medical Imaging 2003: Image Processing.* International Society for Optical Engineering, San Diego, 2003: 1166–1175.

69. Aladl UE, Hurwitz GA, Dey D *et al.* Automated image registration of gated cardiac single-photon emission computed tomography and magnetic resonance imaging. *J Magn Reson Imaging* 2004; **19**: 283–290.

70. Shekhar R, Zagrodsky V, Castro-Pareja CR *et al.* High-speed registration of three- and four-dimensional medical images by using voxel similarity. *Radiographics* 2003; **23**: 1673–1681.

71. Castro-Pareja CR, Jagadeesh JM, Shekhar R. FAIR: a hardware architecture for real time 3-D image registration. *IEEE Trans Inf Technol Biomed* 2003; **7**: 426–434.

72. Osman MM, Cohade C, Nakamoto Y *et al.* Clinically significant inaccurate localization of lesions with PET/CT: Frequency in 300 patients. *J Nucl Med* 2003; **44**: 240–243.

73. Goerres GW, Burger C, Kamel E *et al.* Respiration-induced attenuation artifact at PET/CT: Technical considerations. *Radiology* 2003; **226**: 906–910.

74. Boucher L, Rodrigue S, Lecomte R *et al.* Respiratory gating for 3-dimensional PET of the thorax: Feasibility and initial results. *J Nucl Med* 2004; **45**: 214–219.

75. Casali C, Obadia JF, Canet E *et al.* Design of an isolated pig heart preparation for positron emission tomography and magnetic resonance imaging. *Invest Radiol* 1997; **32**: 713–720.

76. Mäkela TJ, Clarysee P, Sipilä O *et al.* A review of cardiac image registration methods. *IEEE Trans Med Imaging* 2002; **21**: 1011–1021.

77. Sinha S, Sinha U, Czernin J *et al.* Non-invasive assessment of myocardial perfusion and metabolism: Feasibility of registering gated MR and PET images. *Am J Roentgenol* 1995; **164**: 301–307.

78. Mäkela TJ, Clarysee P, Lötjönen J *et al.* A new method for the registration of cardiac PET and MR images using deformable model based segmentation of the main thorax structures. In: Niessen W & Vierrgever MA, eds. *Proceedings of the 4th International Conference on Medical Image Computing and Computer Assisted Intervention (MICCAI 01).* Lecture notes in computer science 2208. Springer-Verlag, Heidelberg, 2001: 557–564.

79. Iida H, Kanno I, Miura S *et al.* A simulation study of a method to reduce positron-annihilation spread distributions using a strong magnetic-field in positron emission tomography. *IEEE Trans Nucl Sci* 1986; **33**: 597–600.

80. Hammer BE, Christensen NL, Heil BG. Use of a magnetic-field to increase the spatial-resolution positron emission tomography. *Med Phys* 1994; **21**: 1917–20.

81. Christensen NL, Hammer BE, Heil BG *et al.* Positron emission tomography within a magnetic field using photomultiplier tubes and lightguides. *Phys Med Biol* 1995; **40**: 691–697.

82. Raylman RR, Hammer BE, Christensen NL. Combined MRI-PET scanner: A Monte Carlo evaluation of the improvements in PET resolution due to the effects of a static homogeneous magnetic field. *IEEE Trans Nucl Sci* 1996; **43**: 2406–2412.

83. Buchanan M, Marsden PK, Mielke CH *et al.* A system to obtain radiotracer uptake data simultaneously with NMR spectra in a high field magnet. *IEEE Trans Nucl Sci* 1996; **43**: 2044–2048.

84. Garlick PB, Marsden PK, Cave AC *et al.* PET and NMR dual acquisition (PANDA): Applications to isolated, perfused rat hearts. *NMR Biomed* 1997; **10**: 138–142.

85. Cherry SR, Shao Y, Siegel S *et al.* Optical fiber readout of scintillator arrays using a multichannel PMT: A high resolution PET detector for animal imaging. *IEEE Trans Nucl Sci* 1996; **43**: 1932–1937.

86. Garlick PB, Medina RA, Southworth R *et al.* Differential uptake of FDG and DG during postischemic reperfusion in the isolated, perfused rat heart. *Eur J Nucl Med* 1999; **26**: 1353–1358.

87. Southworth R, Parry CR, Parkes HG *et al.* Tissue-specific differences in 2-fluoro-2-deoxyglucose metabolism beyond FDG-6-P: A 19F NMR spectroscopy study in the rat. *NMR Biomed* 2003; **16**: 494–502.

88. Shao Y, Cherry SR, Farahani K *et al.* Simultaneous PET and MR imaging. *Phys Med Biol* 1997; **42**: 1965–1970.

89. Slates RB, Farahani K, Shao Y *et al.* A study of artefacts in simultaneous PET and MR imaging using a prototype MR compatible PET scanner. *Phys Med Biol* 1999; **44**: 2015–2027.

90. Marsden PK, Strul D, Keevil SF *et al.* Simultaneous PET and NMR. *Br J Radiol* 2002; **75**: S53–S59.

91. Ziegler SI, Fries O, Pichler B *et al.* Prototype animal PET scanner with avalanche photodiode arrays and LSO crystals. *Eur J Nucl Med* 2001; **28**: 136–143.

92. Pichler B, Lorenz E, Mirzoyan R *et al.* Performance test of a LSO-APD PET module in 9.4 Tesla magnet. *IEEE Nuclear Science Symposium and Medical Imaging Conference.* Albuquerque, 9–15 Nov, 1997: 1237–1239.

93. Pichler BJ, Swann BK, Rochelle J *et al.* Lutetium oxyorthosilicate block detector readout by avalanche photodiode arrays for high resolution animal PET. *Phys Med Biol* 2004; **49**: 4305–4319.

CHAPTER 11

PET and CT in cardiac imaging: Is a paradigm shift from SPECT to hybrid PET/CT inevitable?

Henning Braess & Vasken Dilsizian

Introduction

Over the last three decades radionuclide imaging has continuously expanded its role in non-invasive cardiac diagnostics. This progression can be attributed to parallel advances in SPECT and PET instrumentation, radiopharmaceuticals, and software development for quantitative analysis of myocardial perfusion, function and metabolism. A number of clinical trials have demonstrated the diagnostic and prognostic accuracy of gated myocardial perfusion SPECT, and more importantly, its relevance for patient management. While SPECT continues to be the dominant technology used in clinical practice today, PET has made significant inroads in recent years from being exclusively a research tool to being a clinically viable, and perhaps, superior option to SPECT. The unique capability of PET to quantify myocardial blood flow and metabolism makes it very attractive for study of the effect of risk factors, lifestyle, and medical and interventional treatment.

The recent advent of hybrid PET/CT allows the assessment of myocardial perfusion and coronary anatomy concurrently [1]. Whereas multichannel CT angiography provides information on the presence and extent of epicardial coronary artery narrowing, stress myocardial perfusion PET provides information on the downstream functional consequences of such anatomic lesions. This results in a more refined approach to managing patients with coronary artery disease. Information regarding the size and location of the coronary artery occlusion (CT angiography) combined with the physiologic correlate of extent and severity of myocardial perfusion defect (PET), helps clinicians decide whether interventional or medical therapy is more promising for that particular patient. Distinguishing between isolated coronary occlusions and diffuse atherosclerosis becomes a lot more feasible with the hybrid PET/CT approach.

Advantages in the instrumentation, however, are only relevant if they significantly impact the diagnostic accuracy or the physician's confidence in the results. In this chapter, we will critically review the capabilities and limitations of myocardial SPECT. The assessment will address the sensitivity and spatial resolution of current SPECT scanners, the most important imaging artifacts and correction methods, and the characteristics of typical perfusion tracers. We will then review advantages and disadvantages of PET, CT, and hybrid PET/CT and determine if a paradigm shift from SPECT to PET/CT is inevitable.

Healthcare trend in cardiovascular diseases: prevention

An important driver for cardiac PET comes from a new trend in cardiovascular medicine. The new trend suggests a paradigm shift in cardiovascular medicine from detection and treatment of coronary artery disease to prediction and prevention of coronary artery disease. Current clinical application of myocardial perfusion SPECT is focused predominantly on the identification of isolated lesions,

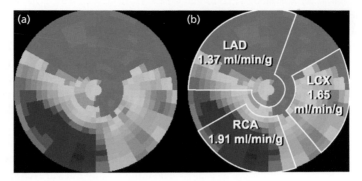

Fig. 11.1 Polar map of myocardial tracer uptake during adenosine vasodilation is shown in a patient with coronary artery disease. (a) relative distribution of the radiotracer (as would be the case with SPECT studies) suggests a single vessel disease in the territory of the left anterior descending (LAD) artery. Quantitative assessment of regional myocardial blood flow reserve with ^{13}N-ammonia PET is shown in (b). In a vascular territory without significant coronary artery stenosis, a normal myocardial blood flow reserve is approximately 3 ml/min/g. As such, quantitative myocardial blood flow assessment identifies abnormal flow reserve in all three vascular territories in this patient; 1.37 ml/min/g in the LAD territory, 1.65 ml/min/g in the left circumflex (LCX) territory, and 1.91 ml/min/g in the right coronary artery (RCA) territory. The clinical implication for the presumed diagnosis of 1-vessel on the evaluation of relative myocardial radiotracer uptake (with SPECT) versus 3-vessel coronary artery disease on quantitative assessment of myocardial blood flow reserve (with PET) is important and not inconsequential. (Figure adapted with permission from: Reference 3, Schindler TH, Schelbert HR. PET quantitation of myocardial blood flow. In: Dilsizian V & Narula J, eds. *Atlas of Nuclear Cardiology, 2nd edition*. Current Medicine, Inc., Philadelphia, 2006: 67–95.)

which can be treated by coronary interventions. As aggressive medical prevention and therapy become effective alternative treatment options for coronary artery disease, the need arises to tailor the medication to the individual needs of patients. This makes quantitative flow reserve measurement with PET very attractive since it allows the most reliable comparison between a baseline study and follow-up studies. PET is the only non-invasive imaging tool to reliably assess coronary endothelial dysfunction, the hallmark of coronary artery disease. By acquiring dynamic, gated myocardial perfusion data, PET studies provide insight into impairment of regional coronary blood flow reserve due to epicardial coronary artery stenosis, microvascular disease, and/or endothelial dysfunction.

The benefit of cardiac prevention is perceived to be so large that according to well accepted guidelines, the number of patients that should be considered for lipid lowering reaches 50 million patients in the United States [2]. The first step in prevention according to these guidelines consists of risk assessment by taking into consideration an individual patient's risk factors (such as lipid levels, smoking, diabetes, high blood pressure, etc). With more

accurate risk assessment, it is possible to adjust medical therapy more closely to the patient's actual needs, thus preventing side effects and unnecessary healthcare costs. Monitoring the response to treatment can help tailor the treatment more appropriately for a particular individual.

Risk assessment based on myocardial perfusion imaging with SPECT relies mostly on the size and severity of reversible and non-reversible perfusion defects, left ventricular ejection fraction, and presence of clinical symptoms during the exercise. It is important to point out, however, that all of these parameters represent endstage coronary artery disease. Detection of early, preclinical atherosclerosis is limited with SPECT. Although the distribution of a radiotracer may be homogeneous throughout the left ventricular myocardium on SPECT, absolute myocardial blood flow may be abnormal (Fig. 11.1) [3]. Quantitative flow reserve assessment with PET may identify the myocardial area of risk even before hemodynamically significant stenosis develops. This risk assessment can justify putting patients on aggressive medical therapy before advanced coronary artery disease ensues. Moreover, because the majority of acute coronary events originate in coronary arteries without distinct angiographic stenosis, identification of preclinical atherosclerosis could prove clinically important. Quantitative measurements of absolute myocardial blood flow with PET might thus identify patients who are at risk for future acute coronary events and thereby provide a strong rationale for aggressive medical and/or therapeutic interventions.

State-of-the-art SPECT

In order to predict the impact of hybrid PET/CT on nuclear cardiology an appreciation of the current clinical routine of stress myocardial perfusion imaging is helpful. With few exceptions, most myocardial perfusion examinations performed currently rely on SPECT imaging with thallium-201 and/or technetium-99m based perfusion tracers [4]. Due to its proven value in patient management (detection of coronary artery disease and prognosis), myocardial perfusion SPECT has become an integral part for the evaluation of patients with suspected coronary artery disease. The most frequent indication for myocardial perfusion SPECT is to determine whether a patient should be referred to coronary angiography for further diagnostics or interventional treatment. One of the largest assets of cardiac SPECT is that cardiologists are familiar with the technology, have used it for patient management decisions for many years (time tested), and have created validated normal databases. All these aspects contribute to the great confidence that cardiologists have in the results of myocardial perfusion SPECT. As such, hybrid PET/CT has to demonstrate a definite advantage over SPECT in order to play a significant role in the clinical care of patients.

When the diagnostic accuracy of myocardial SPECT is evaluated in the literature, most authors measure the sensitivity, specificity, and normalcy rate (in subjects with low likelihood for coronary artery disease who did not undergo coronary angiography) to detect angiographically significant coronary lesions. While the reported values may vary from publication to publication, typical values are approximately 90% sensitivity, 70% specificity, and 90% normalcy rate [5]. Variations in the literature can be explained by patient referral bias, differences in radiotracers, utilization of gated

software, and visual versus semiquantitative data analysis. Nonetheless, the negative predictive value of SPECT has been consistently high in most publications. Some authors argue that the relatively lower positive predictive value is due to the fact that endothelial dysfunction may lead to ischemia, even though there is no anatomically discernible coronary artery stenosis [6].

SPECT Radiopharmaceuticals

The utility of any nuclear technique is determined not only by the instrumentation and physical detection properties of radiotracers but also by the biological characteristics of the radiopharmaceuticals. Until the early 1990s, the potassium-analogue thallium-201 was the only myocardial perfusion tracer available for clinical studies with planar and/or SPECT cameras [7–9]. While the biological properties of thallium were excellent (high extraction fraction, rapid clearance from the blood, and the potential for redistribution), its low photon energy of 80 keV lead to significant attenuation artifacts, especially among patients with large body habitus. In addition, because of its long physical half-life of 73 hours, the amount of thallium administered clinically is confined by its radiation burden. Despite these limitations, thallium continues to be a clinically important radiotracer for the assessment of regional blood flow and myocardial viability. It is currently used in single isotope (thallium stress-redistribution and reinjection) and dual isotope (in combination with Tc-99m perfusion tracers) protocols. Thallium is also being considered for use with other interesting cardiac SPECT tracers that do not primarily depict myocardial perfusion but myocardial innervation, (e.g. ^{123}I-MIBG) or fatty acid metabolism (^{123}I-BMIPP) [10] (Fig. 11.2).

In the 1990s a number of Tc-99m based tracers were developed, of which sestamibi and tetrofosmin have gained both US Food and Drug Administration approval and wide clinical acceptance. Although the extraction fraction of these radiotracers is not ideal (approximately 50–60% when compared to 85% for thallium), the trapping and the short half-life of the ^{99m}Tc perfusion tracers lead to images with superior signal-to-noise ratio when compared to thallium. The higher signal-to-noise level derived with ^{99m}Tc perfusion tracers allowed

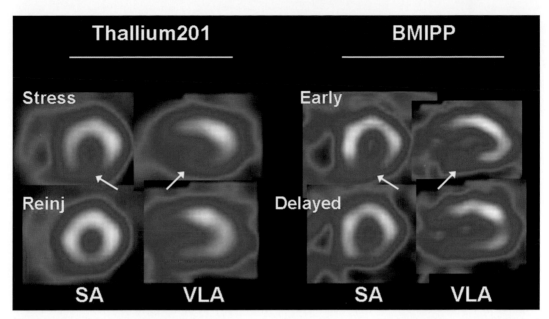

Fig. 11.2 Metabolic imaging with β-methyl-*p*-[^{123}I]-iodophenyl-pentadecanoic acid (BMIPP) can successfully demonstrate the metabolic imprint of a stress induced ischemic episode, also known as *ischemic memory*. Thallium stress and reinjection (reinj) images following treadmill exercise are displayed in the left panel, in the short-axis (SA) and vertical long-axis (VLA) SPECT tomograms. The thallium images demonstrate a severe reversible inferior defect (arrows), consistent with exercise stress induced ischemia. A similar defect is seen on the early BMIPP images in the same tomographic cuts (arrows), with BMIPP injected 22 hours after the stress induced ischemia. These image data suggest that BMIPP detects prolonged postischemic suppression of fatty acid metabolism for up to 22 hours after stress induced ischemia. (Figure adapted with permission from: Reference 10, Dilsizian V, Bateman TM, Bergmann SR *et al.* Metabolic imaging with β-methyl-*p*-[^{123}I]-iodophenyl-pentadecanoic acid (BMIPP) identifies ischemic memory following demand ischemia. *Circulation* 2005; **112**: 2169–2174.)

for combined perfusion and functional SPECT imaging or electrocardiogram (ECG) gated myocardial perfusion SPECT studies. Since the introduction of ^{99m}Tc labeled perfusion agents in combination with gating software, the assessment of wall motion, wall thickening, and ejection fractions have become an essential part of the nuclear cardiology examination. This experience makes cardiac SPECT not only a diagnostic but also a powerful prognostic tool.

Physical limitations of SPECT

The main physical limitations in SPECT acquisition lie in the area of photon detection sensitivity and spatial resolution. The photon detection sensitivity is the primary parameter that determines the noise of the SPECT images. The spatial resolution determines the smallest structures that can be distinguished with the system. These two measures are intimately related as they both depend on the SPECT collimator design. A very tight collimator yields good spatial resolution, however, at the expense of very noisy images. On the other hand, a coarse SPECT collimator results in poor spatial resolution and less noisy images. An additional factor limiting the detection sensitivity with SPECT is the fact that the detector does not cover all angles around the patient. As a result, the sensitivity of a typical dual head SPECT system is in the order of only 0.02%. This means that 99.98% of all emitted photons pass by undetected. The spatial resolution of this set-up is between 10–14 mm, depending on the precise clinical setting.

The limited spatial resolution of over 10 mm with current state-of-the-art SPECT cameras has a number of consequences. The most notable consequence is the so called partial volume effect. This effect causes thicker walls to appear brighter than thinner walls. The wall thickening of the myocardium causes the walls to be brighter during systole than during diastole. Another important consequence of the limited spatial resolution of SPECT systems is the inaccurate measurements of left ventricular volume and ejection fraction measurements, particularly, in hearts with small chambers. Increased visceral and subdiaphragmatic activity, particularly with ^{99m}Tc labeled perfusion agents, becomes quite challenging, if not impossible, to interpret with limited spatial resolution SPECT systems. The signal from extracardiac activity spills over into the myocardium, such that the inferior wall cannot be assessed with confidence.

The other important limitation of the SPECT technology arises from soft tissue attenuation artifacts. These artifacts occur in virtually all patients to some degree. Inhomogeneous attenuation causes artifacts in the anterior or inferior walls. These artifacts look very much like perfusion deficits. A number of techniques have been explored to estimate the attenuation with external devices and to perform attenuation correction. Attenuation correction is considered to be sufficiently mature for its utilization to be generally recommended [11]. However, SPECT attenuation correction does not always rectify the underlying attenuation artifact. More importantly, the attenuation algorithm itself may yield new, artifactual defects that are related to reconstruction problems rather than true underlying myocardial physiology. As a result, it is necessary to review both attenuation corrected and non-corrected SPECT images in order to render an opinion, which of course is time consuming and at times inconclusive. With the exception of a few centers, SPECT attenuation correction is not routinely performed and has not gained widespread acceptance.

State-of-the-Art PET: Technical advantages over SPECT

While both PET and SPECT provide valuable information regarding tomographic distribution of radiotracers, there are a number of physical differences that give PET a clear competitive advantage over SPECT. Namely, PET has high spatial and temporal resolution, reliable attenuation and scatter correction, utilizes short lived positron emitting radiotracers, and offers validated tracer kinetic models for quantifying absolute myocardial blood flow.

From image quality perspective, the biggest difference between SPECT and PET is that the spatial resolution and the detection sensitivity of the PET system are independent. Modern PET scanners have a resolution of 4–6 mm and a sensitivity of a few per cent. The sensitivity depends critically on the precise set-up and the dose of injected tracer. In combination with the short lived tracers, which allows for the injection of large activities of the tracer, PET perfusion images generally have good spatial resolution at acceptable noise levels with short imaging protocols. Because of the superior spatial resolution, the spillover of extracardiac activity into the myocardium is not as much of a problem as in the case of SPECT (Fig. 11.3). Despite the widely acknowledged physical advantages of PET over SPECT, the significantly higher cost of PET studies has limited its widespread use in clinical cardiology.

PET allows attenuation and scatter correction either based on external transmission sources or based on CT images. Unlike SPECT attenuation correction, PET attenuation correction with external sources is so reliable that it is not necessary to review non-corrected PET images during the clinical interpretation. PET attenuation correction drastically increases the specificity of a myocardial perfusion study to as high as 95%. More importantly, such reliable attenuation correction with PET allows for absolute quantification of blood flow [1], metabolism [12], and membrane receptor subtypes [13] in the heart. In the case of attenuation based on CT images there is still some controversy whether respiratory motion will create additional artifacts.

Quantitative analysis with PET is based on dynamic acquisition protocols, which allow assessment of the retention fraction and the wash-out time of the radiotracer. Combining these parameters with the net tracer uptake allows quantitative evaluation of myocardial perfusion (Fig. 11.4). The above procedure makes use of so called compartmental modeling. The most relevant steps of tracer uptake and wash-out, such as tracer diffusion across the cell membrane and metabolic trapping, are modeled by mathematical equations. These equations relate the

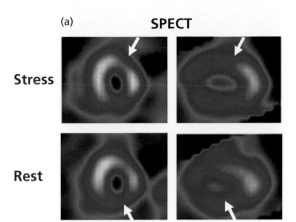

Fig. 11.3 Disparity between myocardial perfusion SPECT and Rubidium-82 PET studies is shown. Clinically indicated adenosine dual-isotope gated SPECT images (a) without attenuation correction show regional Tc-99 m sestamibi perfusion defect in the anterior and inferior regions (arrowhead). On the rest thallium-201 images, the anterior defect became reversible while the inferior defect persisted. Corresponding Rubidium-82 PET myocardial perfusion tomograms performed in the same patient are shown in (b). PET images were acquired on a Gemini PET/CT scanner (Philips Medical Systems) after an infusion of adenosine and 30 mCi of Rubidium-82 (top) and at rest following another 30 mCi infusion of Rubidium-82 (bottom). Rubidium-82 PET images show normal distribution of the radiotracer in all myocardial regions, without evidence for reversible or fixed defects to suggest myocardial ischemia or infarction. Although the high energy positrons of Rubidium-82 degrade spatial resolution and the short half-life increases statistical noise, high quality images free from attenuation artifacts can be produced with Rubidium-82 PET with only 30 mCi injected dose. (Figure adapted with permission from: Reference 1, Lodge MA, Braess H, Mahmood F et al. Developments in nuclear cardiology: Transition from single photon emission computed tomography to positron emission tomography/computed tomography. *J Invasive Cardiol* 2005; **17**: 491–496.)

dynamic behavior of the tracer uptake to the myocardial perfusion. Obviously the values for the myocardial perfusion are only as good as the assumptions made on the tracer kinetics. The most critical model assumption is that the first pass extraction fraction depends in a predictable way on the myocardial perfusion [14]. Assessment of myocardial blood flow at rest and during exercise or pharmacologic stress gives a measure for the flow-reserve, which is the ratio of perfusion during stress and at rest.

PET radiopharmaceuticals

A number of PET tracers, depicting various aspects of myocardial blood flow and metabolism have been studied. Imaging myocardial blood flow has been one of the earliest applications of clinical PET. Cyclotron produced myocardial blood flow tracers include ^{15}O-water and ^{13}N-ammonia, and generator produced tracers include ^{82}Rubidium and ^{62}Copper-PTSM; use of the latter is currently in-

vestigational. PET perfusion tracers can be used to accurately quantify myocardial blood flow in absolute (ml/min/gram of tissue) or relative terms. For purposes of viability assessment, regional myocardial perfusion is usually compared to ^{18}F labeled fluorodeoxyglucose metabolic activity, which is the most commonly used PET radiotracer in clinical practice.

PET myocardial blood flow agents can be divided into two types: freely diffusible and soluble, microsphere-like, extractable tracers. ^{15}O-water is an example of a freely diffusible tracer, the kinetics of accumulation and clearance of which are less complicated than tracers that are extractable. However, by its very nature of rapid physiologic wash-out and clearance from the myocardium, ^{15}O-water does not give clinically meaningful images. Rather one must perform mathematical modeling at each pixel in order to determine parametric images of flow, which often produce quite noisy images. The second type of flow tracers, the so called soluble,

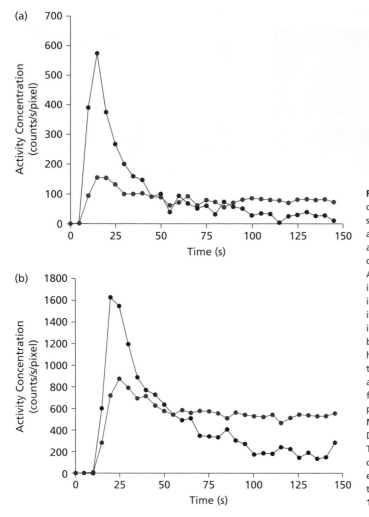

Fig. 11.4 Rubidium-82 time-activity curves at rest (a) and after adenosine stress (b). Solid circles represent the activity concentration in the left atrium and the red circles represent the activity concentration in myocardial tissue. Although the first few minutes after the infusion of Rubidium-82 are not usually included in clinical acquisition protocols, it is precisely this period that is of interest if myocardial perfusion is to be quantified. Dynamic imaging of the heart during this time allows analysis of the Rubidium-82 concentration in both arterial blood and myocardial tissue as a function of time. (Figure adapted with permission from: Reference 1, Lodge MA, Braess H, Mahmood F *et al.* Developments in nuclear cardiology: Transition from single photon emission computed tomography to positron emission tomography/computed tomography. *J Invasive Cardiol* 2005; **17**: 491–496.)

microsphere-like tracers are extractable substances that are trapped in the myocardium. They are usually easier to scan because the radioactivity is fixed in place for a reasonable length of time, and therefore, optimal counting statistics can be obtained. However, the amount of binding may depend on a biochemical interaction and this interaction could change as a function of disease and confound the flow measurement. ^{13}N-ammonia is an example of an extractable tracer, which involves a carrier-mediated transport across the myocardium: the kinetics of accumulation and clearance from myocardium depends on the conversion of ammonia to glutamine via the glutamine synthetase pathway.

The physical half-life of approximately 10 min leads to excellent images after 10–20 min of image acquisition. Absolute quantification requires two- and three-compartment kinetic models that incorporate extraction and rate constants [12, 15, 16]. Thus, ^{13}N-ammonia can be used to produce both high quality clinical images and also quantitative measures of myocardial perfusion.

Rubidium-82 falls more closely into this second category of flow tracers—i.e. the more microsphere-like flow tracers. However, its short half-life (75 s) means that any trapped rubidium quickly disappears from the myocardium by physical decay. This reduces radiation exposure to the patient, and permits repeated studies to be performed. In addition it has been shown (in animal studies) that its extraction fraction does not change significantly over a wide range of metabolic conditions, and is not altered by many drugs, including those which affect sodium-potassium pump function (rubidium retention is of course rapidly affected by cell membrane disruption). Despite its short half-life, rubidium is easily obtained, as it is generator produced. The relatively long lived Sr-82/Rb-82 generator (typically four-week "shelf" life), puts rubidium into the same class as F-18 (physical half-life of 110 min). That is to say, it can be used clinically without the need for an on-site cyclotron. Both ammonia and rubidium have received U.S. Food and Drug Administration (FDA) approval for assessment of myocardial perfusion.

Early detection of coronary artery disease and monitoring medical therapy

A significant advantage of PET over SPECT is its capability to quantify *absolute* regional radiotracer uptake, or at least to do this in some absolute unit that can be compared across patients. Conventional SPECT approaches identify flow-limiting coronary artery narrowing by delineating the *relative* spatial distribution of myocardial blood flow at rest and again during stress. While this approach has been clinically useful, it does not permit comparisons of regional blood flow at rest and during stress, in the same region, quantitatively. Furthermore, it may underestimate balanced reduction in coronary artery blood flow, diffuse non-occlusive luminal coronary artery narrowing, or an occlusive lesion in the region with the highest radiotracer uptake by SPECT. While there is good correlation in the literature between the severity of coronary artery stenosis and myocardial flow reserve assessed by PET [17, 18], a perfect correlation is not to be expected since the flow reserve also depends on other factors, such as collateral flow and endothelial function.

Endothelial dysfunction causes impaired stress induced coronary artery vasodilation, which leads to diminished myocardial blood flow reserve, long before hemodynamically significant coronary artery stenosis develops. Assessment of myocardial blood flow reserve with PET allows early identification of coronary artery disease characterized by endothelial dysfunction. Impaired myocardial blood flow or flow reserve has been shown in asymptomatic patients with elevated cholesterol [19], smoking [20], hypertension [21], and insulin resistance [22], either during pharmaceutical stress or cold pressor test, attributed to underlying endothelial dysfunction. In patients with single vessel CAD undergoing flow-pressure measurements, flow resistance and fractional flow reserve were shown to be abnormal in more than 50% of presumably normal vessels [17]. Endothelial dysfunction is responsible for coronary spasms, leading to ischemia and anginal symptoms. Although there is unequivocal evidence that endothelial dysfunction is a relevant prognostic marker of future cardiac events [23], only a few studies have shown that endothelial dysfunction is a relevant therapeutic target [23, 24].

In patients with advanced coronary artery disease, the main pillars of medical therapy consist of lipid lowering agents, nitrates, ACE-inhibition, and beta blockers. These treatment options have all been shown to improve mortality and morbidity significantly in the appropriate patient groups. Quantitative PET flow measurements have been used to demonstrate improvement in endothelial dysfunction and myocardial ischemia in patients with advanced coronary artery disease after medical treatment (Fig. 11.5) with vitamin C, and a regular exercise program [25–29]. A main advantage of medical therapy is that beyond its beneficial effect on the isolated coronary artery lesion, its systemic effect on all vessels (coronary, carotid, peripheral, etc.) may prevent further progression of atherosclerosis. An example of a patient exhibiting improvement in adenosine-stimulated hyperemia after one year of treatment with 3-hydroxy-3-methylglutaryl coenzyme A reductase inhibitor is shown in Fig. 11.6 [3].

Medical therapy with lipid lowering agents can halt or slow the progression of coronary artery disease. Not only is the coronary morphology affected by lowering lipid levels but the endothelial function also improves. The improved endothelial function prevents paradoxical vasoconstriction, thus reducing ischemia and cardiac symptoms. More importantly, lipid lowering agents may also play a role in preventing plaque rupture, thereby decreasing

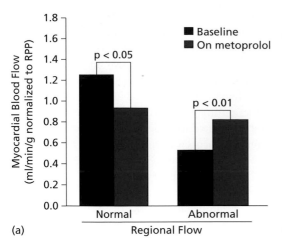

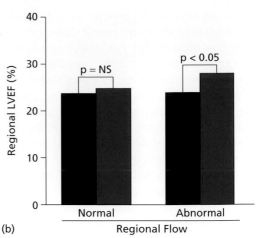

(a) Regional Flow (b) Regional Flow

Fig. 11.5 Quantitative PET flow measurements can be used to study the effects of six months of medical treatment with metoprolol on absolute myocardial blood flow and function in patients with ischemic cardiomyopathy. (a) There is a favorable redistribution of absolute blood flow from normally perfused myocardium to abnormally perfused myocardium from before to after metoprolol therapy. (b) Increased myocardial blood flow is associated with improvement in regional left ventricular ejection fraction (LVEF) in the abnormally perfused regions of myocardium while myocardial regions with normal baseline perfusion show no change in regional left ventricular ejection fraction . The reduction in blood flow in non-ischemic regions by beta blockade most probably reflects the reduction in myocardial oxygen demands induced by the reduction in myocardial contractility and work. On the other hand, the decrease in myocardial oxygen demand of the ischemic area by beta blockade may restore vascular autoregulation and allow the ischemic vasculature to regulate its blood flow. By decreasing myocardial oxygen demand (decrease in heart rate) and increasing myocardial oxygen supply (increased subendocardial blood flow in ischemic myocardium), treatment with metoprolol results in an improvement in oxygen balance of the ischemic myocardium. RPP = rate-pressure product, NS = not significant. (Figure adapted with permission from: Reference 27, Bennett SK, Smith MF, Gottlieb SS *et al.* Effect of metoprolol on absolute myocardial blood flow in patients with heart failure secondary to ischemic or non-ischemic cardiomyopathy. *Am J Cardiol* 2002; **89**: 1431–1434.)

the risk of future cardiac events. The anti-ischemic effect of three to six months of medical therapy has been shown with SPECT and PET perfusion studies [19, 26]. Moreover, a correlation between improvement in myocardial flow reserve after medical therapy and clinical outcome has been shown [19, 30].

In a prospective study, 44 patients who suffered an acute myocardial infarction were randomized to either intensive medical therapy or coronary angioplasty [30]. Myocardial ischemia was quantified with adenosine thallium SPECT at a mean of 4.5 days after the infarction and 43 days after either medical or interventional therapy. The total perfusion defect (and ischemic defect size) was comparably reduced with medical therapy (from $38 \pm 13\%$ to $26 \pm 16\%$; $p < 0.001$) and coronary angioplasty (from $35 \pm 12\%$ to $20 \pm 16\%$; $p < 0.001$). Moreover, the patients who responded to the medical treatment with decreased defect size had better survival compared to those whose defect size did not decrease significantly. Although the correlation between image based response to therapy and prognosis is not surprising, it is not self evident either.

An even closer correlation between clinical outcome and image based response to therapy was shown with ammonia PET [19]. In 15 patients with angiographically documented multivessel coronary artery disease and hypercholesterolemia, dynamic adenosine ammonia PET was performed at two and six months during treatment with fluvastatin lipid-lowering therapy [3]. At six month follow-up, myocardial blood flow reserve increased significantly by 38% from 2.5 ± 0.6 ml/g/min to 3.4 ± 1.0 ml/g/min ($p < 0.05$ versus baseline). Although all patients experienced low density lipoprotein (LDL) improvements, not all patients experienced an improvement in myocardial blood flow reserve.

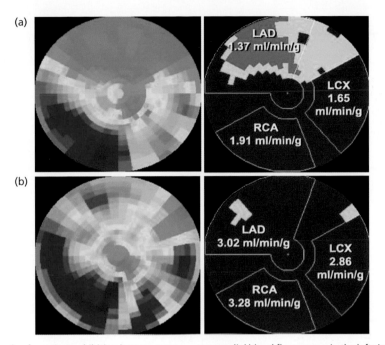

Fig. 11.6 An example of a patient exhibiting improvement in adenosine-stimulated hyperemia after one year treatment with pravastatin. When compared to baseline quantitative myocardial blood flow reserve values with ^{13}N-ammonia PET (a), follow-up polar maps show significant improvement in myocardial flow reserve in all three vascular territories (b). The extent of the stress induced defect decreased from 51% of the left anterior descending (LAD) vascular territory to only 3% one year post medical therapy. Moreover, there is increase and normalization in myocardial blood flow reserve in the left circumflex (LCX) and right coronary artery (RCA) vascular territories, which could only be detected on quantitative measurements of myocardial blood flow but not on the evaluation of the relative radiotracer uptake. (Figure adapted with permission from: Reference 3, Schindler TH, Schelbert HR. PET quantitation of myocardial blood flow. In: Dilsizian V & Narula J, eds. *Atlas of Nuclear Cardiology*. Current Medicine, Inc., Philadelphia, 2006: 67–95.)

The patients were classified as either responders or non-responders on the basis of flow reserve measured with quantitative PET after six months. All responders experienced relief of anginal symptoms and none of the non-responders experienced symptom relief. This correlation is very important, as the precise mechanism for the observed vasoprotection of lipid lowering agents remains unresolved.

Prognostic value of diminished myocardial flow reserve by PET

Quantitative approaches that measure myocardial blood flow with PET identify multivessel coronary artery disease and offer the opportunity to monitor responses to risk factor modification and to therapeutic interventions. Recent studies have shown that diminished myocardial blood flow reserve by PET was also predictive of future cardiovascular out-

come in patents without underlying coronary artery disease [31–33]. Among 51 patients with hypertrophic cardiomyopathy who underwent myocardial blood flow PET studies and were followed for an average of eight years, 16 (31%) had cardiovascular events [31]. The overall accumulative survival (Fig. 11.7, (a)) and cumulative survival free from an unfavorable outcome (Fig. 11.7, (b)) were associated with the level of hyperemic myocardial blood flow achieved during pharmacologic vasodilation. These findings suggest that the degree of microvascular dysfunction of the coronary microcirculation (as reflected by the diminished blood flow observed on PET) was predictive of future cardiovascular outcome.

Similar results were attained among patients with idiopathic dilated cardiomyopathy [32, 33]. Twenty-six patients with dilated cardiomyopathy, of whom 24 had angiographically normal coronary

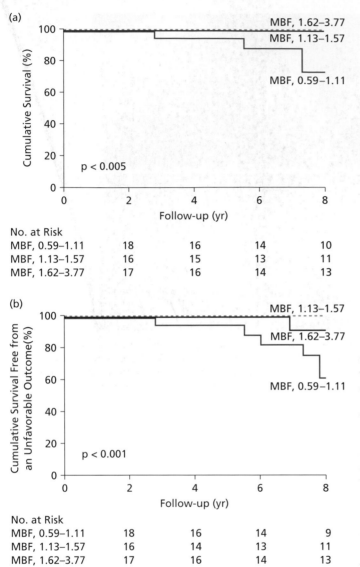

Fig. 11.7 Myocardial blood flow (MBF) values after dipyridamole infusion and long term prognosis are shown in patients with hypertrophic cardiomyopathy. Patients were divided into three equal groups according to MBF after dipyridamole infusion. (a) Shows overall cumulative survival, and (b) shows cumulative survival free from an unfavorable outcome. (Figure adapted with permission from: Reference 31, Cecchi F, Olivotto I, Gistri R *et al*. Coronary microvascular dysfunction and prognosis in hypertrophic cardiomyopathy. *N Engl J Med* 2003; **349**: 1027–1035.)

arteries, underwent myocardial blood flow PET studies and were followed for approximately three years [32]. Nine (35%) patients died during the follow-up period. The overall accumulative three year survival was strongly associated with the spatial heterogeneity of myocardial perfusion derived from the coefficient of variance of absolute regional myocardial blood flow. The probability of three year survival was 33% in subjects whose coefficient of variance was above the median compared with 90% in subjects whose coefficient of variance was below the median (p = 0.01). In a similar study

of 67 patients with dilated cardiomyopathy who underwent myocardial blood flow PET studies and were followed for a mean of three to four years, 24 (36%) patients had major cardiac events: eight cardiac deaths and 16 progression of heart failure [33]. Impaired myocardial blood flow reserve on PET was associated with an increase in relative risk of death or progression of heart failure of 3.5 times over other more common clinical and functional variables (Fig. 11.8).

While assessment of myocardial perfusion with PET has become an indispensable tool in cardiac

(a)

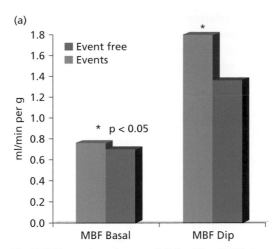

(b)

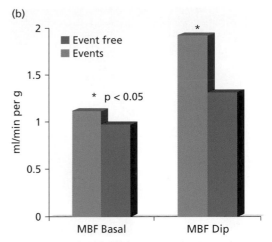

Fig. 11.8 Mean values of myocardial blood flow (MBF) at rest and during dipyridamole vasodilation (MBF Dip) are shown for patients with dilated cardiomyopathy (a) and hypertrophic cardiomyopathy (b). Patients with unfavorable outcome (events) over the ensuing years exhibited impaired MBF with dipyridamole PET when compared to patients with favorable outcome (event free survival). (Figure adapted with permission from: Reference 31, Cecchi F, Olivotto I, Gistri R *et al.* Coronary microvascular dysfunction and prognosis in hypertrophic cardiomyopathy. *N Engl J Med* 2003; **349**: 1027–1035, and with permission from: Reference 33, Neglia D, Michelassi C, Trivieri MG *et al.* Prognostic role of myocardial blood flow impairment in idiopathic left ventricular dysfunction. *Circulation* 2002: **105**: 186–193.)

research, it remains underutilized in clinical practice. The main drawback for the technology is its cost. Not only are the PET cameras expensive, but radiotracers, which require either a cyclotron or an expensive generator for isotope production, are quite expensive to maintain unless maintenance costs are shared with other subspecialties, such as oncology. As PET equipment becomes more widely utilized in cardiovascular disorders, it is expected that the additional clinical benefit of myocardial perfusion PET will be realized.

Hybrid PET/CT scanners

Hybrid PET/CT scanners allow the determination of anatomical and functional information in a single imaging session [34]. CT angiography provides information on the presence and extent of luminal narrowing of coronary arteries, whereas PET provides information on the functional consequence of such coronary lesions in the myocardium. The combination of these two modalities is particularly relevant in patients who have an intermediate finding on either PET or CT. The advantage of the combined scanner is that the corresponding images are spatially aligned and both data sets can be acquired at a single imaging session. An integrated PET/CT cardiac tomogram from a patient with ischemic cardiomyopathy is shown in Fig. 11.9.

Secondary benefits include the improved accuracy with which the heart can be positioned within the PET field of view. In addition, corrections for the energy difference between CT x-rays and annihilation photons of PET have allowed CT images to be used for PET attenuation correction [35]. This has resulted in replacement of Ge-68 or Cs-137 transmission scans (required for PET attenuation correction) with faster CT attenuation correction algorithms, thereby reducing the overall duration of the scanning procedure. However, one potential problem of using fast CT scans for attenuation correction is the motion of the organs during respiration. The CT scanner captures the heart, lungs and liver at one point in the respiratory cycle, while the PET emission provides average data over many respiratory cycles. Various approaches to correct this problem are currently under investigation.

(a)

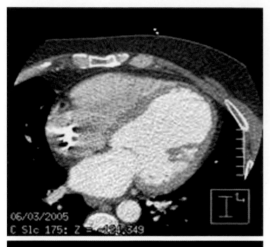

(b)

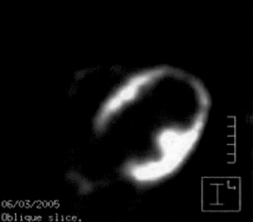

(c)

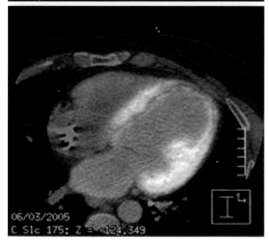

Concordance and discordance between coronary anatomy and myocardial perfusion

The most attractive feature of hybrid PET/CT is that PET perfusion and CT angiography depict complementary aspects of coronary artery disease. Despite rapid developments in CT technology, it is important to point out some limitations of the current technology. Clinically acceptable CT angiography studies require at least a 16-slice CT detector and very careful patient preparation. Among patients who are able to hold their breath for 20 seconds, most proximal sections of the coronary arteries can be assessed. The resolution of CT (0.7–1.0 mm) does not allow visualization of small, distal coronary arteries, which are easily seen on interventional angiography. Arrhythmia, which is common in cardiac patients, can prevent successful cardiac gating. Patient motion and severe coronary artery calcifications are potential sources of error, which can lead to non-diagnostic or inaccurate data. Because the diagnostic accuracy of CT angiography is heart rate dependent, β-adrenergic receptor blockers are often administered to patients to reduce the heart rate (ideally < 60 bpm) during data acquisition.

The success of cardiac nuclear imaging can be attributed to its high sensitivity for detecting coronary artery disease and accurate risk stratification in a variety of patient subsets [36]. Among patients with known or suspected coronary artery disease, stress myocardial perfusion studies are used to guide patient management decisions for cardiac catheterization, revascularization, or medical therapy (Fig. 11.10 and Fig. 11.11). This does not imply, however, that myocardial perfusion SPECT contains all the necessary information to determine whether a patient will benefit from medical therapy or revascularization. There are a number of scenarios where adding CT angiography to myocardial perfusion may lead to a different patient management decision than the results of myocardial

Fig. 11.9 Transverse CT, PET, and integrated PET/CT image of the heart from a patient with ischemic cardiomyopathy is shown. The CT image (a), shows abnormal thinning of the apical and apicolateral regions of the left ventricle, and preserved wall thickness in the septal and lateral regions. The corresponding FDG PET image (b) shows preserved metabolic activity in the septal and lateral regions and relatively decreased metabolic activity in the apical and apicolateral regions. Integrated PET/CT images (c) provide accurate co-registration of the limited spatial resolution metabolic signal of PET with the high resolution anatomic signal of CT. (With permission and courtesy of Dr. Timm Dickfeld).

(a)

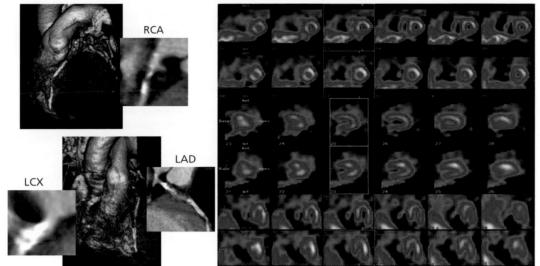

(b)

Fig. 11.10 In this patient example, integrated approach of identifying the presence and extent of epicardial coronary artery narrowing by multidetector CT and downstream functional consequences of such anatomic lesions by myocardial perfusion SPECT is shown. (a) 3D reformatted volume image provides morphologic information of the coronary arteries and surrounding structures. Multiplanar reformatted volume rendering image shows near total occlusion of the proximal right coronary artery (RCA), severe stenosis of the left circumflex (LCX), and moderate stenosis in the left anterior descending (LAD) arteries associated with significant coronary calcification. (b) SPECT myocardial perfusion images show extensive myocardial ischemia in the inferior and inferolateral walls of the left ventricle and preserved myocardial viability in all three vascular territories. (With permission and courtesy of Dr. Jongdae Suh).

(a)

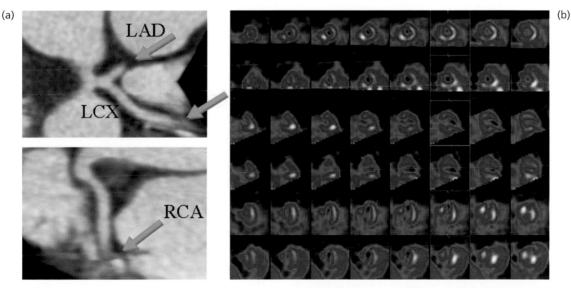

(b)

Fig. 11.11 In this patient example, multiplanar reformatted volume rendering images (a) from multidetector CT angiography show total occlusion of the proximal left anterior descending (LAD) artery and severe stenosis of the proximal left circumflex (LCX) coronary artery. In the absence of corresponding functional image, it is difficult (if not impossible) to predict whether the myocardium subtended by the LAD vessel is viable or scarred. (b) Myocardial perfusion SPECT images demonstrate fixed perfusion defects in the anterior, septal, and apical walls of the left ventricle compatible with prior myocardial infarction. On the other hand, myocardial viability is preserved in the LCX and right coronary artery (RCA) vascular territories. (With permission and courtesy of Dr. Jongdae Suh).

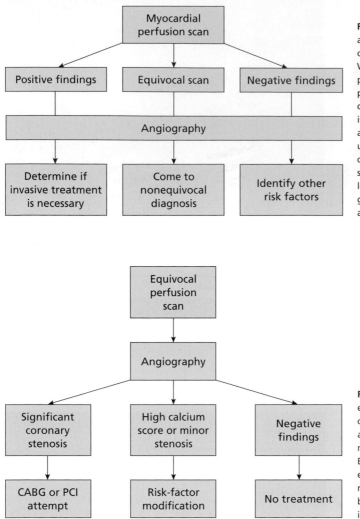

Fig. 11.12 Incremental value of CT angiography to myocardial perfusion on the basis of scan findings is shown. When the myocardial perfusion scan is positive for ischemia, the predominant purpose of CT angiography is to determine whether an invasive therapy is amenable. For equivocal scans, the CT angiography will determine if there is underlying coronary artery lesion. In the case of negative scans, elevated calcium score and insignificant coronary artery lesions detected on CT angiography may guide aggressive risk factor modification and medical therapy.

Fig. 11.13 CT Angiography after an equivocal myocardial perfusion scan. In case of significant stenosis a coronary angiography will follow, after a negative CTA no treatment will follow. But even intermediate findings such as elevated calcium have a prognostic relevance. CABG = coronary artery bypass surgery, PCI = percutaneous intervention.

perfusion alone. Schematic diagrams that provide insight into the incremental value of coronary angiography to myocardial perfusion studies are outlined below (Fig. 11.12, Fig. 11.13 and Fig. 11.14). The incremental value of CT angiography is most obvious in the setting of *equivocal* myocardial perfusion scan (Fig. 11.13).

In the setting of *abnormal* myocardial perfusion scan, the incremental value of CT angiography is that it can determine, non-invasively, whether a revascularization procedure is both amenable and beneficial (Fig. 11.14). Currently, many patients who are triaged to the cardiac catheterization laboratory because of an abnormal myocardial perfusion scan

may not be candidates for revascularization. The main reasons are 1) no significant epicardial coronary artery narrowing is detected despite an abnormal perfusion study (e.g. sequential insignificant anatomic lesions, microvascular, and/or endothelial dysfunction); 2) while there may be evidence for structural disease, percutaneous revascularization of the coronary lesion is not feasible, and 3) revascularization of the coronary disease is unlikely to have beneficial effect on regional or global left ventricular function.

In the setting of a normal myocardial perfusion scan, the incremental benefit of CT angiography is least obvious. Even if the CT angiography shows a

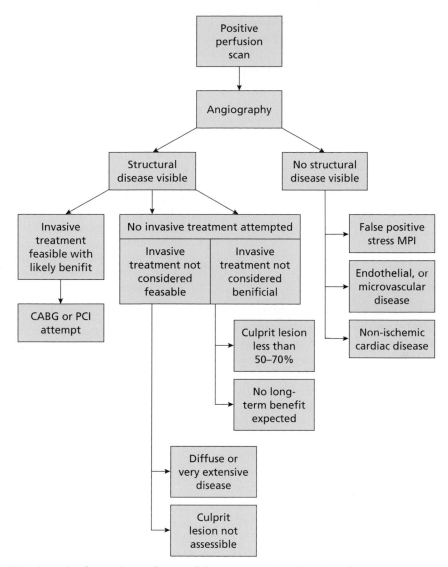

Fig. 11.14 CT angiography after an abnormal myocardial perfusion scan. It is estimated that less than half of the patients who undergo cardiac catheterization after an abnormal perfusion scan are actually candidates for percutaneous coronary intervention. Which means that non-invasive CT angiography may prevent a number of unnecessary cardiac catheterizations. MPI = myocardial perfusion imaging, CABG = coronary artery bypass surgery, PCI = percutaneous intervention.

significant coronary artery lesion, it does not necessarily imply that revascularizaton of that particular lesion is imminent. Endogenous revascularization via collateral vessels may provide adequate perfusion to the myocardium despite the presence of epicardial stenosis [37]. While identification of insignificant coronary artery disease and/or elevated calcium score in the setting of normal myocardial perfusion scan may justify a more aggressive risk-management and preventive medical therapy, this remains hypothetical and untested.

Radiation burden

Using conservative estimates, the radiation burden of multidetector CT angiography is at least twice that of rubidium PET studies using current PET instrumentation. The estimated effective dose of radiation exposure from multidetector CT angiography ranges from 7 to 13 mSv [38], whereas the effective dose for rubidium PET is approximately 5.5 mSv for a maximum allowable activity of 60 mCi at both rest and stress [1]. With current advances in PET instrumentation, diagnostic quality PET images can be acquired using only 30 mCi of rubidium for each of the rest and stress phases of the study. As a result, the effective dose of radiation exposure from rubidium PET falls to 2.75 mSv. These values compare favorably with radiation exposure from SPECT radiotracers, such as 3 mCi of thallium-201 (12.7 mSv) and 30 mCi of Tc-99m sestamibi (4.73 mSv).

Conclusions

Coronary angiography provides information on the presence and extent of arterial luminal narrowing while PET provides information on the downstream functional consequences of such anatomic lesions. With the advent of hybrid PET/CT systems, such complementary information on coronary artery physiology and anatomy can be realized immediately, at the same imaging session. An integrated approach of these two technologies is particularly relevant in patients with an intermediate finding on either PET or CT. The implication of this hybrid PET/CT imaging approach is a decrease in the number of unnecessary cardiac catheterizations and interventions and a more efficient delivery of health care.

References

1. Lodge MA, Braess H, Mahmood F et al. Developments in nuclear cardiology: Transition from single photon emission computed tomography to positron emission tomography/computed tomography. *J Invasive Cardiol* 2005; **17**: 491–496.
2. National Cholesterol Education Program (NCEP) Expert Panel on Detection, Evaluation, and Treatment of High Blood Cholesterol in Adults (Adult Treatment Panel III). Third Report of the National Cholesterol Education Program (NCEP) Expert Panel on Detection, Evaluation, and Treatment of High Cholesterol in Adults (Adult Treatment Panel III). *Circulation* 2002; **106**: 3143–3421.
3. Schindler TH, Schelbert HR. PET quantitation of myocardial blood flow. In Dilsizian V & Narula J, eds. *Atlas of Nuclear Cardiology, 2nd edition*. Current Medicine, Inc., Philadelphia, 2006: 67–95.
4. Dilsizian V. SPECT and PET Imaging: Tracers and Techniques. In: Dilsizian V, Narula J, eds. *Atlas of Nuclear Cardiology 2nd edn*. Braunwald E (series ed) Current Medicine, Inc., Philadelphia, 2006: 35–66.
5. Frans J, Wackers TH. SPECT detection of coronary artery disease. In: Dilsizian V & Narula J, eds. *Atlas of Nuclear Cardiology*. Braunwald E (series ed) Current Medicine, Inc., Philadelphia, 2003: 63–77.
6. Blumenthal RS, Becker DM, Yanek LR et al. Detecting occult coronary disease in a high risk asymptomatic population. *Circulation* 2003; **107**: 702–707.
7. Zaret BL, Strauss HW, Martin ND et al. Non-invasive regional myocardial perfusion with radioactive potassium: Study of patients at rest with exercise and during angina pectoris. *N Engl J Med* 1973; **288**: 809–812.
8. Pohost GM, Zir LM, Moore RH et al. Differentiation of transiently ischemic from infarcted myocardium by serial imaging after a single dose of thallium-201. *Circulation* 1977; **55**: 294–302.
9. Dilsizian V, Rocco TP, Freedman NM et al. Enhanced detection of ischemic but viable myocardium by the reinjection of thallium after stress-redistribution imaging. *N Engl J Med* 1990; **323**: 141–146
10. Dilsizian V, Bateman TM, Bergmann SR et al. Metabolic imaging with β-methyl-ρ-[^{123}I]-iodophenyl-pentadecanoic acid (BMIPP) identifies ischemic memory following demand ischemia. *Circulation* 2005; **112**: 2169–2174.
11. Heller GV, Links J, Bateman TM et al. American Society of Nuclear Cardiology and Society of Nuclear Medicine joint position statement: Attenuation correction of myocardial perfusion SPECT scintigraphy. *J Nucl Cardiol* 2004; **11**: 229–30.
12. Kitsiou AN, Bacharach SL, Bartlett ML et al. ^{13}N-ammonia myocardial blood flow and uptake: Relation to functional outcome of asynergic regions after revascularization. *J Am Coll Cardiol* 1999; **33**: 678–686.
13. Shirani J, Loredo ML, Eckelman WC et al. Imaging the renin angiotensin aldosterone system in the heart. *Curr Heart Fail Rep* 2005; **2**: 78–86.
14. Rimoldi OE, Camici PG. Positron emission tomography for quantitation of myocardial perfusion. *J Nucl Cardiol* 2004; **11**: 482–489.
15. Krivokapich J, Smith GT, Huang S-C et al. ^{13}N-ammonia myocardial imaging at rest and with exercise in normal volunteers. *Circulation* 1989; **80**: 1328–1337.
16. Hutchins GD, Schwaiger M, Rosenspire KC et al. Non-invasive quantification of regional blood flow in the human heart using ^{13}N-ammonia and dynamic positron emission tomographic imaging. *J Am Coll Cardiol* 1990; **15**: 1032–1042.

17. Di Carli M, Czernin J, Hoh CK *et al*. Relation among stenosis severity, myocardial blood flow and flow reserve in patients with coronary artery disease. *Circulation* 1995; **91**: 1944–1951.

18. Muzik O, Duvernoy C, Beanlands R *et al*. Assessment of the diagnostic performance of quantitative flow measurements in normal subjects and patients with angiographically documented coronary artery disease by means of nitrogen-13 ammonia and positron emission tomography. *J Am Coll Cardiol* 1998; **31**: 534–540.

19. Guethlin M, Kasel AM, Coppenrath K *et al*. Delayed response of myocardial flow reserve to lipid-lowering therapy with fluvastatin. *Circulation* 1999; **99**: 475–481.

20. Czernin J, Sun K, Brunken R *et al*. Effect of acute and long term smoking on myocardial blood flow and flow reserve. *Circulation* 1995; **91**: 2891–2897.

21. Masuda D, Nohara R, Tamaki N *et al*. Evaluation of coronary blood flow reserve by 13N-NH3 positron emission computed tomography (PET) with dipyridamole in the treatment of hypertension with the ACE inhibitor (Cilazapril*). Ann Nucl Med* 2000; **14**: 353–360.

22. Prior JO, Quinones MJ, Hernandez-Pampaloni M *et al*. Coronary circulatory dysfunction in insulin resistance, impaired glucose tolerance, and type 2 diabetes mellitus. *Circulation* 2005; **111**: 2291–2298.

23. Modena MG, Bonetti L, Coppi F *et al*. Prognostic role of reversible endothelial dysfunction in hypertensive postmenopausal women. *J Am Coll Cardiol* 2002; **40**: 505–510.

24. Cohn JN, Quyyumi AA, Hollenberg NK *et al*. Surrogate markers for cardiovascular disease. *Circulation* 2004; **109**: IV31–IV46.

25. Czernin J, Barnard RJ, Sun KT *et al*. Effect of short term cardiovascular conditioning and low fat diet on myocardial blood flow and flow reserve. *Circulation* 1995; **92**: 197–204.

26. Baller D, Notohamiprodjo G, Gleichmann U *et al*. Improvement in coronary flow reserve determined by positron emission tomography after six months of cholesterol lowering therapy in patients with early stages of coronary atherosclerosis. *Circulation* 1999; **99**: 2871–2875.

27. Bennett SK, Smith MF, Gottlieb SS *et al*. Effect of metoprolol on absolute myocardial blood flow in patients with heart failure secondary to ischemic or non-ischemic cardiomyopathy. *Am J Cardiol* 2002; **89**: 1431–1434.

28. Schindler TH, Nitzsche EU, Munzel T *et al*. Coronary vasoregulation in patients with various risk factors in response to cold pressor testing: Contrasting myocardial blood flow responses to short and long term vitamin C administration. *J Am Coll Cardiol* 2003; **42**: 814–822.

29. Gould KL, Martucci JP, Goldberg DI *et al*. Short term cholesterol lowering decreases size and severity of perfusion abnormalities by positron emission tomography after dipyridamole in patients with coronary artery disease. *Circulation* 1994: **89**: 1530–1538.

30. Dakik HA, Kleinman NS, Farmer JA *et al*. Intensive medical therapy versus coronary angioplasty for suppression of myocardial ischemia in survivors of acute myocardial infarction. *Circulation* 1998; **98**: 2017–2023.

31. Cecchi F, Olivotto I, Gistri R *et al*. Coronary microvascular dysfunction and prognosis in hypertrophic cardiomyopathy. *N Engl J Med* 2003; **349**: 1027–1035.

32. Shikama N, Himi T, Yoshida K *et al*. Prognostic utility of myocardial blood flow assessed by ^{13}N-ammonia positron emission tomography in patients with idiopathic dilated cardiomyopathy. *Am J Cardiol* 1999; **84**: 434–439.

33. Neglia D, Michelassi C, Trivieri MG *et al*. Prognostic role of myocardial blood flow impairment in idiopathic left ventricular dysfunction. *Circulation* 2002; **105**: 186–193.

34. Townsend DW, Carney JPJ, Yap JT *et al*. PET/CT today and tomorrow. *J Nucl Med* 2004; **45**: 4S–14S.

35. Koepfli P, Hany TF, Wyss CA *et al*. CT attenuation correction for myocardial perfusion quantification using a PET/CT hybrid scanner. *J Nucl Med* 2004; **45**: 537–542.

36. Suh J, White CS, Mittal V *et al*. Prevalence of heart disease in patients referred for pulmonary embolism: Evaluation with multidetector CT angiography and myocardial perfusion SPECT. *J Nucl Med* 2004; **45**: 241P.

37. Dilsizian V, Cannon RO, Tracy CM *et al*. Enhanced regional left ventricular function after distant coronary bypass via improved collateral blood flow. *J Am Coll Cardiol* 1989; **14**: 312–318.

38. Hunold P, Vogt FM, Schmermund A *et al*. Radiation exposure during cardiac CT: Effective doses at multidetector row CT and electron beam CT. *Radiology* 2003; **226**: 145–152.

Index